The History of the World in 100 Pandemics, Plagues and Epidemics

The History of the World in 100 Pandemics, Plagues and Epidemics

From Prehistory to COVID-19

Paul Chrystal

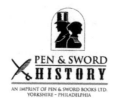

PEN & SWORD
HISTORY

AN IMPRINT OF PEN & SWORD BOOKS LTD.
YORKSHIRE ~ PHILADELPHIA

First published in Great Britain in 2021 by
Pen & Sword History
An imprint of
Pen & Sword Books Ltd
Yorkshire – Philadelphia

ISBN 978 1 39900 542 5

Printed and bound in the UK by CPI Group (UK) Ltd, Croydon, CR0 4YY.

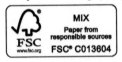

MIX
Paper from
responsible sources
FSC® C013604

Pen & Sword Books Limited incorporates the imprints of Atlas, Archaeology, Aviation,
Discovery, Family History, Fiction, History, Maritime, Military, Military Classics,
Politics, Select, Transport, True Crime, Air World, Frontline Publishing, Leo Cooper,
Remember When, Seaforth Publishing, The Praetorian Press, Wharncliffe Local
History, Wharncliffe Transport, Wharncliffe True Crime and White Owl.

For a complete list of Pen & Sword titles please contact

PEN & SWORD BOOKS LIMITED
47 Church Street, Barnsley, South Yorkshire, S70 2AS, England
E-mail: enquiries@pen-and-sword.co.uk
Website: www.pen-and-sword.co.uk

Or
PEN AND SWORD BOOKS
1950 Lawrence Rd, Havertown, PA 19083, USA
E-mail: Uspen-and-sword@casematepublishers.com
Website: www.penandswordbooks.com

'Gentlemen, it's the microbes which will have the last word.'
—Louis Pasteur, 1822–1895

'He wanted to do what all those around him were doing, apparently believing that the plague can come and go without the hearts of men being changed…they all returned home …apparently triumphing over the plague, forgetful of those who had also arrived by the same train but had found no one and were preparing in their homes to have confirmation of fears already born in their hearts out of a long silence. For them, the ones who now had only their brand new sorrow for companion, and for others who were at that moment contemplating the memory of a lost loved one, things were very different and the feeling of separation had reached its peak. For such people, mothers, husbands, wives and lovers, who had lost all happiness with the being who was now buried in some anonymous pit or had dissolved into a pile of ashes, the plague was still there.'
—Albert Camus. *The Plague*, 1947

For Anne, Rachael, Michael and Rebecca –
key workers all

Table of Contents

Pandemics, plagues and epidemics in world history

PREHISTORY, PLAGUE IN THE NEOLITHIC AGE, THE CLASSICAL PERIOD, BYZANTIUM, ANCIENT CHINA AND JAPAN

THE MIDDLE AGES

THE 20TH CENTURY

THE 21ST CENTURY

List of Plates

1. The Reconstruction of Myrtis. (*Photographer: Tilemahos Efthimiadis. Licensed under the Creative Commons Attribution-Share Alike 2.0 Generic license*)

2. The angel of death knocking on a door during the plague of Rome. (*Engraving by Levasseur after J. Delaunay. From the Wellcome Library, http://catalogue.wellcomelibrary.org/record=b1158081*)

3. Michael Sweerts' 'Plague in an Ancient City' (ca. 1652–54). (*Los Angeles County Museum of Art*)

4. St Sebastian pleading for the life of a gravedigger afflicted with plague during the Plague of Justinian, AD 541–549. (*Josse Lieferinxe (–1508) Walters Art Museum, Baltimore*)

5. Tsukioka Yoshitoshi, 'Driving Away the Demons'.

6. Sitala Mata.

7. A child infected with smallpox in Bangladesh, 1973.

8. Edward Jenner vaccinating patients against smallpox. (*Wellcome Collection, V0011069*)

9. *Encephalitis lethargica.*

10. Dr. Simmonds injecting his curative serum in a plague patient during the outbreak of bubonic plague in Karachi, 1897. (*Contained in an album of photographs which show the work of the Karachi Plague Committee in 1897. Library reference: ICV No 29763 Photo number: V0029287. Full Bibliographic Record: http://catalogue.wellcomelibrary.org/record=b1187933, Wellcome Library. Photograph probably by R. Jalbhoy*)

11 & 12. Washing away the plague in Bombay 1896–1905. (*Capt. C. Moss, Wellcome Library*)

13. Flagellants at Doornik in the Netherlands scourging themselves in atonement, believing that the Black Death is a punishment from God for their sins, 1349.

14. The rat incinerator in Sydney.

15. Rat catchers with a pile of dead vermin in Sydney in 1900. Rats were fetching up to 6d a head during the outbreak.

16. A heap of rats in Sydney; about 600 of them.

17. Sydney's Sutton Forest Butchery at 761 George Street; the meat preparation area was clearly less than ideal and probably contributed to the mortality figures. (*Pictures 14–17 courtesy of the Mitchell Library, State Library of New South Wales, [FL1087836; FL1064108; FL1064109; FL1087816]*)

Preface

'the UK's preparedness and response, in terms of its plans, policies, and capability, is currently not sufficient to cope with the extreme demands of a severe pandemic that will have a nationwide impact across all sectors.'

– Findings of the report on Exercise Cygnus,
suppressed for four years

The aim of this book is to show how pandemics and epidemics have influenced and changed the course of history – from Neolithic times to the current 21st century scourge that is COVID-19. However, this is not just yet another arid list of pestilential events, enumerating mortality and morbidity statistics although these figures are, of necessity, included. The book differs from others in that it qualifies and contextualises such statistics with significant characteristics relating to each of the episodes, thus enabling them to usefully progress our knowledge of disease management and pandemic-epidemic planning. In other words, it spoon feeds for policy makers the lessons from history which we need to learn if we are to be better equipped to deal with the next contagion event which, sorry to say, is probably not going to be far behind COVID-19 if and when COVID-19 is finally reduced to socially tolerable levels of morbidity and mortality.

The need to learn is pivotal and paramount. So far, for the past 2,500 years or so, we have – despite the ongoing sterling efforts of scientists and medical specialists, doctors, nurses and care home workers – so far we have largely elected to ignore or dismiss what pandemic after epidemic has shown us clearly needs to be done if we are to mitigate the next one. The pestilences will keep on coming, just as night follows day. There have been exceptions where lessons have been learnt, for example after the Manchurian plague and the Italian plague, but these flashes of enlightenment and perspicacity are few and far between; short termism, expediency, lack of vision and selectively 'following the science' are usually what follows. For example in the UK, the government's decision in 2019 to scrap the Cabinet-led Threats, Hazards, Resilience and Contingency Committee just months before (the anticipated) arrival of COVID-19 was short-sighted in the extreme. I say 'anticipated' because the government had until October 2020 suppressed publication of a multi-organisation drill focused on a hypothetical H2N2 influenza pandemic, which took place in October 2016 (Exercise Cygnus) highlighting shortages of intensive care beds, PPE, ventilators and mortuary space. The government insisted that all the recommendations had been implemented but later events were to prove that this was not the case.

The government might protest 'but we have the Scientific Advisory Group for Emergencies (SAGE)', and indeed we have, but SAGE is an ad hoc committee with a brief wider than COVID-19 management and control. Pandemics are a huge long term problem: we need a long term advisory group that looks at pandemics from a long-term perspective, whose advice is impartial, is totally free from government interference and is based on the best science and research available at the time.

Apart from the disappointing revelation that managing Brexit was deemed more important than girding us up for a pandemic that has so far killed over 127,000 people and has wrecked the economy, that fateful decision exemplifies the myopia shared by most governments around the globe.

It is perhaps naïve to think that this book will change very much, if anything. However, if it further educates policy makers and makes them think more progressively and proactively then it will have achieved its aim in helping to mitigate the next terrible pandemic.

The literature on the subject is truly prodigious; for that reason I have, in the hope that it will help the reader, included up to four references for each chapter specific to that chapter; this is followed at the end of the book by further reading of a more general nature.

Personally speaking, researching and writing this book has been more experiential than usual, researched and written as it was during the highly dynamic and unpredictable COVID-19 pandemic. The book has inevitably been defined to some extent by this colossal and disruptive world event and the real world undertones have made the book's message all the more poignant and urgent: we must learn from the past and plan for the future, now. History is watching us and history will judge us.

Paul Chrystal, York, May 2021

Acknowledgements

Thanks to Anne Drayton, Librarian at the State Library of New South Wales for permission to use the photographs of the Sydney plague, and Guardian Newpapers Ltd for various short extracts. My thanks too to Phil Sidnell and his colleagues at Pen & Sword for taking on this intractable and important project. I should also mention all the key workers in the health professions, education, social care, sanitation, communications, hospitality, retail and the food industry as well as the scientists and clinicians who have tirelessly worked to deliver the progress in therapies and vaccine development which we have clearly made. Not least, I must remember *all* the 127,000 or so families and their friends who have lost loved ones too soon to the most capricious and versatile of diseases.

About the author

Paul Chrystal attended the Universities of Hull and Southampton where he took degrees in Classics. For the next thirty-five years he worked in medical publishing, much of the time as an international sales director for one market or another, while latterly creating medical educational programmes for the global pharmaceutical industry for family doctors and hospital doctors.

He has been history advisor to local visitor attractions such as the National Trust in York and written features for national newspapers and broadcasting on local BBC, on the Radio 4 PM programme and on the BBC World Service.

He is a contributor to a number of history and archaeology magazines and the author of over 120 books published since 2010 on a wide range of subjects including classical history, British social and military history, confectionery, the history of pubs and beverages, the Cold War and The Troubles.

He is a regular reviewer for and contributor to 'Classics for All', editorial advisor for Yale University Press and a contributor to the classics section of 'Bibliographies on Line' published by Oxford University Press. In 2019 he was guest speaker for Vassar College, New York's London Programme in association with Goldsmith University. In 2020 he took over as History Editor for the Yorkshire Archaeological Journal. In 2021 he assisted with the research for an episode of *Who Do You Think You Are?* to be aired in 2022.

paul.chrystal@btinternet.com
www.paulchrystal.com

By the same author:

British Army of the Rhine (2018)
Northern Ireland: The Troubles: From The Provos to The Det, 1968–1998 (2018)
Women at War in the Ancient World (2020)
War in Greek Myth (2020)
War in Roman Myth and Legend (2020)
The History of Sweets (2021)
A Historical Guide to Roman York (in press 2021)
Factory Girls, Climbing Boys and Munitionettes (in press 2021)
Whitby: Historic Walks (in press 2021)
Bioterrorism (in press 2021)
The Book in Ancient Greece & Rome (in press 2022)

For a complete list please visit www.paulchrystal.com

Introduction

Between 1999 and 2001 from a passage grave at Frälsegården, 185 miles south-west of Stockholm, an international multi-disciplinary research team from France, Denmark and Sweden, including archaeologists from the University of Gothenburg using advanced DNA sequencing techniques, revealed the world's oldest traces of the plague bacterium's DNA. It was 5,000 years old.

On Friday, 21 March 2020 the eighth cohort of front line medical workers from Inner Mongolia boarded a Chinese Air Force plane covering the 723 miles to fight COVID-19 in Wuhan, Hubei Province.

If proof were needed of the fact that disease, contagion, pestilence or whatever else we call it is a constant in human civilisation, and that it has been our lethal and unwelcome companion over at least 5,000 years, then these two simple actions prove it beyond any doubt. The two events describe the scope of the book – a history of the world as defined by 100 or so pandemics, epidemics and outbreaks from the Neolithic age 5,000 years ago to AD 2021, taking in infectious disease epidemics and pandemics from around the globe – all with one thing in common – they killed, and continue to kill by the tens of thousands, hundreds of thousands and millions.

Being so powerful, lethal, evasive and destructive it is hardly surprising that many of these catastrophic public health nightmares turned the tide of history in numerous ways, dictating the outcome of wars, effecting political and religious change, wrecking economies, decimating populations, disrupting societies, culture and education. But, on a positive note, pandemics have challenged and galvanised scientific and medical research, which, in the case of COVID-19, propelled it forward into largely uncharted waters in which time consuming protocols were swept aside and truly international cooperation reached new heights. However, what pandemics also did was repeatedly expose a blizzard of international shortcomings when it came to heeding and acting on all those warnings from pestilences past – from ancient Greece to the present day. We can sum this all up as the serial failure or inability to ring-fence pre-emptive pandemic budgets, half-hearted pandemic preparation and an abject failure to either 'follow the science' properly, or consistently, or to exert rigorous, decisive and efficient management programmes for pandemics and epidemics.

It is, of course, easy to be wise with nearly 2,500 years of hindsight; moreover, no rational society is going to compromise the treatment of a diabetes or cancer patient today while saving up money to deal with the next pandemic – health budgets are largely spent on the here and now, at the point of need. We could, though, with some validity, question why those budgets do not, to some extent at least, permit us to do both: when that next pandemic descends upon us, it will, as COVID-19 is clearly doing now, disrupt and seriously weaken and shred social and economic fabric the world over whatever happens. Money raised, ring-fenced and spent prudently would surely mitigate the effect of future disease disasters and economic meltdowns, and would be money well spent.

As part of 'a wider consolidation of Cabinet sub-Committees' in order to focus on Brexit negotiations the UK Prime Minister, Boris Johnson, impetuously scrapped the Cabinet ministers' pandemic team – the Threats, Hazards, Resilience and Contingency Committee (a subcommittee of the National Security Council). He did this soon after taking office and just six months before coronavirus hit Britain: the committee was disbanded without any formal agenda for further discussion. The appointment of an interim minister with (limited) special responsibility for vaccine roll out goes some way to redress the misjudgement, but the UK really needs to take on board the reality that pandemic planning requires much more than a stop-gap minister with conflicting cabinet responsibilities and to appreciate the inevitability of another pandemic which will do its best to wreck us again, economially and socially, in the next few years.

We hear all the time about how 'we are in unprecedented times'; often it is a feeble excuse, perhaps, for dilatoriness and procrastination and mismanagement. While COVD-19 is certainly a novel virus with its own unique and specific characteristics and scientific challenges, including (magnificent) vaccine development and roll out programmes, many of the non medico-scientific characteristics and best practice responses to them are well documented. Moreover, the briefest of glances at the history books and the copious scientific-medical literature will demonstrate that we are not 'in unprecedented times'. Nothing like it. This book proves that fact 100 times over: each of the pandemics, epidemics and outbreaks described here have – as well as leaving a trail of death and destruction – endowed the nations of the world with a lesson to take with us to mitigate the next calamity. All we had and have to do was, and is, listen to and learn from these sonorous lessons, adapt and implement them.

The journey this book makes takes us back to the Neolithic Age, through classical and Byzantine history, into the Middle Ages and the Renaissance, then to the discovery and ravaging of the New World, through early modern history, the slave trade, colonialism and finally into the 21st century. We embark on a truly world wide journey, into the Americas and Canada, throughout Europe and Russia, into Africa and the Middle East, the Indian subcontinent and the Pacific, over to southeast Asia, Japan and China, then down to Australia and New Zealand. Table 1 lists the guilty diseases in question: they include the usual horror stories like plague, malaria, cholera, influenza, AIDs, polio, yellow fever, TB, leprosy, Ebola and smallpox, but also some less well-known (but often just as virulent) or forgotten 'pathogens' that have wreaked their own insidious havoc; these include psittacosis, sweating disease, dance plague, diphtheria and *Encephalitis lethargica*.

Along the way we discover the deathly vectors which pass on the diseases so effectively: we all perhaps are familiar with the horse-shoe bat, the anophelese mosquito and the plague-giving Oriental rat flea (*Xenopsylla cheopis*); but what about the dromedary camel, the flying squirrel, racoon dogs, masked civets, macaque monkeys and all manner of exotic birds? We describe the world-changing vaccines of earlier epidemics and we examine the ground-breaking preventative measures developed, for example, after the Manchurian plague epidemic and by Ragusa, and the city of Ferrara after the Italian plague in 1629. We travel on the ineffably foul slave ships, we stay on the equally squalid coffin ships and in the bleak fever sheds; sometimes we recover in a quarantining *lazaretto.*

Plagues and pandemics have often given rise to civil unrest so the reader inevitably gets embroiled in the Moscow plague riots and in unrest in Bombay, Guinea and Sierra Leone. We witness violent attacks on health workers and see the blame game in repellent action with Jews, numerous indigenous nations and gypsies persecuted or wiped out. Nasty prejudice prevails to this day against people with leprosy and AIDS. These pandemics and epidemics also expose the worst in human society as we uncover instances of genocide in Canada, ethnic cleansing in the US and in the Pacific islands, often with the annihilation of whole indigenous tribes and populations. The atrocities committed in the slave trade and in the name of colonialism, in an age when black lives clearly could not matter less, still resonate and shock today despite them being half-excused as 'of their time'. Racism, scapegoating and marginalisation: they all rear their ugly heads with disturbing frequency. The horrors of bioterrorism have been with us since time immemorial but some infectious agents today are teeing themselves up as potential weapons of mass destruction if they fall into the wrong hands. Nowadays the world temperature is rising – in more than one sense – Extinction Rebellion is raising the profile of irrefutable climate change which is undoubtedly complicit in fostering epidemics and pandemics, while Black Lives Matter do similar work for the world's BAME communities disproportionately represented as they are in mortality statistics. All of this in a time of pestilence when the plague riots of history are substituted by the storming of the Capitol in Washington DC by those seeking to overturn democracy in January 2021.

Just as importantly we chart the early, more enlightened developments in pandemic-epidemic management: from Thucydides' mission to educate in order to benefit future generations in 430 BC, through communicable disease recording in early China and Japan, quarantining, timely personal protective equipment provision, self-isolation, safe funeral rites, dignified disposal of bodies, social distancing, border control, hand and respiratory hygiene and the rest. These, of course, are the very lessons, with a few laudable exceptions, we have clearly failed to heed to any viable degree.

Here is a list of the diseases which make up the pandemics, epidemics and outbreaks covered here:

Table 1: The Diseases

NAME	CAUSATIVE AGENT	VACCINE	PREVENTION
AIDS	Caused by Human Immunodeficiency Virus (HIV).	No	Safe sex; needle exchange programmes. Anti-retroviral treatment can slow the course of the disease and may lead to a near-normal life expectancy.
CHOLERA	An infection of the small intestine by some strains of the bacterium *Vibrio cholerae*.	Yes	Best prevention: vaccine, sanitary water supplies and sewage treatment; early treatment with fluid replacement and, in severe cases, antibiotics.
COVID-19	Caused by a novel strain of coronavirus.	Yes	Vaccination; testing, tracking and tracing. Social distancing, hand hygiene, masking, rigorous compliance with official restrictions, respiratory etiquette, shielding.
DANCING PLAGUE	Cause unknown	n/a	
DIPHTHERIA	Caused by *corynebacterium diphtheria* that makes toxin.	Yes	Airborne and direct contact transmission.
EBOLA VIRUS	Ebola virus disease (EVD) or Ebola haemorrhagic fever (EHF), is a viral haemorrhagic fever of humans and other primates caused by ebola viruses.	Yes VSV-EBOV vaccine	Community engagement is key to successfully controlling outbreaks; infection prevention and control practices, surveillance and contact tracing, a good laboratory service, safe and dignified burials.

ENCEPHALITIS LETHARGICA	An atypical form of encephalitis. Also known as 'sleeping sickness' or 'sleepy sickness' (as distinct from tsetse fly-transmitted sleeping sickness).	No	The disease attacks the brain, leaving some victims in a statue-like condition, speechless and motionless.
INFLUENZA OR 'FLU'	A viral respiratory illness caused by an influenza virus. Three of the four types of influenza viruses affect humans: Type A, Type B, and Type C.	Yes	Best prevention: annual vaccination for seasonal flu.
LEGIONNAIRES' DISEASE	Caused by *Legionella* bacterium; it is a severe form of pneumonia.	No	
MALARIA	A mosquito-borne infectious disease caused by single-celled micro-organisms of the Plasmodium group most commonly spread by an infected female Anopheles mosquito.	No, but the recommended treatment is a combination of antimalarial medications that includes artemisinin.	Prevention: mosquito nets and insect repellents or with mosquito-control measures such as spraying insecticides and draining standing water.
MEASLES	A highly communicable airborne viral respiratory disease caused by a virus in the paramyxovirus family, Measles morbillivirus.	Yes. MMR	

(continued)

Table 1: The Diseases

NAME	CAUSATIVE AGENT	VACCINE	PREVENTION
MERS	Middle East respiratory syndrome is a viral respiratory disease caused by a novel zoonotic coronavirus (MERS coronavirus, or MERS-CoV).	No	General hygiene measures, including regular hand washing before and after touching animals, and avoiding contact with sick animals.
PLAGUE (bubonic, septicemic and pneumonic)	Caused by *Yersinia pestis* bacterium	Yes	
POLIOMYELITIS	A highly infectious viral disease caused by the poliovirus. It is highly contagious via the faecal-oral (intestinal source) and the oral–oral (oropharyngeal source) routes.	Yes	
PSITTACOSIS	A zoonotic infectious disease caused by *Chlamydia psittaci* and contracted from infected parrots and many other species of birds.	No	Treatment is with antibiotics.
SARS	Severe acute respiratory syndrome is a viral respiratory disease caused by a SARS-associated coronavirus known as SARS CoV.	No	Prevention as with COVID-19.
SMALLPOX	Caused by the *variola* virus.	Yes	Except for laboratory stockpiles, the variola virus has been eliminated.

SWEATING DISEASE	Cause a mystery although an unknown species of hantavirus may have been responsible. Sewage, poor sanitation and contaminated water supplies might have harboured the source of infection.		
YELLOW FEVER	An acute viral haemorrhagic disease transmitted by the bite of an infected female mosquito, often Aedes aegypti. The virus is an RNA virus of the genus Flavivirus.	Yes	Prevention: vaccination and as malaria.
ZICA Virus	Zika is spread mostly by the bite of an infected *Aedes* species mosquito (*Ae. aegypti* and *Ae. albopictus*).	No	Prevention: seek travel health advice, and as malaria; pregnant women should be especially cautious.
LEPROSY (Hansen's Disease)	A chronic, progressive bacterial infection caused by the bacterium *Mycobacterium leprae*. It primarily affects the nerves of the extremities, the skin, the lining of the nose, and the upper respiratory tract. Leprosy is also known as Hansen's disease.	No vaccine, but treatable with MDT.	Avoid close contact with untreated sufferers

(continued)

Table 1: Continued

NAME	CAUSATIVE AGENT	VACCINE	PREVENTION
TUBERCULOSIS	Tuberculosis (TB) is an infectious disease most often caused by *Mycobacterium tuberculosis* (MTB) bacteria which usually affects the lungs, but can also affect other parts of the body. Most infections are asymptomatic when it is known as latent tuberculosis. About 10% of latent infections progress to active disease which, if left untreated, kills about half of those affected.	No vaccine: treatment requires multiple antibiotics over a long period. Antibiotic resistance is a growing problem with increasing rates of multiple drug-resistant tuberculosis (MDR-TB) and extensively drug-resistant tuberculosis (XDR-TB).	Prevention: stop smoking, moderate alcohol intake; avoid close contact with untreated sufferers.

Pandemics are never just pandemics: they have always brought in their wake colossal ancillary problems and crises. It should not be necessary but here are just a few indirectly related factors which nations must always be mindful of and redress if they are to avoid making subsequent pandemics even worse than they need to be:

1. Disease surveillance must be maintained and ramped up for all notifiable infectious diseases but particularly for novel infectious agents such as AIDS and variations on SARS, influenza and COVID-19 which could, will and do mutate and engulf us repeatedly.
2. War – the notorious bedfellow of epidemics down the years which can intensify and amplify all the usual effects of a pandemic with the destruction of communications, IT, sanitation, health care, vaccination production and roll-out, and insecticide production and distribution (sparking another bedfellow, famine).
3. As we are finding out with COVID-19, mutation is a vital weapon in any virus' armoury – familiar pandemic diseases such as measles or plague could re-emerge fitter and more resilient, with heightened morbidity and mortality, resistant to current therapies and vaccines. Robust and constant monitoring of the efficacy and versatility of vaccines is therefore paramount as is pharmacovigilance to ensure the highest levels of vaccine safety.
4. Immunosuppression (suppression of the immune system and its ability to fight infection) – caused either through side effects of planned drug development and the deliberate use of

drugs in various cancers and bone marrow and other transplantations, also triggered through adverse drug reactions to routine therapies for other conditions, or occurring naturally through disease such as HIV-AIDS or lymphoma.

5. Climate change. The causes of climate change can foster pandemics: for example, deforestation is the largest cause of habitat loss worldwide. Loss of habitat gives animals, birds and insects no choice but to migrate into neighbouring populations and potentially contact other strange animals or people and exchange their germs. These newly infected creatures in turn can infect virgin human populations in new locations spreading zoonotic infections. Temperature changes can encourage the spread of vectors – for example, for malaria – into previously non endemic areas making them endemic and introducing pathogens to new hosts. Climate change also encourages migratory flux in human populations in a bid to avoid parasites and encroaching disease by moving to cooler regions leading to more potential infections.

The statistics generally are grim: 18 April 2021 saw the total deaths from COVID-19 exceed 3 million worldwide. The UK accounts for 4.23% of those; the UK population is equivalent to 0.87% of the total world population. As with recording casualties of war or in natural disasters it will be easy for the reader to become blasé and inured very quickly to the number of deaths in each of the bleak episodes the book covers so that the zeros at the end of the mortality statistics are rendered virtually meaningless. Indeed, with the classical authors in particular we should exercise caution because the mortality figures quoted are often nothing more than nice round figures designed to convey 'a big number'.

Nevertheless, we should remember that many of the mortality figures quoted represents a death with all the profound impact that inflicts on family members. Taking COVID-19 as an example, these figures also always conceal another secondary toll – the many thousands who have suffered or died because health care systems, such as they are, have, because of a preoccupation with COVID, been unable to proceed with what we might call routine business in the treatment of, for example, cancer and a myriad of other, non-pandemic conditions.

Ask the 127,000 or so families of the those who have died from COVID-19 in the UK up to April 2021; then go and ask their friends. We owe it to the bereaved to be mindful of the social significance and psychological ramifications of all pandemic related deaths. Mortality statistics are much more than just big numbers; each one of them conceals a personal tragedy and profound grief.

The Background: Pandemics, plagues and epidemics – definitions and what usually happens, or doesn't happen

'Marginal groups such as immigrants, Jews, gypsies, Chinese and black people often took the blame, as usual and were persecuted accordingly.'
>   –The central thesis of Rana Hogarth's
>   'Medicalising Blackness' (2020)

Before the advent of biomedical laboratory sciences, before the development of modern healthcare systems and before the upsurge in global transportation and communication first through ships, railways, motor transport, aeroplanes and printing and then the internet, before all this, pandemics and epidemics were poorly understood and experienced largely through an ineffective mishmash of folk medicine, superstition and quackery. The lethal arrival and spread of diseases like bubonic plague, cholera, yellow fever and smallpox with their concomitant morbidity and mortality caused disruption and dislocation on a prodigious scale, stopping people going about their daily lives – preventing them from earning a living, putting food on the table, getting an education, worshipping their god and having a dignified funeral.

The sick were sometimes left to fend for themselves because pestilence was often accompanied by stigma and a massive exodus of the population; the authorities took over the task of burying the dead and attending to the sick and needy. Depopulation could lead to burglaries of abandoned properties, robberies in the streets and an upsurge of quacks and charlatans who thought nothing of exploiting and harming frightened and vulnerable fellow citizens. Marginal groups such as immigrants, Jews, gypsies, Chinese and black people often took the blame and were persecuted accordingly. Those people who remained in the cities and towns were often subject to mandatory evacuation but there was no shelter when they reached their strange new destinations.

Amazingly, it was not quite all dystopian and hopeless. Just taking South and Central America as an example, sometimes, on the city streets after dark, disease-defiant residents would light bonfires in a bid to smoke out the contagions. They also gathered in the *pulperías* (gaucho bars), inns and tenements to sing and drink to banish the epidemic. In Mexico, epidemics like cholera, smallpox and typhoid, provoked similar scenes in which sectors of the population could find themselves demonstrating against government authorities. Most positively, though, in Brazil the arrival of yellow fever in 1849–1850 triggered a much-needed and overdue national debate about sanitation.

Nevertheless, there was and is an underlying sense of foreboding as a cloak of fear, uncertainty, loss of community and routine, and the virtual extinction of society as people knew it, exacerbated radical departures from normal aspects of normal life. Sudden widespread death worsened this grave new world of chaos. Thucydides, an eyewitness and disease sufferer during the Plague of Athens in 430 BC, described how the unsuspecting city panicked as it struggled to deal with the rapidly spreading, devastating disease. Moreover, he stressed a theme that has relevance today – namely, that fear and panic made the disruption of society worse, adding to the psychological impact on the individual. Moreover, fear exaggerated the spread of disease. The destructive nature of fear has remained a characteristic feature of pestilences that have, down the ages, caught ill-prepared societies off-guard, such as Bubonic plague in medieval times, AIDS in the 1980s, Ebola and COVID-19 today.

Your god, of course, had a lot to do with initiating pestilence, spreading it and causing the death and destruction that ensued. Time and time again throughout the ages we will witness the epidemiological hand of god in pandemic after epidemic – from classical Greece to the present day. Illness generally was the price you had to pay for annoying the gods or god – sin and hubris would not be tolerated. The Christian god, for example, was the 'divine physician', diagnosing egregious behaviour, prescribing and dispensing unspeakable suffering, death and destruction on a global scale according to the sin perpetrated by fickle and feckless man and woman. Moreover, there was never any shortage of zealots to stoke the fear of god. Sexual incontinence was penalised particularly harshly: leprosy, syphilis and plague sufferers were cruelly ostracised, victimised and marginalised. Just look at today's persisting prejudices against those with leprosy and HIV. Moral rectitude apart there was, is, another way to save your soul: the Christian Seven Corporal Works of Mercy include visiting the sick and burying the dead as given in Matthew 25, 31-46: do this and you get to heaven; don't and you burn in hell. No wonder, with such heavy moral responsibilites, the clergy, monks and nuns are often amongst the most badly hit in pandemics.

Most people comply with the often desperate and last minute efforts to restrict and mitigate a pandemic and there are legions of compassionate and unselfish people who make it their business to help one another, particularly the less well off, the vulnerable and the elderly. We, in the developed world at least, benefit from all the fantastic 21st-century innovation and sophistication of molecular virology, epidemiological modelling and accelerated vaccine design – but sadly, human behaviour and official attitudes have sometimes been reluctant to move on. In 2020 a kind of panic (or was it just pure selfishness) manifested in some with supermarket trolleys overfilled with toilet rolls and there is little sign that many countries have heeded the warnings from the past and COVID-19 has demonstrated that they have not made anything like the necessary or adequate provision for pandemic planning across all sectors, but notably in health care facilities, care homes, disease management and vaccine research – the importance of which the previous epidemics and pandemics so vocally warned us.

COVID-19 has introduced the non scientific amongst us to a completely new lexicon. Here are some definitions with which, embroiled in and fatigued by coronavirus, we have become all too familiar:

Cluster refers to an aggregation of cases grouped in place and time that are suspected to be greater than the number expected, even though the expected number may not be known.

Contagion: the communication of disease from body to body by direct contact; a plague or pestilence. First reference AD 1535.

Endemic refers to the constant presence and/or usual prevalence of a disease or infectious agent in a population within a geographic area.

Epidemiology: the branch of medicine which deals with the incidence, distribution, and possible control of diseases and other factors relating to health.

Epidemic: a disease prevalent amongst a specific community or country. This presumes only infectious agents, but non–infectious diseases such as diabetes and obesity exist in epidemic proportion in many countries. The US Centers for Disease Control and Prevention defines epidemic as: 'the occurrence of more cases of disease, injury, or other health condition than expected in a given area or among a specific group of persons during a particular period. Usually, the cases are presumed to have a common cause or to be related to one another in some way.' Hippocrates medicalised what was originally a Homeric word *epidemios* (*epi* [on] plus demos [*people*],[1] in his *Epidemics* when the word denoted a collection of clinical syndromes, such as coughs or diarrhoeas, occurring and propagating in a given period at a given location. Thucydides[2] gives us our first account of an epidemic when he describes the the Great Plague of Athens.

Exogenous: having an external cause or origin.

Immunity: the ability of an organism to resist a particular infection or toxin by the action of specific antibodies or sensitized white blood cells.

Outbreak: The WHO defines a disease outbreak as 'the occurrence of disease cases in excess of normal expectancy. The number of cases varies according to the disease-causing agent, and the size and type of previous and existing exposure to the agent'. Experts agree that the term be restricted to smaller events as acknowledged in *Stedman's Medical Dictionary*.

Mortality and **Morbidity** – the number of deaths; the number of infections.

Pandemic: The WHO defines a pandemic as 'an epidemic occurring worldwide, or over a very wide area, crossing international boundaries and usually affecting a large number of people'.

Pestilence: any fatal epidemic disease affecting man or beast and destroying many victims; specifically bubonic plague.

Plague: a pestilence, infection, affliction, calamity, scourge; a general name for any malignant disease afflicting man or beast; an epidemic with great mortality (1548); the Bubonic plague (1601).

Pox: the name for different diseases characterised by pocks or eruptive pustules on the skin; smallpox (1819); syphilis (1503).

Sporadic refers to a disease that occurs infrequently and irregularly.

Vaccine: a substance used to stimulate the production of antibodies and provide immunity against one or several diseases, prepared from the causative agent of a disease, its products, or a synthetic substitute, and treated to act as an antigen without inducing the disease.

Vector: (epidemiology), an agent that carries and transmits an infectious pathogen into another living organism.

Virus: an infective agent that typically consists of a nucleic acid molecule in a protein coat, and is able to multiply only within the living cells of a host.

1. Homer, *Odyssey* 1, 194, 230
2. *History of the Peloponnesian War*

Zoonosis is an infectious disease caused by a pathogen (an infectious agent, such as a bacterium, virus, or parasite) that has jumped from a non-human animal (usually a vertebrate) to a human.

Martin P., 2,500-year Evolution of the Term Epidemic. Emerging Infectious Diseases. (2006) 12, 976–980.
Hogarth, Rana, A., Medicalizing Blackness: Making Racial Difference in the Atlantic World, 1780–1840 (2020)

Globalization, the Columbian Exchange; the Four Horsemen

Globalization is one of the main characteristics and facilitators of a pandemic. The Columbian Exchange, named after Christopher Columbus (1451–1506), was the extensive transfer of plants, animals, culture, human populations, technology, ideas and *diseases* between the Americas, West Africa, and the Old World in the 15th and 16th centuries. It can also refer to European colonization and trade for centuries following Christopher Columbus's 1492 voyage. And we all know that it was never just commodities which criss-crossed the oceans in the holds of ships: infected human cargo and the cargoes themselves were vectors of infectious disease year in year out.

Invasive species, including communicable diseases, were a by-product of the Columbian Exchange. The changes in agriculture significantly altered global populations. The most significant immediate impact of the Columbian exchange was the cultural exchanges and the transfer of people (both free and enslaved) between continents. The most deleterious was unfettered importation of infectious disease from the Old World to the New.

Globalization today, of course, remains one of the key factors in the spread of infectious disease creating pandemics out of epidemics, wreaking death with no regard for political or natural borders. The only difference from the spread of disease in the Middle Ages is that now transmission is far more efficient and fast, hitching a ride on jet planes, fast trains and speeding cars and lorries as distinct from slow boats to China, horses and beasts of burden.

Crosby, Alfred, *The Columbian Exchange: Plants, Animals, and Disease between the Old and New Worlds* (New York, 2009)
Crosby, Alfred, *The Columbian Exchange: Biological and Cultural Consequences of 1492.* (Westport, 2003).
Nunn, Nathan; 'The Columbian Exchange: A History of Disease, Food, and Ideas'. *Journal of Economic Perspectives.* 24 (2010): 163–188

We have John of Patmos to thank for what is a cautionary tale to end all cautionary tales; he was supremely well qualified to write the book of Revelation: according to Tertullian (c. AD 155 – c. AD 240, a prolific early Christian author from Carthage) in *The Prescription of Heretics*, John was banished from Rome by the emperor Domitian after being plunged into boiling oil and walking away none the worse for his immersion.

Revelation 6 describes a scroll in God's right hand that is sealed with seven seals. The Lamb of God/Lion of Judah opens the first four of the seven seals to reveal four beings that ride out on white, red, black, and pale horses. In Zechariah's version they are described as 'the ones whom the Lord has sent to patrol the earth'. Ezekiel has them as 'sword, famine, wild beasts, and plague'.

In John's revelation, the first horseman is on a white horse, carrying a bow, and wearing a crown, riding forward as a figure of Conquest, invoking Pestilence, Plague Christ, or the Antichrist. The second carries a sword and rides a red horse and is the bringer of War. The third is a food merchant riding on his black horse, symbolizing Famine. The fourth and final horse is pale green, and ridden by Death accompanied by Hades, god of the Underworld. Revelation tells us 'They were given authority over a quarter of the earth, to kill with sword, famine, and plague, and by means of the beasts of the earth.'

The Christian apocalyptic vision is that it was the Four Horsemen who set a divine end time on the world as harbingers of the Last Judgment.

The most lethal triad: war, famine and pestilence

'The horseman on the white horse was clad in a showy and barbarous attire. ... While his horse continued galloping, he was bending his bow in order to spread pestilence abroad. At his back swung the brass quiver filled with poisoned arrows, containing the germs of all diseases.'

–Vicente Blasco Ibáñez (1916).
The Four Horsemen of the Apocalypse (ch V)

It is impossible to read very far into the book you are now reading before being struck by the ubiquity of references to pestilence, specifically in its close association with war and famine. Cartwright and Biddiss describe this catastrophic coalition as follows: 'Pestilence, famine and war interact and produce a sequence. War drives the farmer from his fields and destroys his crops, destruction of the crops spells famine; the starved and weakened people fall easy victims to the onslaught of pestilence. All three are diseases. Pestilence is a disorder of the human. Famine results from disorders of plants and cattle, whether caused by inclement weather or more directly by insect or bacterial invasion. Even war may be regarded, though more arguably, as a form of mass psychotic disorder,' – Frederick Cartwright, *Disease and History* (1994)

Famine had the added disadvantage of encouraging the stockpiling of food reserves in towns and villages which in turn attracted plague-infected rodents.

Although by no means universal, we will, nevertheless, witness this dreadful three-way alliance time and time again throughout history, evident as it is in numerous contagions and geographical regions. The association of the three, of course, was, as noted above, given lurid and eternal publicity by the Four Horseman of the Apocalypse as featured in the Christian Bible and other religious works where pestilence, famine and war conspire to introduce death to the party. For centuries god-fearing people all around the globe and in many religions, cultures and civilisations have believed, and have been encouraged to believe, that their wars were holy (and justifiable) wars and that famine and disease were the just rewards for living a life of sin and going against their gods.

The horsemen ride into our lives in the New Testament's final book, Revelation, as well as in the Old Testament's prophetic Book of Zechariah, and in the Book of Ezekiel, where they are named as harbingers of punishments from an angry and vengeful God. The Four Horsemen have been firmly lodged in the recesses of our collective memory by believers and non-believers ever since.

Beale, G.K., 1999, *The Book of Revelation* (3rd ed.). Grand Rapids, MI

Ibáñez, Vicente Blasco, 1916, *The Four Horsemen of the Apocalypse*

Lenski, Richard Charles Henry, 2008, *The Interpretation of St. John's Revelation*. Augsburg Fortress Publishers

Morris, Leon, 1988. *The Book of Revelation: An Introduction and Commentary* (2nd ed.). Leicester

PREHISTORY, PLAGUE IN THE NEOLITHIC AGE, THE CLASSICAL PERIOD, BYZANTIUM, ANCIENT CHINA AND JAPAN

Plague in the Neolithic Age

'And this strain has all the genetic components we know of that are needed for the bubonic form of the disease. So plague, with the transmission potential that we know today, has been around for much longer than we thought.'
– Kirsten Bos, Max Planck Institute,

Our story begins some 5,000 years ago in the late Neolithic Age (10,000 BC – 4,500 BC) in a grave at Frälsegården outside Falköping in Gökhem, 185 miles south-west of Stockholm. Here, as noted in the Introduction, between 1999 and 2001 an international multi-disciplinary research team from France, Denmark and Sweden, including archaeologists from the University of Gothenburg using advanced DNA sequencing techniques, revealed the world's oldest traces of the plague bacterium's DNA. The team also suggests that the discovery incidentally may have identified the first pandemic in history which ravaged across Europe in to Asia by way of new trade and transportation routes in the very early days of globalisation.

In the very beginning, human beings tended to live up in the mountains and hills, or on extensive plains. Population density was very low for the hunter gatherer with little if any of what you could call crowding. But things were about to change when the hunter gatherer came down onto the plains seeking more space and fertile land in what we term as the Agrarian Revolution. The only problem, and it was a monumental one, was that once settled our hunter gatherer had to defend that land, his livestock and family against competing interests in the guise of others with the same lifestyle, aspirations and objectives. There was safety in numbers so the Neolithic Age eventually saw the first populations coexisting in what we call proto-urban civilizations: crowded settlements which permitted and encouraged specialised occupational groups, hierarchies and social classes, the economic exploitation of surpluses, public buildings and writing and reading. Ironically, when these urban centres started to develop more sophisticated methods of sanitation they ran the risk of creating another conduit for disease transmission when water supplies became polluted; it was rarely a problem for their hunter-gatherer forebears who had relied on running freshwater streams or ad hoc cess pits in a secluded copse or wood. These new civilisations provided, for the first time in human history, ideal conditions for the proliferation and spread of infectious diseases, or crowd diseases; give an infectious disease to a certain number of susceptible people and that disease will thrive, often exponentially. The formation of crowds was essentially one of the vehicles for infectious disease transmission and the graduation into epidemic then pandemic status.

The new settled, increasingly domesticated life also brought man closer to the earth; the soil he and she cultivated was teeming with bacteria and what diseases they didn't contract from the soil they caught from their animals. Neolithic man was, of course, blithely unaware that both soil and animals – his primary source of food and therefore survival – were at the same time capable of killing him. With animals came the zoonoses and with them zoonotic disease. And so began the ongoing battle of disease versus man with man's immune system in perpetual conflict with agents of disease which fight to circumvent that system.

Animals, domesticated and otherwise have a lot to answer for down the years: six out of every ten infectious diseases in people are zoonotic; here are some examples, with the culprits: tuberculosis comes from cattle and birds, anthrax from grazing herbivores, leprosy from mice, rabies from dogs, foxes and bats, chicken pox from chickens, measles from canine distemper or rinderpest, the common cold from horses. Moreover, certain occupations rendered Neolithic man particularly susceptible if he was a butcher, tanner or farmer. Table 2 shows the alarming number of diseases we can catch from our animal neighbours.

Some Neolithic civilisations, for example the Cucuteni-Trypillia culture (c. 5500 BC to 2750 BC) which extended from the Carpathians to Ukraine, just vanished for unknown reasons: could a devastating plague provide a reasonable enough explanation for its annihilation? Even earlier, excavations at Çatalhöyük in modern Turkey have yielded evidence of malaria and respiratory disease from around 7000 BC and possibly even plague and enteric dysentery; with its population of around 10,000 it was a reservoir of infection.

The Swedish grave referred to above contained 78 skeletons which had been dumped in a disorderly heap. Astonishingly, those DNA studies have concluded that this population had been afflicted by a variant of the plague, not bubonic but pulmonary. Specifically, when scientists re-examined DNA from two of the teeth of a young woman they discovered genetic sequences from *Yersinia pestis*, the bacterium that causes plague. Hitherto scientists thought the disease had originated thousands of miles away to the east in Asia; its appearance so far west, in Sweden, and so long ago, was a defining moment in palaeopathology. The origins of plague are being re-evaluated after this truly significant discovery.

Nicolás Rascovan, a genetics researcher at Aix Marseille Université, reports that the bacteria from the woman's teeth might be the earliest evidence of a continent-wide epidemic, one that explains a contemporary sudden and mysterious collapse in the European population.

When he found *Yersinia pestis* in the woman's teeth, Rascovan examined the other 78 skeletons from the people who were buried around the same time, suggesting a surge in deaths that could have been caused by a virulent epidemic. Indeed, a young man in the tomb also exhibited fragments of plague bacteria in his teeth. The strain of *Yersinia pestis* in this grave site was distinct from all others ever sequenced: crucially the team believe that it diverged from other known strains 5,700 years ago.

Scientists are turning their focus to the pathogens the migrants and traders carried and how they died. Some believe that is a step toward understanding how plague –

Table 2: Zoonotic diseases found in the UK

Disease	Organism	Main reservoirs	Usual mode of transmission to humans
ANTHRAX	Bacillus anthracis	livestock, wild animals, environment	direct contact, ingestion, inhalation
ANIMAL INFLUENZA	Influenza A viruses	pigs, other livestock, humans	direct contact
AVIAN INFLUENZA	Influenza A viruses	poultry, ducks	direct contact
BOVINE TUBERCULOSIS	Mycobacterium bovis	cattle	unpasteurised milk, exposure to tuberculous animals
CAMPYLOBACTERIOSIS	Campylobacter spp.	poultry, farm animals	direct animal contact, raw meat, milk
CAT SCRATCH FEVER	Bartonella henselae	cats	bite, scratch
COWPOX	Cowpox virus	rodents	direct contact (usually with cats)
CRYPTOSPORIDIOSIS	Cryptosporidium spp	cattle, sheep, pets	contaminated water, direct contact
CYSTICERCOSIS/ TAENIASIS	Taenia spp.	cattle, pigs	raw/ undercooked meat
ERYSIPELOID	Erysipelothrix rhusiopathiae	pigs, fish, environment	direct contact, fomites, environment
FISH TANK/SWIMMING POOL GRANULOMA	Mycobacterium marinum	fish	contact with fish or contaminated water
GIARDIASIS	Giardia spp	humans, wildlife	contaminated water, ingestion
HAEMORRHAGIC COLITIS AND HAEMOLYTIC URAEMIC SYNDROME (HUS)	Shiga toxin- producing E. coli	ruminants	direct contact, foodborne

(continued)

Table 2: Continued

Disease	Organism	Main reservoirs	Usual mode of transmission to humans
HANTAVIRUS SYNDROMES	Hantaviruses	rodents	aerosolised excreta
HEPATITIS E	Hepatitis E virus	pigs, wild boar, deer	undercooked animal meats
HYDATID DISEASE	Echinococcus granulosus	dogs, sheep	ingestion of eggs excreted by dog
LEPTOSPIROSIS	Leptospira spp	rodents, ruminants	urine-contaminated water or direct contact
LISTERIOSIS	Listeria spp.	cattle, sheep, soil	dairy produce, meat products
LOUPING ILL	Louping ill virus	sheep, grouse	direct contact, tick bite
LYME DISEASE	Borrelia burgdorferi	ticks, rodents, deer, sheep, small mammals	tick bite
LYMPHOCYTIC CHORIOMENINGITIS	Lymphocytic choriomeningitis virus (LCMV)	rodents	direct contact
ORF	Orf virus	sheep, goats	direct contact
OVINE CHLAMYDIOSIS	Chlamydia abortus	sheep, farm animals	direct contact, aerosol
PASTEURELLOSIS	Pasteurella spp	dogs, cats, many mammals	bite/scratch, direct contact
PSITTACOSIS	Chlamydia psittaci	psittacine birds, poultry, ducks	aerosol, direct contact
Q FEVER	Coxiella burnetii	cattle, sheep, goats, cats	aerosol, direct contact, products of conception, fomites
RABIES	Rabies virus and other lyssaviruses	bats only in the UK	Bite or scratch

RAT BITE FEVER	Streptobacillus moniliformis	rats	bite/scratch, milk, water
RINGWORM	Dermatophyte fungi	many animal species	direct contact
SALMONELLOSIS	Salmonella spp.	poultry, farm animals	direct animal contact, raw meat, other raw foods
STREPTOCOCCAL SEPSIS	Streptococcus suis	pigs	direct contact, meat
STREPTOCOCCAL SEPSIS	Streptococcus zooepidemicus	horses	direct contact
TOXIOCARIOSIS	Toxocara canis/catis	dogs, cats	ingestion
TOXOPLASMOSIS	Toxoplasma gondii	cats, ruminants	ingestion of faecal oocysts, meat
ZOONOTIC DIPHTHERIA	Corynebacterium ulcerans	cattle, farm animals, dogs	direct contact, milk

Source: https://www.gov.uk/government/publications/list-of-zoonotic-diseases/list-of-zoonotic-diseases

and other pathogens – became deadly. According to Simon Rasmussen, a metagenomics researcher at the Technical University of Denmark and the University of Copenhagen, 'We often think that these superpathogens have always been around, but that's not the case,' he says. 'Plague evolved from an organism that was relatively harmless. More recently, the same thing happened with smallpox, malaria, Ebola and Zika'.

Despite its huge historical and modern impact and significance, the origin and age of bubonic plague are still not well understood. Crucially, exactly when and where *Y. pestis* acquired the virulence profile that allows it to colonize and transmit through the flea vector remains unclear. A 2018 analysis of two 3,800-year-old *Y. pestis* genomes by an international team of researchers led by the Max Planck Institute for the Science of Human History in Jena, Germany suggests a Bronze Age origin for bubonic plague. The strain identified by the researchers was recovered from individuals in a double burial in the Samara region of Russia, who both exhibited the same strain of the bacterium at death. The study, published in *Nature Communications*, shows that this strain is the oldest sequenced to date containing the virulence factors characteristic of the bubonic plague, and is a precursor to the strains that caused the Justinian Plague, the Black Death and the 19th century plague epidemics in China.

In the study, the researchers analyzed nine individuals from tombs in Samara. Two were infected with *Y. pestis* at the time of their deaths; they were buried together in a single grave and were approximately 3,800 years old. Analysis of the human DNA showed that the individuals were likely from the Samara-region Srubnaya-culture, which chimes with the archaeological evidence. 'Both individuals appear to have the same strain of *Y. pestis*,' says Kirsten Bos of the Max Planck Institute. 'And this strain has all the genetic components we know of that are needed for the bubonic form of the disease. So plague, with the transmission potential that we know today, has been around for much longer than we thought.'

The researchers used the data collected in combination with previously sequenced *Y. pestis* strains to calculate the age of their newly identified lineage at around 4,000 years. This pushes back the proposed age of the bubonic plague by 1,000 years. 'Our *Y. pestis* isolates from around 4,000 years ago possessed all the genetic characteristics required for efficient flea transmission of plague to rodents, humans and other mammals,' according to Maria Spyrou of the Max Planck Institute, lead author of the study.

Spyrou, Maria A. et al, 2018 Analysis of 3800-year-old *Yersinia pestis* genomes suggests Bronze Age origin for bubonic plague, *Nature Communications*

Andrades Valtueña, Aida; 'The Stone Age Plague and Its Persistence in Eurasia'. *Current Biology*: CB. 27 (23) (2017): 3683–3691

Chapter 1

Hamin Mangha to the Middle Ages

As we have noted, on Friday, 21 March 2020 the eighth cohort of front line medical workers from Inner Mongolia were on a Chinese Air Force plane covering the 723 miles to fight COVID-19 in Wuhan, Hubei Province. Wuhan, as we all now know, is the epicentre and starting point of the global coronavirus epidemic which ravaged the world from December 2019.

With malevolent irony the world of contagion and pestilence had come full circle, for it is in China that we have discovered some of the earliest evidence for the existence of plague, the atrocious disease that has been slaying populations the world over since around 5,000–4,000 BC. Then, an unassuming village called Hamin Mangha in Inner Mongolia – long dead and deserted – played host to one of the first manifestations of plague, much later known as the Black Death and scourge of populations everywhere, even to this day.

Between the winter of 2011 and summer of 2015, archaeological excavations by a team from the prestigious Jilin University in Changchun made a dramatic and profound discovery that would change our perception of world history in general and palaeopathology in particular: the archaeologists unearthed a Neolithic village site comprising 29 one-room houses with doors and hearths. In addition in the 2011 dig there were other signs of thriving activity such as ten ash pits, three tombs and one surrounding moat, from which more than 100 shards of potteries, jades, stone implements and artifacts made of bone, horn and shell were excavated. The excavation at the Hamin Mangha site in 2012 yielded semi-subterranean house foundations, 19 ash pits, six burials, two surrounding moats, from which over 500 pieces of artifacts including pottery, jades and implements made of stone, bone and shell were unearthed.

The population was probably no more than a few hundred, yet it lost nearly 100 villagers over a few days or weeks at most. In the village were the incinerated remains of 97 skeletons unceremoniously dumped in the middle of the floor of a 210 square feet hut – crisis burials. Half were aged between 19 and 35, and the rest were younger; none was older. This world-changing, disorganised pile of bones indicates that the surviving villagers were anxious to be rid of their dead and to quarantine them hastily and as effectively as possible.

Anthropologists contend that the villagers probably died of an unknown but virulent lethal infection and that the speed of mortality created so much fear that the usual funerary rituals were dispensed with in a panicked attempt to rid the village of and escape from the pestilence. It is reasonable to assume that they brought out the dead, set fire to the hut causing the thatched roof to collapse and fled their village never to return. The victims lay undisturbed until the arrival of the archaeologists in the winter of 2011.

The ages of the victims at Hamin Mangha coincide largely with those found in another prehistoric mass burial unearthed in modern-day Miaozigou in northeast China; the researchers noted, 'This similarity may indicate that the cause of the Hamin Mangha site was similar to that of the Miaozigou sites. That is, they both possibly relate to an outbreak of an acute infectious disease,' wrote team leaders Ya Wei Zhou and Hong Zhu. It is also similar to a northeast China site at Lajia.

According to Owen Jarus in *Live Science* July 27, 2015 'The team has published a second study, in Chinese, in the *Jilin University Journal* – Social Sciences edition, on their finds. (A brief English-language summary of their results is available on the American Association of Physical Anthropologists website.)

While the exact pathology of this putative infection remains unknown, what is clear is the role that climate change had in its spread. Hamin Mangha is not the only Neolithic site in the region where we see a similar pattern of epidemics, mass burials and abandoned sites, albeit it at different times. The one common factor is the warm period called the Holocene Climate Optimum which gave increases of up to 4°C near the North Pole. The Hamin Mangha epidemic occurred at the end of this warm climatic period which had lasted from ca. 7,000 BC to 3,000 BC and would have had a more pronounced impact that was harder to survive in an inland and relatively high altitude area like Inner Mongolia, than in places that stayed relatively warm like coastal or Southern China.

During the Holocene Climate Optimum, 'Current desert regions of Central Asia were extensively forested due to higher rainfall and the warm temperate forest belts in China and Japan were extended northwards.' It appears that this civilization collapsed due to the rapid encroachment of northern deserts into its territories, maybe forcing its people to migrate to the south. Interestingly, or worryingly, we are today in another period of climate change and the world is again a warmer place than hitherto.

Aruna Li, 2015, The excavation of the Neolithic site at Hamin Mangha in Horqin Left Middle Banner, Inner Mongolia in 2011, *Chinese Archaeology* 14

Colledge, Sue, 2019, 'Neolithic population crash in northwest Europe associated with agricultural crisis' *Quaternary Research*: 1–22

Downey S.S., 2016, European Neolithic societies showed early warning signals of population collapse. *Proc. Natl. Acad. Sci.* 113, 2016; 9751–9756

Leafloor, Liz (27 July 2015) 'Prehistoric Disaster: Nearly 100 Bodies Found Stacked in Ancient House in China'. *Ancient Origins.* 9 May 2020.

The Bible, Greece, Rome and China

'Empires are big and microbes small, but both have shaped history by conquering territories and bodies, leaving death, disease, and devastation in their wake.'

– Peter C. Perdue, FP.com 4 July 2020

Before the Bible

The Bible is not that old in terms of available records of disease: the Old Testament was written down between the 6th and 1st centuries BC, well after 8th century Homer and Hesiod; records of infectious diseases exist on ancient Egyptian stele, tomb paintings and on papyri and Akkadian tablets. They extend far beyond the Near East to India and China. The first recorded epidemic in human history was 'a great pestilence' that occurred in Egypt in the reign of Pharaoh Mempses in the First Dynasty, 3180 BC. Manetho, the third century BC Egyptian priest and historian, noted in his list of pharaohs, 'Mempses, for eighteen years. In his reign many portents and a great pestilence occurred.' This is our first example of public health surveillance, a discipline which dates back to this the first recorded epidemic.

Our first record of precautions being taken to avoid or mitigate infectious disease comes on an Akkadian tablet from 1770 BC when King Zimri-Lim had occasion to tell his scribe to send a note to Queen Shiptu regarding measures she should take to avoid being infected by a servant called Nanna who was displaying lesions. The king, with remarkable good sense and a heightened awareness of infection control, advised his queen not to share cups with Nanna, and not to sit on or use chairs or beds used by Nanna.

Rabies is first described in a Babylonian legal document, the Eshnunna Code (2300 BC), advising that the bite of a dog could be fatal and that the guilty animal's owner will be subject to a fine. Interestingly, the fine for biting a 'man' and causing his death was 40 shekels of silver, that for infecting and killing a slave was the cut rate of 15 shekels.

Biblical Plague

Apparently, one of the things we remember most from childhood readings of the Bible is mankind's brushes with numerous plagues – one of the members of that unholy trinity constituted of disease, famine and war. Amongst the more famous are the Plagues of Egypt as found in the Book of Exodus; they are an expression of God's displeasure towards the Egyptians who foolishly declined to let his people (the Israelites) go. They are as follows:

> *Turning river waters to blood: Ex. 7:14–24*
> *Frogs clogging up the Nile: Ex. 7:25–8:15*
> *Lice or gnats harming livestock: Ex. 8:16–19*
> *Wild animals or flies: Ex. 8:20–32*

Pestilence of livestock: Ex. 9:1–7: God said: Let my people go, so that they may worship me. If you refuse to let them go and continue to hold them back, the hand of the LORD will bring a terrible plague on your livestock in the field—on your horses and donkeys and camels and on your cattle and sheep and goats.

Boils: Ex. 9:8–12: The LORD said to Moses and Aaron, 'Take handfuls of soot from a furnace and have Moses toss it into the air in the presence of Pharaoh. It will become fine dust over the whole land of Egypt, and festering boils will break out on men and animals throughout the land.'

> *Thunderstorm of hail and fire: Ex. 9:13–35*
> *Locusts: Ex. 10:1–20*
> *Darkness for three days: Ex. 10:21–29*
> *Death of firstborn children: Ex. 11:1–12:36*

Plague, of course, is used in a generic sense here but clearly two of them are directly plagues of a medical or veterinary nature. Others have indirect significance – arthropod-borne and arthropod-caused diseases – as they would lead to famine (locusts, flies, lice and gnats). Although these were not precise historical events they do at one level illustrate quite vividly early eschatological beliefs relating to sin and punishment, judgement, heaven and hell. On another level some scholars believe the plagues to be metaphors for natural disaster caused by climate change over a period of time and focused on the city of Pi-Ramesses in the Nile delta. As an example, the reign of Rameses II (1279 BC – 1213 BC) was witness to an unusually warm and wet period followed by a marked drop in temperature which led the Nile to dry up and become a semi-stagnant area of mud flats around its delta; such conditions are ideal for the formation of algae called Burgundy Blood algae (*Oscillatoria rubescens*) which, when it dies, stains the water red taking on the appearance of blood. Another theory names *chromatiaecea* bacteria as the culprit. Whatever, the algae would have attracted lice and flies while causing the frogs to flee the river in search of new habitats; their absence would have allowed mosquitos to thrive while the three days of darkness could have been the consequence of volcanic activity in the region.

1 Samuel tells that in 1141 BC the Israelites lost 40,000 men in a battle with the Philistines; not to be outdone they orchestrated another battle, this time parading their Ark of the Covenant, and promptly lost a further 30,000 men. Worse still, the Philistines captured the Ark from the Israelites but, for their troubles, endured an outbreak of 'tumours' (Hebrew ophal), an affliction which followed them as they moved the Ark from city to city (Ashron, Gath and Ekron). It did not take long for the Philistines to work out that the Ark was the vector for this ongoing disaster, so the leaders decided to return it to the Israelites along with a guilt offering of five golden tumours and five golden rodents (akbar). But soon after in Beth-shemesh 70 Israelites died there while a further 50,000 later succumbed throughout Israel. Some scholars have concluded that the outbreak was bubonic plague, with its associated buboes.

Deuteronomy 28 has a chilling warning: 'If thou wilt not observe to do all the words of this law that are written in this book, that thou mayest fear this glorious and fearful name, The Lord Thy God; Then the Lord will make thy plagues wonderful, and the plagues of thy seed, even great plagues, and of long continuance, and sore sicknesses, and of long continuance. Moreover he will bring upon thee all the diseases of Egypt, which thou wast afraid of; and they shall cleave unto thee. Also every sickness, and every plague, which is not written in the book of this law, them will the Lord bring upon thee, until thou be destroyed.'

To these we can add: God promised judgment if the people of Israel turned against the Lord. Part of God's judgment included plagues (Leviticus 26:25).

Numbers 21: 6,8 and Deuteronomy 8:15 both refer to a fiery serpent, possibly guinea worm which causes dracunculiasis, a parasitic infection caused by drinking infected water and detected in mummies from the period.

God sent a three-day plague to wipe out 70,000 men after King David sinned by numbering the people of Israel (2 Samuel 24:10–17).

Amos prophesied that God would send several judgments against the nation of Israel, including plagues.

Israel, including plagues similar to those Egypt endured (Amos 4:10).

God sent several judgments against the nation of Judah, including a plague, when he sent King Nebuchadnezzar to sack Jerusalem (Jeremiah 21:7, 24:10, 29:17).

Ehrenkranz, N. Joel, 2008, Origin of the Old Testament Plagues: Explications and Implications, *Yale J Biol Med*. 81(1): 31–42.

Freemon, Frank R., 2005, Bubonic plague in the Book of Samuel, *J R Soc Med*. 2005 Sep; 98(9): 436

Greifenhagen, F.V. 2000. 'Plagues of Egypt'. In Freedman (ed.). *Eerdmans Dictionary of the Bible*. *Amsterdam*, p. 1062.

Overall there are almost 100 references to plague in the Bible, mainly in the Old Testament. As we know, plagues get a mention in the New Testament's Book of Revelation with reference to the end of the world and the second coming of Jesus Christ as foreshadowed with prophetic warnings of plague, pestilence and economic collapse.

Revelation 11 reads: 'These witnesses have power to shut the sky so that no rain will fall during the days of their prophecy, and power to turn the waters into blood and to strike the earth with every kind of plague as often as they wish.'

Revelation 18: 'Therefore her plagues will come in one day – death and grief and famine – and she will be consumed by fire, for mighty is the Lord God who judges her.'

Plague is also mentioned in the Book of Hosea 13 in the Hebrew Bible: 'I will ransom them from the power of Sheol; I will redeem them from Death. "Where O Death, are your plagues? Where, O Sheol, is your sting?"'

Jesus warned in Matthew 24: 'Take heed that no man deceive you. For many shall come in my name, saying, I am Christ; and shall deceive many. And you shall hear of wars and rumours of wars: see that you be not troubled: for all these things must come to pass, but the end is not yet. For nation shall rise against nation, and kingdom against kingdom: and there shall be famines, and pestilences, and earthquakes, in various places. All these are the beginnings of sorrows.'

A biblical plague often forms part of God's judgment against sin. Sometimes, God sent plagues or pestilences against unbelievers as above when Egypt enslaved and oppressed the people of Israel. At other times, God sent a plague against his own people to judge their sin. God sent many prophets to the people of Judah, but they still did not turn from sin. So Jeremiah reports God's Word when he said, 'Though they fast, I will not hear their cry, and though they offer burnt offering and grain offering, I will not accept them. But I will consume them by the sword, by famine, and by pestilence.' (Jeremiah 14:12).

Greece and Rome

Our pursuit of infectious diseases, viruses and pandemics in the classical world is literally plagued by a lack or an absence of detailed information and analysis by the extant historians, encyclopedists or physicians whom we might have expected to record them. Nevertheless, what does exist in Hippocrates (ca 470 BC – 360 BC), Thucydides (c. 460 BC – 400 BC, Pliny the Elder (AD 23 – 79), Soranus (fl. 1st-2nd century AD) and Galen (AD 129 – AD 210) to name the most informative, does provide some viable information which allows us to piece together to varying levels of certainty, the course, symptoms of and socio-economic and political consequences of the pandemics and epidemics which scourged the Greek and Roman worlds. Frustratingly, though, we are not always able to identify the actual micro-organisms involved and so, in some cases cannot be sure that this plague, pestilence or contagion is, for example, bubonic plague, smallpox, Ebolavirus or typhus.

Hippocrates was the first physician to believe that diseases were caused naturally, and not because of superstition and the gods. As Roy Porter elegantly put it 'he plucked disease from the heavens and brought it down to earth'.[1] *The Hippocratic Corpus* is a collection of around seventy early medical works some of which may have been written by Hippocrates. [1]

Hippocrates and his acolytes knew about many of the infectious diseases which interest us, including septicaemia, tuberculosis, malaria and possibly polio and influenza. On malaria he was *au fait* with the link to stagnant water and familiar with quartan and tertian malaria – (fever every third day, fever on alternate days). In short, the Hippocratic Corpus tried to treat every known disease in a systematic and rational manner. Some argue that malaria was not introduced into Greece before 500 BC. According to Nobel prize winner for medicine, Sir Ronald Ross (1857–1932), in his article, Malaria in Greece, 'malaria fell like a blight on many fertile districts' ruining health, depopulating lands essential for economic survival and from the Hellenistic period to the early 20th century was ever present and was 'the decisive factor in the fall of classical civilisation'.

---

1. Porter, Roy (1997), The Greatest Benefit to Mankind: A Medical History of Humanity from Antiquity to the Present, London, pp. 53–54

Malaria (*plasmodium falciparum*) was widespread in many parts of Italy and other parts of the empire despite attempts to improve drainage of marshlands and river plains. In a 5th century AD cemetery near Lugnano in Umbria almost all of the 47 graves contained either infants, neonates or foetuses. The foetuses were from miscarriages, particularly from *primigravidae* mothers, caused by the immune suppression common in women in the final two trimesters of pregnancy, brought on by malaria. The female anopheles mosquito is thought to be attracted to certain chemical receptors found in the placenta of pregnant women. Empedocles (c.494 BC– c.434 BC) blocked off a gorge in Acragas, Sicily, because it was found to be a funnel for a southerly wind bringing in mosquitoes which introduced placental malaria. Pliny the Elder quotes Icatidas, a Greek doctor who taught that malaria in men is cured by having sex with a woman just starting her period.

In imperial Rome, diseases were a fact of life, due largely to the crowded conditions in the cities and the opportunities for contagion afforded, paradoxically, by the sophisticated sewage sytems and the public baths. Deforestation exaggerated disease transmission in marshlands due to the rising water tables it caused. What with all those public baths, latrines with washing facilities, sewer systems, fountains and clean drinking water from aqueducts you would think that the Romans (at least the comfortably off ones) would have enjoyed a reasonable level of personal hygiene and were largely free from chronic stomach upsets, infectious and intestinal disease generally. Not a bit of it; research led by Piers Mitchell from the Department of Archaeology and Anthropology at the University of Cambridge, and published in the journal *Parasitology*, found that baths and the like did nothing to protect the Romans from those annoying, embarrassing parasites.

Mitchell and his team rolled up their sleeves and used archaeological evidence from cesspits, sewer drains, rubbish pits, burials and other sites to assess the impact of parasites across Roman Europe, the Middle East and North Africa. Unfortunately for the Romans analysis of all of the above plus ancient latrines, human burials and coprolites (fossilized faeces) clearly demonstrated that, instead of decreasing as expected, intestinal parasites actually increased compared with the preceding Iron Age.

'The impressive sanitation technologies introduced by the Romans did not seem to have delivered the health benefits that we would expect,' Mitchell said. He found that the most widely spread intestinal parasites in the Roman Empire were whipworm (Trichuris trichiura) and roundworm (Ascaris lumbricoides) which are transmitted by the contamination of food with faeces. 'It could have been spread by the use of unwashed hands to prepare food or by the use of human faeces as crop fertilizer,' Mitchell concluded. Also prolific was Entamoeba histolytica, a protozoan that causes dysentery, with bloody diarrhoea, abdominal pain and fevers. It is contracted by drinking water contaminated by human faeces.

Ectoparasites such as lice and fleas were as common among Romans as in later Viking and medieval populations, where bathing was not so widely practised. Excavations in York in the main sewer shows that despite all their regular bathing and flushing latrines the Romans systematically undid all that good public health work by routinely using as a substitute for toilet paper and for solo hand washing… communal sponges on a stick. These, of course, were breeding grounds for dysentery, diarrhoea and parasites.

Pliny the Elder's most famous extant work is the 37 book *Historia Naturalis*, an encyclopedia which includes material on dermatologic disease, the efficacy of 'lichen', and leprosy, sourced from a myriad of earlier and contemporary authors.

Soranus provides a remarkable description of pthisis, tuberculosis:

'The sputa are at first bright red, then muddy, then bluish or greenish and finally white and purulent, and either sweet or salt. The voice is either hoarse or high pitched, breathing laboured, cheeks flushed and the rest of the body, ashen colored. The patient is emaciated. In some cases there is a hissing sound or wheezing in the chest.'

Galen is easily antiquity's most prolific author in Greek: his works formed the basis of medical education in the Byzantine empire and in Europe for many centuries. Galen became a specialist in malaria: many of the patients Galen diagnosed with 'fever' would have suffered from this. Significantly in the history of medicine, to Galen fever was not a symptom but a disease which meant recurrent paroxysms of shivering, rigor, sweating, burning heat, and a characteristic pulse. Galen also waged war on smallpox, as we will see in our coverage of the Antonine Plague below.

Doctors were the preserve of the wealthy; the less well-off would have stuck with their traditional folk and sometimes phoney remedies and put their faith in the gods, the magicians and the quacks. Pliny the Elder said it very well when he declared that thousands of people lived without doctors, but not without medicine.

Superstition was by no means unusual; it was rife and omnipresent. In a world where it was considered unpropitious for a black cat to enter your house or a snake to fall from the roof into your yard, where it was unlucky if a statue of a god was reliably seen to sweat blood, where a horse was born with five legs, a lamb with a pig's head and a pig with a human head, where a rampant bull ran up three flights of stairs and a cow talked, and where a statue laughed uncontrollably, a horse cried hot tears – in a world where it was inauspicious to sneeze in the presence of a waiter holding a tray or to sweep the floor when a guest was standing up – where it was *de rigueur* to whistle when lightning flashed – in such a world it should come as no surprise to hear that you should cut your nails only on market days, and then starting with the forefinger and doing it in silence – but never while at sea. In certain Italian towns it was forbidden by law for women to walk through the streets carrying a spindle, a true badge of Roman womanhood.

But it is important to put this into some sort of context and remember that the Romans were probably no more superstitious than other cultures and societies. Indeed, if we look at the old wives' tales recounted by George Orwell from a rural childhood around 1900 in *Coming Up for Air*, can we say that they are any less rational than the Romans'? Take for example:

'…swimming was dangerous, climbing trees was dangerous…all animals were dangerous…horses bit, bats got in your hair, earwigs got into your ears, swans broke your leg…bulls tossed you…raw potatoes were deadly poison, and so were mushrooms unless you bought them at the grocer's…if you had a bath after a meal you died of cramp...and if you washed your hands in the water eggs were boiled in you got warts...raw onions were a cure for almost anything.'

Before the Greeks and Romans strains of influenza repeatedly ravaged the then centres of dense population, Central Asia, Mesopotamia and Southern Asia, in the reign of Tiglath–Pileser I (1114 BC – 1076 BC) and Nebuchadnezzar (630 BC – 562 BC). The virus also afflicted ancient Babylon in 1103 BC. There was an epidemic in Nineveh during the reign of Sargon II, King of Assyria (r. 722 BC – 705 BC).

We have a number of pestilences in Greek and Roman literature before the account of the Plague of Athens given by Thucydides (c. 460 BC – 400 BC) in his *History of the Peloponnesian War*,[2] going back to the dawn of western literature. They include: Homer (c.750 BC)[3], when, at the very start of the epic *Iliad*, Apollo unleashes a 'foul plague' (νουσον κακην) on the Greek armies because Agamemnon, their commander, refused to return Chryseis, daughter of Chryses, whom he had appropriated. This was a zoonotic disease which started in the tenth year of the Trojan War with mules and dogs spreading it to the Greek warriors after they had been inoculated with the disease by Apollo's well-aimed arrows. Herodotus[4] reveals how Cretan warriors returning home from the Trojan War imported a pestilence which infected men and cattle leading to the desertion of the island – perhaps these two were connected? Sophocles, *Oedipus Rex* 25ff, describes a disease in Thebes which affected crops, cattle and men – including unborn babies. Thucydides[5] tells how pestilence was one of many catastrophes in the historian's day, along with earthquakes, famine and drought.

Plague was present right at the very start of Roman civilisation when mythical Aeneas and his men, defeated in the Trojan War, were sailing around the Mediterranean looking for the place at which they were to found Rome. In the early days of Rome, Livy tells us how Tullus Hostilius (r.673 BC – 642 BC), the legendary third king of Rome, negligent in his duty to respect the gods, died in 642 BC of the plague. Towards the end of his reign, Rome was beset by bad omens: a shower of stones fell on the Alban Mount; a supernatural voice boomed out complaining that the Albans had failed to show due devotion and a plague struck Rome. Tullus was so intent on proceeding with war that he initially refused to stand down the army during the pestilence, thus causing much death, distress and enmity. Tullus himself fell ill with the plague. Hubris got you nowhere.

Livy mentions plague and pestilence a number of other times including: 437 BC at 4, 20, 9 (*pestilentia, inopia frugum*); 437 BC at 4, 21, 2 *(quia pestilentia populum invasit)*; 436 BC at 4, 21, 6 (*pestilentior inde annus*). In fact, between books 2 and 5 Livy records 16 occasions when one disease or another infected Rome. For Livy disease is comparable with war and famine as the worst evils that a state could suffer, and he concludes that people attributed these calamities to *ira deum*, the wrath of the gods.

---

2. 2, 47–55; 59, 1–2; 61, 3–4; 64, 1

3. *Iliad*, 1, 50

4. 7, 171, 1–2

5. 1, 23

Roughly three years before the plague at Athens, Livy tells us that Rome was similarly affected with a two year long contagion.[6] Was this possibly the same plague which later raged in Athens, brought to Greece on Carthaginian and other trade routes?

In 412 BC it seems there was a flu pandemic. We hear of it from Hippocrates when it scourged northern Greece, and from Livy as it ravaged the city of Rome. First Hippocrates:

'In Thasus (an island in the north Aegean)...severe fevers occurred in a few instances, and these very mild, being rarely attended with hemorrhage, and never proving fatal. Swellings appeared about the ears, in many on either side, and in the greatest number on both sides, being unaccompanied by fever so as not to confine the patient to bed; in all cases they disappeared without giving trouble ... without inflammation or pain, and they went away without any critical sign. They seized children, adults, and mostly those who were engaged in the exercises of the palestra and gymnasium, but seldom attacked women. Many had dry coughs without expectoration and accompanied with hoarseness of voice. In some instances earlier, and in others later, inflammations with pain seized sometimes one of the testicles, and sometimes both; some of these cases were accompanied with fever and some not; most were attended with much suffering. In other respects they were free of disease, so as not to require medical assistance. ... many of those who had been gradually declining, took to bed with symptoms of phthisis (pulmonary tuberculosis)...Many, and, in fact, most of them, died; and of those confined to bed, I do not know if a single individual survived for any considerable time; they died more suddenly than is common in such cases.'

– Hippocrates, *Of the Epidemics* 1, 1-2 adapted from
the translation by Francis Adams

Now Livy:

'After this year [412 BC-411 BC]...a pestilence broke out, which, though it threatened more than it killed, made men think less of the Forum and politics than of their homes and the care of the sick...The state had escaped with very few deaths, considering the great number of those who had fallen ill, when the year of pestilence was succeeded...by a scarcity of corn, owing to diminished harvesting in such times.'

– Livy 4, 52, 3–5

Livy (5, 42) tells of a pestilence, probably malaria, in 390 BC during the Gallic sack of Rome. The Gauls were now camped in a cauldron of a valley where conditions fell well short of salubrious: it was dry, very hot and dusty – the complete opposite to the climate and environment they were used to back in Gaul. They were soon plagued by an epidemic, exacerbated, no doubt, by the putrefying corpses of the unburied dead.

---

6. 4, 25, 3–7

Alexander the Great (356 BC – 323 BC) reputedly died of flu in the temple of Nebuchadnezzar II. However, there is whole host of other claimants on his life: they include: malaria and typhoid fever (both prevalent in Babylon at the time) while a paper in the *New England Journal of Medicine* attributed his death to typhoid fever complicated by bowel perforation and ascending paralysis.[7] Other suggestions are pyogenic (infectious) spondylitis or meningitis. Other illnesses fit the symptoms, including acute pancreatitis and West Nile virus. If nothing else the speculation gives a clear picture of the diseases prevalent at the time.

The Greek historian Diodorus Siculus records (14, 41, c.90 BC – c.30 BC) a raging pestilence in 592 BC with Carthaginians in Libya suffering headache, coma and death. At the Siege of Syracuse in 396 BC plague struck, again helped by questionable hygiene on marshy grounds and malaria.[8] Numerous soldiers and sailors succumbed to the disease, burial parties were overwhelmed, bodies were hastily buried, new burials were almost impossible and the stench of decaying bodies filled the air. Fear of infection may have prevented proper care being given to the sick. The cause of the contagion was attributed to the Carthaginians' and their desecration of Greek temples and tombs. If the Carthaginian general, Himilco, took any measures to combat the plague they were ineffective; Carthaginian morale plummeted because of the disease, along with combat effectiveness.

The Greek god of medicine, Asclepius, was imported from Epidaurus into the Roman pantheon in 293 BC, on the advice of the *Sibylline Books* consulted in some panic during an outbreak of plague. A snake slithered out of the temple at Epidaurus and took up residence on the mast of the ship which was to bring a statue of the god to Rome – hence the familiar British Medical Association logo which survives today. At the Epidaurus temple supplicants habitually carved cures on the walls or erected monuments to help subsequent sufferers of various ailments. The snake jumped ship, landing on Insula Tiberina where a temple to Asclepius was promptly built: the plague soon subsided and the temple became a clinic attended by the sick and dying, its reputation constantly enhanced by reports of miraculous cures. The insular site may actually have been chosen because it facilitated the quaranteening of infectious diseases.

Grmek, Mirko, D.,1983, *Diseases in the Ancient Greek World*, Baltimore

Ross, Ronald, Malaria in Greece, 1906, *Jnl Trop.Med.* 9, 341–7

Scheidel, Walter (2009) Disease and Death in the Ancient City of Rome, *Princeton/ Stanford Working Papers in Classics*

Smith, Christina A., Plague in the Ancient World: A Study from Thucydides to Justinian, *The Loyola University History Department Student Historical Journal* 28.

---

7. Oldach, DW et al; June 1998. 'A mysterious death'. *N. Engl. J. Med.* 338 (24): 1764–69
8. Diodorus 14, 70–71; Livy 25, 26

Schistosomiasis (bilharziasis) and other ancient infectious diseases

There are records of other diseases which were prevalent in the ancient world. Schistosomiasis (bilharziasis) is a parasitic infection that has evolved hand in hand with the march of human civilisation from earliest times. We have evidence for it in ancient Egyptian medical papyri while Assyrian medical texts reported signs and symptoms that could well be schistosomiasis; similarly, there are passages in the Bible which describe an epidemic (a 'curse') that is believed to be associated with the spread of schistosomiasis in Mesopotamia. Today, schistosomiasis still affects more than 200 million people worldwide and it is a stark reminder of how hard it is to prevent, control and treat intransigent tropical diseases.

It is caused by flatworms (flukes) of the genus Schistosoma; the most important species for human pathology are *S. haematobium* (responsible for urogenital disease), *S. mansoni*, and *S. japonicum* (both responsible for intestinal/hepatic disease). *S. haematobium* is endemic in Africa and Middle East; *S. mansoni* in Africa, Middle East, Central and South America and *S. japonicum* in eastern Asia. In 2018 Stefano di Bella reported that 'with more than 700 million people living in endemic areas and increasing migratory flux to non-endemic areas, 200 million people worldwide are at risk for urogenital and intestinal/hepatic schistosomiasis. Despite medical progress, liver fibrosis and bladder cancer remain oppressive complications of the chronic infection sustained by Schistosoma spp.'

Schistosomiasis is considered 'the most important water-based disease from a global public-health perspective' reflecting the fundamental role of water in its spread. Water and life have always been interconnected, so it is unsurprising that schistosomiasis has been present in ancient civilizations over the centuries. Its origins take us all the way back more than 6,000 years when human skeletal remains were found in Tell Zeidan in an early settlement of farmers in northern Syria (5800–4000 BC). It is believed that schistosomiasis had spread to Egypt through the importation of monkeys and slaves during reign of the fifth dynasty of pharaohs (~2494 BC – 2345 BC).

Schistosomiasis is mentioned in Egyptian medical papyri 22 times from 1500 BC suggesting it was not uncommon, and tells of a disease characterized by discharge from the penis. To prevent it the ancient Egyptians were advised to avoid polluted water, and fishermen, farmers and others in regular contact with the river were advised to wear penile linen sheaths.

Since the early 2000s advances in molecular biology technology have allowed us to research specific fragments of DNA. Before that in 1910, Marc Armand Ruffer, professor of bacteriology, president of the Sanitary, Maritime and Quarantine Council of Egypt (Alexandria), published a paper in *The British Medical Journal*, reporting his studies on Egyptian mummies of the twentieth dynasty (1250–1000 B.C.): 'in the kidneys of the two mummies of the twentieth dynasty I have demonstrated in microscopic sections a large number of calcified eggs of Bilharzia haematobia, situated, for the most part, among the straight tubules.' This paper prompted the foundation of the Manchester Egyptian Mummy Project in 1973 and information about mummies held in collections all over the world began to be recorded.

In 1990, Deelder et al. detected a schistosome circulating anodic antigen in the cheek, gut and shin of Egyptian mummies known to be infected with *S. haematobium*; a similar study in 1992 used samples of desiccated skin and brain from 23 mummies recovered from Nubia (AD 350–AD 550); 65 per cent had schistosomiasis.

In 2014, with the benefit of molecular biology techniques scientists found *S. mansoni* and *S. haematobium* DNA from the liver of the Nekht-Ankh mummy and *S. haematobium* DNA from intestinal samples from the Khnum-Nakht mummy.

Polio virus may account for the slender femur shaft (and paralysis) of a 40-year-old male from Lerna, south of Argos. Some researches believe they have identified traces of smallpox on Egyptian mummies. Tuberculosis may account for the spinal deformation found in an exhumed Iron Age Greek lady.

Di Bella et al., 2018, History of schistosomiasis (bilharziasis) in humans: from Egyptian medical papyri to molecular biology on mummies, *Pathogens and Global Health*, 268–273.

Mahmoud, Adel A.F. 2004, Schistosomiasis (bilharziasis): from antiquity to the present, *Infect Dis Clin North Am*, 207–218

Ziskind, Bernard, 2009, Urinary schistosomiasis in ancient Egypt. *Nephrology Therapy*, 658–661 [Article in French]

Infectious disease in Ancient China

Our understanding of ancient Chinese infectious disease is dogged by problems of interpretation, not least because traditional Chinese medicine does not lend itself to translation into western tongues and because Chinese writing did not attain its modern form until the 3rd century BC. Records in much earlier chronicles, oracle bones and grave goods are written in pictograms with all the imprecision that brings. Notwithstanding, attempts have been made to quantify the epidemics, for example, by William McNeil who comes up with 99 between 243 BC and the time of the Black Death in the 14th century.

The oldest records appear on oracle bones from the Shang Dynasty (c. 1600 BC-1046 BC) written on scapulae and bits of tortoise shell; many diseases feature but what concerns us are the various lethal seasonal epidemics and cases of schistosomiasis. The Yueh Ling (Monthly Ordinances) reveal seasonal diseases with autumn fever indicating malaria and typhus and tetanus prevalent in winter. Later we find evidence of tuberculosis and leprosy.

Ancient India

Suśruta was an ancient Indian physician and the main author of the treatise *The Compendium of Suśruta* – one of the most important surviving ancient treatises on medicine and is one of the foundational texts of Ayurveda. It covers all aspects of general medicine and probably dates from around 500 AD. In its extant form, in 184 chapters it contains descriptions of 1,120 illnesses, 700 medicinal plants, 64 preparations from mineral sources and 57 preparations based on animal sources.

The text is strong on surgical techniques. Our first mention of leprosy (kushta) is described in Suśruta Samhita. Cholera and, of course, malaria were well known.

Sharma, P. V., 1992. History of medicine in India, from antiquity to 1000 A.D. New Delhi
Yi Zeng, Infectious Disease in China, https://www.jst.go.jp/astf/document2/45pre.pdf

Ancient Japan

In very early Japan disease was thought to be sent by the gods or conjured up by evil spirits. Treatment and prevention were based largely on religious rites, such as prayers, incantations, and exorcism; at a later date drugs and bloodletting were also deployed.

From AD 608, when aspiring young Japanese physicians were sent to China for extensive study, Chinese influence on Japanese medicine was huge. In 982, Tamba Yasuyori completed the 30-volume Ishinhō, the oldest extant Japanese medical work. This covers diseases and their treatment, classified mainly according to the affected organs. It is based entirely on older Chinese medical works, with the concept of yin and yang underlying the theory of disease causation.

Kampō medicine (漢方医学) is the study of traditional Chinese medicine in Japan following its introduction then adapted and modified to suit Japanese culture and traditions. Traditional Japanese medicine uses most of the Chinese therapies including acupuncture and moxibustion, and traditional Chinese herbology and traditional food therapy.

Y. Motoo, 2011, 'Traditional Japanese medicine, Kampo: its history and current status'.
Chinese Journal of Integrative Medicine. 17 (2): 85–87.
Yamada, Terutane, 1996, 'The Tradition and Genealogy of the Kampo Medicine'. *Japanese Journal of Oriental Medicine* 46 (4): 505–518.

'You can't pin it down but the ancient world does give us a bit of an insight into how plague and pandemic have been incorporated into people's experience.'

– Mary Beard, *The Times*, 8 May 2021

Chapter 2

The Plague of Athens 430 BC

'I shall simply set down its nature, and explain the symptoms by which perhaps it may be recognized by the student, should it ever ever break out again. This I am qualified do, as I had the disease myself, and have watched its course in others.'
— Thucydides, *History of the Peloponnesian War*, 2, 48

Thucydides' description of the plague in Athens is a shocking and vivid account of a public health disaster, the like of which the city, nor any Greek city had ever suffered before. Its appearance so soon after the stirring and patriotic Funeral Oration delivered by Pericles gives it a sharper focus and imbues it with even more realism and horror in its depiction of the fragility of human life.

The Plague of Athens (Λοιμὸς τῶν Ἀθηνῶν) was an epidemic that devastated the city-state of Athens during the second year of the Peloponnesian War against the Spartans; this was at a time when Athens was under siege by Sparta, although an Athenian victory was still a real possibility. In the next three years most of the population was infected and perhaps as many as 75,000 to 100,000 people, 25 per cent of the city's population, died. The epidemic broke in early May 430 BC, with subsequent waves in the summer of 428 and in the winter of 427–426[1]. It lasted almost five years. Thucydides is our main source; Plutarch is less useful. Up until Thucydides it was commonly believed that it was the gods who visited plagues on mankind in punishment for disrespect, hubris or ungodly behaviour. We see this in Herodotus, as well as in the *Book of Exodus* and, as already noted, in the *Iliad*:

> 'And which of the gods was it that set them on to quarrel? It was the son of Jove and Leto; for he was angry with the king and sent a pestilence upon the host to plague the people, because the son of Atreus had dishonoured Chryses his priest.'
> — Homer, *Iliad*, I, 9–11

Significantly, Thucydides had no time for intervention by the gods in his history. This is particularly evident in his account of the Athenian plague. Thucydides thereby initiated an historiographical tradition which would become the model for future historians.

---

1. Thucydides 3, 87

Pericles, leader of the Athenians, had delivered the customary funeral oration the year before: the purpose of the speech was to boost morale among military and citizenry alike in a city at war; it eulogises Athens and glorifies Athenian achievements. If Pericles' stirring speech was a force for the good in war-torn Athens, then what was to follow the next year had completely the opposite effect. What no one – Spartan or Athenian – could have predicted was the devastating impact an outbreak of plague had on the course of their war.

In 430 BC that plague struck Athens, spreading relentlessly and remorselessly through the packed, stifling city and in the port of Piraeus. The king of Sparta, Archidamus II (r. 476–427 BC), had from the start been determined to deflect a war so he now dispatched a new delegation to Athens with a brief to get the significantly weakened and preoccupied Athenians to submit to Sparta's demands. The delegation, however, was refused entry to Athens. A frustrated Archidamus now invaded Attica only to find, to his amazement, the place empty of Greeks. Pericles, in pursuit of a strategy of retreat, had anticipated Archidamus's plans for devastation and evacuated the entire population from the land to within the walls of Athens – in effect a massive migration flow from the Attic countryside into an already very overcrowded city. The disastrous effect was to exaggerate the already insufferable and insanitary conditions, while adding to the chronic shortages, inadequate food and water supplies and no doubt a corresponding increase in migratory insects, lice, rats and refuse. It is easy to underestimate just how huge a life-changing move this was for the displaced farmers and landowners around Athens. They had to leave everything they had to the prey of the Spartans in exchange for a new, highly unappealing, life in a packed urban Athens; not surprisingly there was much discontent.

Due to the crowded conditions, the total inability to socially distance and its poor hygiene Athens was a breeding ground for disease. Shanty towns sprang up on waste ground or in temples or around the fortifications; life-saving rain tanks soon became fouled.

War-time Athens' cramped, hellish conditions were notorious, with comic play-wright Aristophanes joking that residents even lived in casks, crevices and dovecots, blinded with smoke.[2] Thucydides reports 'dying men lay tumbling one upon another in the streets...'[3] And Sophocles seems to allude to the plague, when, in the opening scene of *Oedipus Rex* (ca. 430 BC–423 BC), the Priest of Zeus vividly compares Thebes with what Athens must have been like at the time:

'For the city...can no longer lift her head from beneath the angry waves of death. A blight has fallen on the...land... and the flaming god, the malign plague, has swooped upon us, and ravages the town...'[4]

---

2. *Knights* 795
3. 2.52.2
4. lines 22–30

This plague was a major contributory factor in Athens' defeat: it exterminated highly trained sailors and first line soldiers as well as generals, including Pericles and his sons, Paralus and Xanthippus. It weakened Athens' military power and left her morale in tatters.

What of Pericles' death? Thucydides[5] merely says: 'He lived after the war began two years and six months,' i.e. until 429 BC. It is only from Plutarch, writing some 500 years later, that we learn 'the plague laid hold of Pericles' along with 'not a few of his intimate friends', his sons Xanthippus and Paralus, his sister, many other family members, and 'those who were most useful to him in his administration of the city...'[6]

Plutarch's sources are rather murky, however, and it seems the biographer is either simply guessing as to Pericles' cause of death or is guilty of spreading fake news.

Between one-third and two-thirds of the Athenian population died. Athenian manpower was drastically depleted and even foreign mercenaries refused to hire themselves out to a city reduced to its knees with rampant plague. Sparta went so far as to abandon its invasion plans of Attica for fear of contagion. The effect of the disease on Athens' military and civilian population was apparently devastating, based on the mortality figures Thucydides provides. In the summer of 430 BC, when Athens 'made war upon the Chalcideans...and...Potidaea...,' the disease 'devoured the army' and 'Agnon...came back with his fleet, having, of 4,000, in less than forty days, lost 1,050 to the plague.'[7]

Later, after reporting the disease's resurgence (427/426 BC), the historian writes: '... the number that died of it of men of arms enrolled were no less than 4,400 and horsemen, 300; of the other multitude, innumerable'.[8] Even more troubling, the plague was not the only current concern. There were also earthquakes in Athens, Euboea and Boeotia.[9]

On the origins of the disease Thucydides tells of a contagion emanating from Ethiopia and passing through Egypt and Libya into the Greek and Persian worlds then spreading throughout the wider Mediterranean; the plague is believed to have entered Athens through Piraeus, the city's bustling port and only source of food and supplies. Much of the eastern Mediterranean was also afflicted, although to a lesser extent. It was a plague so virulent that no one could remember anything like it; doctors working in the infancy of medical science had no experience of such a ruthless epidemic and were not only helpless but died in droves as they had the most contact with the infected. According to Thucydides, not until 415 BC had Athens recovered sufficiently to mount a major new offensive, the disastrous Sicilian Expedition.

Thucydides tells us that symptoms included people previously in good health all of a sudden attacked by violent headaches and conjunctivitis; the throat or tongue

---

5. 2.65.6
6. Pericles. 36.1, 3, 4; 38.1
7. 2.58.3
8. 3.87.3
9. Thuc. 3.87.4

became bloody, emitting an abnormal and fetid breath… followed by sneezing and hoarseness, after which the pain soon reached the chest and produced a hard cough. The victims then coughed up blood and suffered from extremely painful stomach cramping, followed by vomiting and attacks of 'ineffectual retching'. (hiccups?) When the contagion settled in the stomach, it caused diarrhoea. There were discharges of all kinds of bile known to doctors, blisters, ulcers, low mood, necrosis of the extremities, brain damage, loss of memory…

> 'Most places were full of the corpses of those who had just died there; as the crisis spiralled out of control, men, not knowing what was going to happen to them, became equally contemptuous of the gods' property and what was due to the gods. All customary burial rites were totally contravened as people buried the bodies as best they could. Many… resorted to the most shameless tombs: taking advantage of those who had raised a pile of corpses, they threw their own dead body on a stranger's pyre and lit it; sometimes they tossed the corpse they were carrying on the top of another that was burning and just walked off.
>
> Though many lay unburied, carrrion and beasts would not touch them, or if they did, died after eating them …the bodies of dying men lay one on top of another, and half-dead creatures reeled about the streets and thronged round all the fountains in their thirst for water…'

There have been various suggestions as to what the Athenian plague actually was; thirty pathogens have been suggested including Ebola haemorrhagic fever, glanders, typhus, typhoid, anthrax, measles and toxic shock syndrome or smallpox. Glanders is a zoonotic infectious disease found primarily in equines but can be contracted by other animals, such as dogs, cats and goats. Humans can catch it through close contact with these animals.

Such speculation is, of course, pointless – as Thucydides himself declares:

> 'All speculation as to its origin and its causes, if causes can be found adequate enough for so great a calamity, I leave to other writers, whether amateur or professional; for myself, I shall simply set down its nature, and explain the symptoms by which perhaps it may be recognized by the student, should it ever ever break out again. This I am qualified do, as I had the disease myself, and have watched its course in others.'[10]

In January 1999, the University of Maryland devoted their fifth annual medical conference which celebrates notorious case histories, to the Plague of Athens. They concluded that the disease that killed the Greeks was typhus. 'Epidemic typhus fever is the best explanation,' said David Durack, consulting professor of medicine at Duke University. 'It hits hardest in times of war and privation, it has about 20 per cent mortality, it kills the victim after about seven days, and it sometimes causes a striking complication: gangrene

---

10. Thucydides 2, 47–55

of the tips of the fingers and toes. The Plague of Athens had all these features.' In typhus cases, progressive dehydration, debilitation and cardiovascular collapse ultimately cause the patient's death.

Another strong candidate is viral haemorrhagic fever (VHF): Thucydides refers to the increased risk experienced among health care workers which is more characteristic of the person-to-person contact spread of viral haemorrhagic fever (such as Ebola virus disease or Marburg virus) than typhus. Thucydides' description further invites comparison with VHF in the character and sequence of symptoms developed, and of the usual fatal outcome on about the eighth day. Some scientists have interpreted Thucydides' expression 'lygx kenē' (λύγξ κενή) as the unusual symptom of hiccups, which is now recognized as a common presentation in Ebola virus disease.

Haemorrhagic fever aetiology is supported by the Roman Epicurean philosopher Lucretius (b.94 BC). He characterized the Athenian plague as having 'bloody' or black discharges from orifices. Lucretius cited and was a follower of two scientific predecessors in Greek Sicily, Empedocles and Acron, a physician and author. While none of the original works of Acron are extant, it is reported that he died c.430 BC after travelling to Athens to fight the plague; here he ordered large fires to be started in the streets to purify the air and provide some relief to the sick. Superstition reigned, especially in the peddling of old oracles.[11] To Lucretius, the plague exemplified not only human vulnerability, but also the futility of religion and belief in the gods.[12]

The Athenian plague was a totally unpredictable and unforeseen event that resulted in one of the largest recorded losses of life in ancient Greece as well as a breakdown of Athenian society. Thucydides describes the collapse of social morality, adding that people stopped obeying the law since they believed they were already living under a death sentence. Similarly, citizens started spending money indiscriminately rather than saving prudently as they used to; social strata were disrupted when poor people unexpectedly became rich when affluent relatives died. Generally, the Athenians began behaving immorally because most did not expect to live long enough to be rewarded by the gods for living a pious life.

The temples themselves were now wretched, ungodly places, filled with homeless refugees from the Athenian countryside. Soon they were filled with the dead and dying. Innate Greek superstition played its part: the Athenians saw the plague as evidence that the gods favoured Sparta, and this was supported by an oracle that Apollo himself (the god of disease and medicine) would fight for Sparta: but when Apollo was asked by the Athenians 'whether they should go to war, he answered that if they put their might into it, victory would be theirs, and that he would himself be with them.'[13] Alarmingly, an earlier oracle had warned that 'A Spartan war will come and bring a pestilence with it.'

The plague diminished Athens' international power and its ability to develop alongside its rivals. Many of the surviving Athenians were metics (foreign workers

---

11. 2, 54
12. *De Rerum Natura* 11
13. Thuc. 2.54.4

with limited citizenship) who had forged their documentation or had bribed officials to hide their original status. A number of these were reduced to slaves when caught. This resulted in stricter laws dictating who could become an Athenian citizen, reducing both the number of potential soldiers available to the state and hastening a decline in treatment and rights for metics in Athens.

The plague then dealt a huge military, economic and social blow to Athens two years into the Peloponnesian War, from which it never recovered. Athens would then go on to be defeated by Sparta and lose its place as a major superpower in ancient Greece.

'It was a disaster of epic proportions that altered not only the Peloponnesian War, but the whole of Greek, and consequently world, history. While the war would not end for nearly 26 years after the first wave of sickness, there is little doubt that the Great Plague changed the course of the war (being at least in part responsible for Athens' defeat) and significantly shaped the peace that came afterward, planting the seeds that would weaken and then destroy Athenian democracy.'

—Katherine Kelaidis, Resident scholar at the National Hellenic Museum and a visiting assistant professor in Classical Studies at Loyola University Chicago, What the Great Plague of Athens Can Teach Us Now, *The Atlantic*, 23 March 2020

Kelaidis goes on to explain the significance of Thucydides' 'visceral' account, born of first hand experience as a victim:

'Thucydides has been called the "father of political realism" …as few others have before or since, Thucydides understood the ways in which fear and self-interest, when they are submitted to, guide individual motives, and consequently the fate of nations… Thucydides looks frankly at the practical and moral weaknesses that the disease was able to exploit. He sharply notes how crowding in Athens, along with inadequate housing and sanitation, helped the disease spread more quickly and added to the number of casualties. He is aware that a lack of attention to important public-health and safety measures allowed the Plague to take root and made its effects much worse than they would have otherwise been.'

Excavations during 1994–95 just outside Athens' ancient Kerameikos cemetery unearthed a mass grave and nearly 1,000 tombs, dated between 430 and 426 BC. The shaft-shaped grave contained a total of 240 individuals, at least ten of them children; skeletons were haphazardly placed with no layers of soil between them, without any of the usual care and dignity that ancient Greeks usually showed for the dead and their burial.

Archaeologist Efi Baziotopoulou-Valavani, of the Third Ephoreia of Antiquities, reported that:

'The mass grave did not have a monumental character. The offerings we found consisted of common, even cheap, burial vessels; black-finished ones, some small red-figured, as well as white lekythoi (oil flasks) of the second half of the 5th century

BC. The bodies were placed in the pit within a day or two. These [factors] point to a mass burial in a state of panic, quite possibly due to a plague.'

Myrtis is the name bestowed by archaeologists on an 11-year-old girl from Athens, whose remains were discovered in 1994–95 in a mass grave during work to build the metro station at Kerameikos. Forensic analysis showed that Myrtis and two other bodies in the mass grave had died of typhoid fever during the Plague of Athens.

Mitchell Berger, 2015, Influenza, not Ebola, More Likely the Cause of 430 BCE Athenian Outbreak, *Clin Infect Dis* 61, 1492–3

Morens, David et al., 1992, 'Epidemiology of the Plague of Athens', *Transactions of the American Philological Association 122*, 271–304.

Papagrigorakis, M.J., 2006, 'DNA examination of ancient dental pulp incriminates typhoid fever as a probable cause of the Plague of Athens.' *International Society for Infectious Diseases*, 10, 206–14.

Papagrigorakis, M.J., 2011, Facial Reconstruction of an 11-year-old Female Resident of Athens, *Angle Orthodontist* 81

Pestilence and other diseases in the Roman Empire

The eruption of Vesuvius in AD 79 is famous for its destruction, and conservation, of Pompeii and Herculaneum. Much less known is the epidemic which overran the Campagna region in the wake of the devastation apparently killing 10,000. Scholars believe that it may well have been fulminating malaria possibly accompanied by an outbreak of anthax.

In 2000 when Richard Stothers (National Aeronautics and Space Administration Goddard Institute for Space Studies, NASA, in Cleveland, Ohio) statistically examined the occurrences of plagues that have been recorded throughout western history, he uncovered a curious coincidence. Many of these pandemics occurred soon after a volcano underwent a huge eruption. He tells us that:

'Volcanoes have been known to spew sulfurous gases into the stratosphere, where the sulfur combines with water vapor to form sulfuric acid aerosols. These aerosols screen out some of the radiation coming from the Sun and so cool off the Earth's surface... these eruptions were followed by stratospheric dry fogs that dimmed the Sun's light, chilled the atmosphere, and led to an increase in the amount of precipitation. In each case, many food crops failed and a fatal pandemic, originating from a focus in Asia or Africa, spread throughout the Mediterranean area within one to five years after the eruption. It is believed that in at least five instances the contagion responsible for the mass mortality was true plague..'

The 5th century Spanish historian Orosius speaks of a plague which engulfed Numibia (mainly Algeria with bits of Libya and Tunisia) and Utica (modern Tunisia) in AD 125 killing 800,000 and 200,000 respectively (an exaggeration). This was preceded by a plague of locusts whose depradations caused significant famine on the north African littoral with disease and famine spreading over into Italy.

Disease was an inevitable and devastating aspect of life in the Roman empire. There were a variety of possible causes which included the sewage systems, the public bathing houses, sanitation and litter, the diet of citizens as well as environmental issues such as deforestation. Chopping down trees to facilitate urban sprawl provoked high rates of transmission due to a chain reaction in the marshes from the rising water table that stemmed from such deforestation and resulted in marshlands. This in turn attracted larva which harboured diseases borne by blood-sucking bugs. Mosquitoes and other vectors, of course, were carriers of various diseases, such as malaria. We have seen above how malaria was an incessant problem for the Romans and how children's skeletons unearthed at Lugnano proved to be reservoir for malaria.

The skeletons of a pair of twins excavated in a pomegranate store in Oplontis near Pompeii show what were almost certainly the signs of congenital syphilis. If correct, this torpedoes the long-held belief that the repellent disease was introduced to Europe from the New World by Christopher Columbus the 15th century.

In 2015, about 45.4 million people worldwide were infected with syphilis with six million new cases that year. During 2015, it brought about 107,000 deaths, down from 202,000 in 1990. The availability of penicillin in the 1940 saw deaths plummet but rates of infection have since increased since 2000 in many countries, often in combination with human immunodeficiency virus (HIV).

Mentagra was a Roman disease thought to be spread by kissing. It was a skin disease usually starting in the chin before spreading over the entire face and sometimes other body parts. While it caused few medical complications, it was aesthetically off putting, to both the patient and the observer. Romans went so far as having scar-inducing cauterizations to rid them of the abhorrent disease.

Respiratory diseases, in particular anthracosis, were common due to high levels of pollution in Roman homes, according to Professor Luigi Capasso. Carbon was constantly emitted from lamps, cooking, and fireplaces. The carbon produced lesions on the Roman's lungs which have been detected in bone studies and a study on a Roman mummy. Periostitis or periostalgia, is a usually chronic medical condition caused by inflammation of the periosteum, a layer of connective tissue that surrounds bone. It is indicated by tenderness and swelling of the bone, and by pain.

Capasso, Luigi, 2000. 'Indoor pollution and respiratory diseases in Ancient Rome. *The Lancet*. 356 (9243): 1774.

Gigante, Linda. 'Death and Disease in Ancient Rome.' *Innominate Society*.

O'Sullivan, Lara. 2008. 'Deforestation, Mosquitoes, and Ancient Rome: Lessons for Today'. *BioScience*. 58 (8): 756–760

Stothers, R.B., 1999. Volcanic dry fogs, climate cooling, and plague pandemics in Europe and the Middle East. *Climatic Change* 42, 713–723.

Vuorinen, Heikki S., 2010. 'Water, toilets and public health in the Roman era'. *Water Supply*. 10 (3): 411–415

Chapter 3

The Antonine Plague, AD 165–180

'*The Antonine Plague was the first of three highly destructive pandemics, the others being the Plague of Cyprian (AD 249–AD 262) and the Justinian Plague (AD 541– AD 542), which rocked the Roman Empire to the core due to their high mortality rates.*'
–Kyle Harper, 2017, *The Fate of Rome: Climate, Disease, and the End of an Empire*

It was never only the booty which victorious troops returning from war brought back to the homeland and their families and friends. Sexually transmitted infections and other diseases were sometimes incubating in the soldiers and infecting their baggage trains, only too ready to spread into new populations. The Antonine Plague, or the Plague of Galen, which was probably smallpox, took hold during the golden reign of Marcus Aurelius Antoninus (r. AD 161-AD 180), devastated the Roman army and may have killed over 5 million people in the Roman empire after the army came home from the war in Parthia (161–166). It has even been suggested that a quarter to a third of the entire population of the empire perished, estimated at 60–70 million.

The Antonine Plague was in fact the western flank of the pandemic which originated in China's Han dynasty in AD 200; it is acknowledged that it precipitated the Western Empire's decline and eventual fall some 300 years later.

The plague may have claimed the life of emperor Lucius Verus, who died in 169 and was co-emperor with Marcus Aurelius Antoninus. In 168, as Verus and Marcus Aurelius returned to Rome from the field, Verus fell ill with symptoms consistent with food poisoning, dying after a few days. However, scholars now believe that Verus may have succumbed to smallpox. Some also believe that Marcus Aurelius himself died from this plague some eleven years later.

A blend of legend and historical fact give two different explanations as to how the plague developed to infect the human population. In one Lucius Verus is said to have opened a closed tomb in Seleucia during the sacking of the city and in so doing released, Pandora-like, the disease. This suggests that the epidemic was considered a supernatural punishment because the Romans violated an oath to the gods not to pillage the city. In the second story, a Roman soldier opened a golden casket in the temple of Apollo in Babylon allowing the plague to escape. Two different 4th-century sources, *Res Gestae* by Ammianus Marcellinus (c.AD 330 – AD 400)[1] and the biographies of Lucius Verus and

---

1. 23,6, 24 & *Verus* 8,1, 1–2

Marcus Aurelius in the famously unreliable *Historia Augusta*, ascribe the outbreak to a sacrilege by the Romans when violating the sanctuary of a god. Other Romans preferred to blame Christians for angering the gods by refusing to worship them, believing that angry gods sent the plague as a punishment.

Marcus Aurelius accordingly embarked on a programme of persecutions against Christians but these backfired when the tenets of Christianity started to exert themselves: Christians of course felt an obligation to help others in time of need, including those suffering from a lethal illness, and to 'love thy neighbour'. Therefore, they made themselves available to provide the most basic needs, food and water, for those too ill to fend for themselves. This not only helped the needy but it inculcated good feelings between Christians and their pagan counterparts. Christians stayed to help while pagans fled. At an eschatological and existential level Christianity offered meaning to life and death in times of crisis and an assurance of life after death. Those who survived gained solace in knowing that loved ones, who died as Christians, could receive their reward in heaven. This promise of salvation in the afterlife triggered a spike in recruitment to the faith which, in the longer term, facilitated the acceptance of Christianity as the sole, official religion of the empire in the reign of Constantine I.

We should also mention the pestilence (νόσος λοιμῶδες) vividly described by the orator Aelius Aristides (AD 117 – AD 181) in his *Sacred Tales* (*Hieroi Logoi*) which erupted in the suburbs of Smyrna in the summer of AD 165.[2] This suggests that the smallpox plague hit before any post-war military movements, indicating that the Parthian campaign contributed to and exacerbated an outbreak of pestilence which was already established in the East, rather than being the primary cause and driver of the epidemic. In 165 AD, Aristides fell ill with the plague but survived; in AD 171 he composed the *Sacred Tales* in which he recorded the numerous omens and insights he had received from Asclepius in his dreams over nearly thirty years.

It seems that the Antonine Plague found its way to the Roman empire along the Silk Road from China, festering in Ctesiphon, Seleucia and other urban centres, and on trading vessels sailing from the east. Rafe de Crespigny speculates that the plague may have also broken out in Eastern Han China before 166 because of notices of plagues in Chinese records. It first emerged as a Roman public health problem during the siege of Seleucia in Mesopotamia (a major city on the Tigris River) as prosecuted by the Romans in the winter of 165–166. All sources agree that Verus' troops brought disease back west with them on their victorious return. Rome and the provinces were all affected, and the army was particularly badly hit; a concern with compromised Roman manpower is noted in many sources, for example Ammianus Marcellinus[3] and Orosius[4] and Eutropius[5] who reports that the plague was so severe that, 'in Rome and throughout Italy and the provinces most people, and almost all

---

2. Aelius Aristides, *Orations.* 48, 38–45
3. 23,6,24
4. 7,15,5
5. *Breviarium* 8,12

soldiers in the army, were afflicted by weakness'. This was especially problematic since the empire was now under threat along its north-eastern frontiers, and had some difficulty mobilising sufficient forces for the Marcommanic Wars at the end of the AD 160s. Marcellinus records that the plague rampaged through the western empire to Gaul and to the legions stationed along the Rhine and as far north as Hadrian's Wall.

The spread of the contagion through the armed forces would have been accelerated by soldiers and sailors who had been on leave returning to active duty and infecting other legionaries and crews. Twenty-eight legions totalling approximately 150,000 highly and expensively trained men were exposed to the virus: many succumbed. As a result Marcus Aurelius was desperate to recruit any able-bodied man who could fight: freed slaves, prisoners of war, criminals and gladiators were all signed up. Fewer gladiators meant fewer games in Rome and around the empire, which antagonised the Roman people who demanded more, not less, entertainment during a time of intense national stress. The resulting poorly trained and ill-disciplined army failed badly: in AD 167, Germanic tribes crossed the Rhine for the first time in more than 200 years. Such enemy successes served to expedite the decline of the Roman military, which, along with economic crises, were early steps in the decline and fall of the Empire.

Eutropius[6] stated that a large population died throughout the empire. According to Cassius Dio[7] the disease broke out again nine years later in AD 189 and led to up to 2,000 deaths a day in Rome, one quarter of those who were infected. The total death count has been estimated at 5 million, and the disease killed as much as one third of the population in some areas and again devastated the ranks of the Roman army.

This prodigious death toll severely reduced the number of people paying tax and contributing to the state's coffers, so government revenues plummeted. It diminished recruits for the army, candidates for public office, businessmen and farmers. Production on the farms fell as fewer farmers meant that so much more land was uncultivated with a further adverse effect on tax revenues. Crop shortages led to inflation and steep price increases along with decreasing food supplies. Fewer craftsmen and artisans also meant a downturn in productivity which impacted local economies. Workforce shortages led to higher wages for those who survived the epidemic and fewer businessmen, merchants, traders and financiers caused profound interruptions in domestic and international trade.

So, a long term effect of the Antonine plague was to set off a gradual progression to the decline of the Roman Empire in the west: Hanna, in *The Route to Crisis* would have it that 'Roman culture, urbanism, and the interdependence between cities and provinces' helped the spread of infectious disease thus creating the basis for the collapse of the empire. Overcrowded cities, poor diet and malnutrition, and a lack of sanitary measures made Roman cities cess pits for disease transmission. The contagions spread unchecked along the land and sea trade routes which connected the cities to the outlying provinces.

---

6. 31, 6, 24
7. 72, 14, 3–4

Harper (*The Fate of Rome*) suggests that 'the paradoxes of social development and the inherent unpredictability of nature, worked in concert to bring about Rome's demise'. Climate change at the end of a favourable climate period allowed the introduction of new, catastrophic diseases including the Antonine Plague which introduced smallpox to the world. Harper argues that the Antonine Plague was the first of three highly destructive pandemics, the others being the Plague of Cyprian (AD 249 – AD 262) and the Justinian Plague (AD 541 – AD 542), which rocked the Roman Empire to the core due to their high mortality rates. They rendered the empire helpless and enfeebled when trying to maintain the strength and integrity of the Roman army, the very extent of the empire, the extensive, lucrative trade networks and the size and number of Roman cities.

Our major sources for the Antonine Plague include Galen who listed some of the symptoms of the pestilence in *On the Natural Faculties* and the *Letters* of Marcus Cornelius Fronto, who was a tutor to Marcus Aurelius. Galen's Περὶ Ἀλυπίας *(De indolentia)* contains two references to the plague. In AD 166 Galen travelled from Rome back to his home in Pergamum: in his *Methodus Medendi, or, the Description and Treatment of the Principal Diseases incident to the Human Frame*, he describes fever, diarrhoea and inflammation of the pharynx, along with dry or pustular eruptions of the skin after nine days; it is these symptoms which have led scholars to conclude the disease was most likely smallpox.

The earliest outbreak of this plague recorded in Jerome's *Chronicle*, the universal chronology he compiled in the late fourth-century, is listed for AD 168, when, 'A plague (*lues*) took hold of many provinces, and affected Rome.' Four years later things were even worse, 'There was such a great plague throughout the whole world that the Roman army was reduced almost to extinction.' Dio alleges that death by disease was augmented by mass scale poisoning, performed by paid criminals equipped with sharp needles and a deadly compound in what to him was the worst plague he had ever come across and that 'two thousand often died in a single day' in Rome.[8]

Herodian confirms that there was a severe plague outbreak in Rome around AD 190.[9] All Italy was affected and infected; 'great destruction of both men and livestock resulted'. Doctors advised Commodus, the emperor at the time, to flee Rome to a safer place, and recommended those who remained in the city to make good use of incense and other aromatics. This would either keep the corrupt air out of their bodies, or overcome any that did manage to enter. The remedy failed for both humans and the animals they shared their living space with.

A second wave struck during the reigns of Decius (AD 249–251) and Gallus (AD 251–253). This plague broke out in Egypt in 251, and from there infected the whole of the Roman empire. Again, its mortality rate severely depleted the ranks of the army,

---

8. Dio, *Epitome* 73, 14,3
9. Herodian 1,12, 1–2

and caused massive labour shortages. According to Zosimus[10] the plague was still raging in 270, when it claimed the emperor Claudius Gothicus (268–270).

Based on demographic studies, the average mortality rate during the Antonine plague was probably 7–10 per cent and possibly 13–15 per cent in cities and armies.[11]

Marcus Aurelius was deeply concerned by what he saw going on all around, with his subjects resorting to hubris, peddling fake news, anarchy and lawlessness. He expressed his anxiety in a passage in his *Meditations*:

> Real good luck would be to abandon life without ever encountering dishonesty, or hypocrisy, or self-indulgence, or pride. But the 'next best voyage' is to die when you've had enough. Or are you determined to lie down with evil? Hasn't experience even taught you that—to avoid it like the plague? Because it is a plague—a mental cancer—worse than anything caused by tainted air or an unhealthy climate. Disease like that can only threaten your life; this one attacks your humanity.
>
> - Meditations, 9, 2

For evidence that the Antonine Plague reached as far as Hadrian's Wall and other

Bruun, Christer, 2007, 'The Antonine Plague and the "Third-Century Crisis"' in Olivier Hekster (ed.), Crises and the Roman Empire, Leiden/Boston (Impact of Empire, 7), 201–218.

Gilliam, J.F., 1961, 'The Plague under Marcus Aurelius'. *American Journal of Philology* 82, 225–251

Harper, Kyle, 2017, *The Fate of Rome: Climate, Disease, and the End of an Empire*, Princeton University Press

Littman, R.J., 1973, 'Galen and the Antonine Plague'. *American Journal of Philology*, 94243–255.

Tomlin, R.S.O., 2014, 'Drive away the cloud of plague': a Greek amulet from Roman London. In Collins, Rob, *Life in the Limes: Studies of the people and objects of the Roman frontiers*, Oxford, 197–205.

---

10. *New History* I, 26, 37 and 46
11. *New History* Littman 1973, 254–55

Chapter 4

The Han Dynasty Smallpox Epidemic, AD 200

It was a 'harbinger of something much more ominous'.
– Raoul McLaughlin, Rome and the Distant East referring to the Roman trade
mission to the Han Dynasty in AD 166.

The Han Dynasty (漢朝) was the second imperial dynasty of China (202 BC–220 AD), established by the rebel leader Liu Bang and ruled by the House of Liu. Spanning over four centuries, the Han dynasty was a golden age in Chinese history, and has influenced the identity of the Chinese civilization ever since.

Smallpox reached China somewhat later than it attacked the Mediterranean region. Before the epidemic the Han dynasty had a population of 60 million, then by AD 400 after the Han collapsed due to a combination of disease, the Yellow River area drought and internal political turmoil, they had lost 10 million people. A hospital specializing in infectious diseases, called An Lu, was built for victims. By the time of the Northern and Southern Dynasties, the isolation method of hospitalization had developed into a formal system. This may be the first public temporary epidemic hospital in Chinese history and one of the first in the world.

When Emperor Huan died in AD 168, an 11-year-old boy from the dynasty was made Emperor Ling. He was seen as a weak and corrupt ruler and his reign was marked by rebellions and protests. One of the most dangerous was the Yellow Turban Revolt of 184 – a peasant rebellion, triggered by multiple outbreaks of a lethal plague throughout the 170s and 180s. The more fatalities, the more survivors began to blame the emperor, believing he had the power to end their suffering. But Ling had no cure for the plague, and to make matters worse he also imposed heavy taxes on his people. So the peasants turned to faith healers in their quest for magical cures. One of these, Zhang Jue, was very popular and built up a huge following. By 184, Zhang Jue turned his movement into a violent uprising and led his followers to revolt against the Han. The army was able to defeat the rebels, but peasant rebellions continued to flare up over the next decade.

Although Ge Hong was the first writer of traditional Chinese medicine who accurately described the symptoms of smallpox, the historian Rafe de Crespigny mused in the 1930s that the smallpox plagues afflicting the Eastern Han Empire during the reigns of Emperor Huan of Han (r. 146–168) and Emperor Ling of Han (r. 168–189) – with outbreaks in 151, 161, 171, 173, 179, 182, and 185 – were possibly connected to the Antonine plague on the western fringes of Eurasia. De Crespigny suggests that 'it may be only chance' that the outbreak of the Antonine plague in 166 coincides with the Roman embassy of 'Daqin' (the Roman Empire) landing in Jiaozhi (northern Vietnam) and visiting the Han court of Emperor Huan, claiming to represent 'Andun' (安敦; a transliteration of Marcus Aurelius Antoninus or his predecessor Antoninus Pius.)

Raoul McLaughlin wrote that the Roman embassy visiting the Han Chinese court in 166 could have ushered in a new era of Roman Far East trade, but it was also a 'harbinger of something much more ominous'. McLaughlin argues that the origins of the plague lay in Central Asia, from some isolated population group, which then spread to the Chinese and the Roman worlds. The plague caused 'irreparable' damage to the Roman maritime trade in the Indian Ocean as proven by the archaeological record spanning from Egypt to India as well as significantly damaging Roman commercial activity in Southeast Asia.

de Crespigny, Rafe, 2007. *A Biographical Dictionary of Later Han to the Three Kingdoms (23–220 AD)*. Leiden, 600

Hill, John E., 2009. *Through the Jade Gate to Rome: A Study of the Silk Routes during the Later Han Dynasty, First to Second Centuries CE*, 27.

Liangsong, Li, 1997, Brief view on arrangement of infectious diseases and hospital for infectious diseases in ancient China, *Chin J Med History*, 1,34–37

McLaughlin, R., 2010, *Rome and the Distant East: Trade Routes to the Ancient Lands of Arabia, India, and China*, London, 59

Pulleyblank, Edwin G., 1999, 'The Roman Empire as Known to Han China'. *Journal of the American Oriental Society*. 119 (1), 71–79.

Chapter 5

The Plague of Cyprian: AD 250–AD 271

*'All were shuddering, fleeing, shunning the contagion, impiously exposing their own
friends, as if with the exclusion of the person who was sure to die of the plague, one could
exclude death itself as well.'*

— Pontius of Carthage, *Life of Cyprian*

The Third Century Crisis also goes by the names Military Anarchy or the Imperial Crisis; it was a disaster of the first magnitude, lasting from AD 235 to 284 and involved military and economic catastrophe as well as plague.

In AD 250 the Roman Empire was losing its way, badly. The Imperial Crisis exploded when the Roman Empire was destabilised by a seemingly endless series of barbarian invasions, rebellions and imperial pretenders queuing up to wrest power from the man in charge. It all began with the assassination of Severus Alexander by his own troops in 235 who then proclaimed Maximinus Thrax the new emperor, commander of one of the legions. Maximinus (regarded as a peasant by the senate) was the first of the so-called barrack room emperors – rulers who were elevated by their troops even though they lacked any of the traditional aristocratic Roman qualifications for the job: political experience, a supporting faction, money, distinguished ancestors, or a hereditary claim to the imperial throne. The assassination ignited a 50-year period during which there were at least 26 claimants to the title of emperor, mostly prominent Roman army generals, who assumed imperial power over all or part of the Empire.

The catastrophic Year of the Six Emperors came in AD 238 during which all of the original claimants (Maximinus Thrax; Gordian I; Gordian II; Pupienus, half-British Balbinus and Gordian III) met their deaths.

By 268, the empire had splintered into three competing states: the Gallic Empire, the Palmyrene Empire (including the eastern provinces of Syria Palaestina and Aegyptus) and the Italian-centred independent Roman Empire proper. And then matters became much, much worse: plague began to ravage the empire. The Plague of Cyprian originated in Ethiopia around Easter of AD 250. It reached Rome in the following year, eventually spreading to Greece and further east to Syria.

We have seen how the Antonine Plague in the previous century drained the Roman armies of manpower, skills and experience and wrecked the Roman economy. From AD 249 to AD 262, the Plague of Cyprian also laid waste the Roman Empire to such an extent that some cities, such as Alexandria, experienced a 62 per cent decline in population from something like 500,000 to 190,000, although not all of these may have died of plague: some may have just fled in panic. The Bishop of Alexandria claimed that:

> 'This immense city no longer contains so many inhabitants, from infants to those of extreme old age. As for those aged from 40 to 70, they were then so much more numerous than they are now though we have counted and registered as everyone entitled to the public food ration [the public grain dole] from 14 to 80; those who look the youngest now are no more numerous than the oldest men.'

The plague greatly hampered the Roman Empire's ability to ward off barbarian invasions, not helped by additional problems such as famine, with many farms abandoned and unproductive as farmers sought refuge in the cities. The absence of consistent leadership and the further dilution of the army during all the political instability, plus the ineptitude of a long succession of short-lived emperors all incapable of stemming the contagion – two of them died from the plague, Hostilian in 251 and Claudius II Gothicus in 270 – just added to the parlous state the empire was in.

Named after St. Cyprian, a bishop of Carthage who saw the epidemic as signaling the end of the world, the Plague of Cyprian was estimated to be killing 5,000 people a day in Rome alone. What disease caused the pandemic? It may well have been smallpox, pandemic influenza or viral haemorrhagic fever, the Ebola virus. However, none of the sources describe the full-body rash that is the distinctive feature of smallpox. Eusebius, in his church history written in the early fourth century, describes an outbreak that was more like smallpox in AD 312–13. Eusebius called this a 'different illness' than the Plague of Cyprian and also distinctly described the typical pustular rash. The putrescent limbs and permanent debilitation of the Plague of Cyprian are not consistent with smallpox.

Bubonic plague does not fit the pathology, seasonality, or demographics. Cholera, typhus, and measles are remote possibilities, but each is problematic. The two-generation hiatus between the smallpox epidemic under Commodus and the Plague of Cyprian means that the entire population would have been infectable again.

Pandemic influenza is a possibility and was well known in the ancient world although descriptions of flu epidemics and pandemics are thin on the ground. The Cyprian pestilence presented as an acute-onset disease with burning fever and severe gastrointestinal disorder; its symptoms included conjunctival bleeding, bloody stools, oesophageal lesions and necrosis in the extremities. These signs are consistent with an infection caused by a virus that induces a fulminant haemorrhagic fever.

In 2014 things started to look up on the identification front when working at the Funerary Complex of Harwa and Akhimenru in the west bank of the ancient city of Thebes (modern-day Luxor) in Egypt, the team of the Italian Archaeological Mission to Luxor (MAIL) found the bodies of plague victims. Attempts had been made to quell the spread of the disease by covering the corpses with lime as well as by burning the bodies. The Italians also uncovered three lime kilns and the remains of the incinerated plague victims. Attempts to extract DNA from the remains proved futile as the Egyptian climate causes the complete destruction of DNA.

Whatever it was, the Cyprian Plague destroyed whole populations throughout the empire causing widespread shortages in manpower, food production and army recruitment – just as the Antonine Plague had done in the previous century. Its effect was to severely weaken further the empire during the Crisis of the Third Century.

St Cyprian's biographer, Pontius of Carthage, described its terrible effect in Carthage:

> 'Afterwards there broke out a dreadful plague, and excessive destruction of a hateful disease invaded every house in succession of the trembling populace, carrying off day by day with abrupt attack numberless people, every one from his own house. All were shuddering, fleeing, shunning the contagion, impiously exposing their own friends, as if with the exclusion of the person who was sure to die of the plague, one could exclude death itself as well.'
>
> – Pontius of Carthage, *Life of Cyprian*. Trans. Ernest Wallis, 1885. Available online at *Christian Classics Ethereal Library*.

The usual scapegoating ran riot: the 'Decian persecution' was blamed on the Christians. Fifty years later, a North African convert to Christianity, Arnobius, defended his new religion from pagan demonisation:

> '…that a plague was brought upon the earth after the Christian religion came into the world… but pestilences, say my opponents, and droughts, wars, famines, locusts, mice, and hailstones, and other damaging things, by which the property of men is assailed, the gods bring upon us, incensed as they are by your wrong-doings and by your transgressions.'
>
> – Arnobius of Sicca, *Adversus Gentes* 1, 3. Online at Christian Classics Ethereal Library

Cyprian, ever moralizing and desperate to reassure his flock who were no more immune for being Christian than anyone else the plague encountered, gives graphic descriptions of the horrible physical symptoms in his *De Mortalitate*:

> 'The pain in the eyes, the febrile attacks, and the aching in all the limbs are the same among us and among the others, so long as we share the common flesh of this age… These are proof of faith: that, as the strength of the body dissolves, the bowels dissipate in a flow; that a fire that begins in the inmost depths burns up into wounds in the throat; that the intestines are shaken with continuous vomiting; that the eyes are set on fire from the force of the blood; that the infection of the deadly putrefaction amputates the feet or other extremities of some; and that as weakness prevails through the failings and losses of the bodies, you go lame, deaf or blind.'
>
> – Cyprian, *De Mortalitate*. Adapted from Harper, *The Fate of Rome*.

The relentless march of the disease through every corner of the empire saw Christians ennobling it by comparing the suffering it caused with the excruciating pain endured by martyrs while others, grappling with anxiety and panic, believed the contagion to be spread through 'corrupted air' that pervaded the empire or that the disease was transmitted through the clothes or simply by being looked at by an infected person.

All the while the Third Century Crisis rumbled on and the barrack emperors persisted with their corrupting policies, bribing armies to ensure their support in the civil wars, debasing the coinage, igniting rampant inflation and generally wrecking the economy. The people resorted to a black market economy, thus depriving the treasury of essential taxes; taxes were paid in kind in food or goods.

The various armies were so distracted by their own differences and battling that they ignored the incursions on their borders by the Carpians, Goths, Vandals and Alamanni on the Rhine and Danube with raids by the Sassanids in the east. Climate change in what are now the Low Countries caused sea levels to rise forcing the displacement of inhabitants there in search of new land to settle.

The plague was still raging in AD 270 when an incident involved the death of Claudius II Gothicus. According to the Historia Augusta:

> 'In [AD 270] the favour of heaven furthered Claudius' success. For a great multitude, the survivors of the barbarian tribes, who had gathered in Haemimontum [in the Balkans] were so stricken with famine and pestilence that Claudius now scorned to conquer them further... during this same period the Scythians attempted to plunder in Crete and Cyprus as well, but everywhere their armies were likewise stricken with pestilence and so were defeated.'

The crisis, aided and abetted by the plague, forced wholesale changes in the military – the Romans, if anything, were going to learn from this perfect storm, chaos and mayhem to try and prevent it from recurring. The army had failed singularly to deal with the many external threats and it had been misused for personal gain and benefit. Under Gallienus (r. 253–268), senators were barred from serving in the army: this had the dual benefit of reducing the likelihood of senatorial insurrection against Gallienus and eliminating the old hoary aristocratic hierarchy in the military. Officers would now have to work their way up through the ranks, no longer reliant on their privileged status. The result was a much more experienced and rigorous officer corps. To win his victories over the Gallic and Palmyrene secessionists, Aurelian deployed fleet cavalry rather than the usual infantry. Diocletian increased even further the cavalry element to ensure speedy and flexible deployment wherever armies were required. Diocletian reigned from the regions as well as Rome so that his fast reaction forces were nearer to potential trouble spots. He held sway from cities in the East, forming the Tetrarchy, a system of four consecutively reigning emperors, who each ruled from a region close to the previously porous borders.

Harper, Kyle, 2017, 'Solving the Mystery of an Ancient Roman Plague'. *The Atlantic*

Harper, Kyle, 2015, 'Pandemics and Passages to Late Antiquity: Rethinking the Plague of c. 249–70 described by Cyprian,' *Journal of Roman Archaeology* 28, 223–60

Stathakopoulos, D. Ch., 2007, *Famine and Pestilence in the late Roman and early Byzantine Empire*, 95

The *Chronicle* of Hydatius

Hydatius or Idacius (*c*. AD 400–*c*. AD 469) was bishop of Aquae Flaviae in Roman Gallaecia (modern Chaves, Portugal). He compiled a contemporary chronicle that gives us, among other things, our best record of parts of Hispania in the fifth century and the only detailed source written about the fifth-century barbarian invasions and settlements. Hydatius starts off in the year AD 379, using four parallel chronological and historical sources. Given his aim to paint a picture of the deepening dissolution of society in the western Roman empire and in Hispania in particular, it is not surprising that what emerges is a very bleak, doom-laden account of fifth-century life. The fact that he had read the apocryphal letter of Christ to Thomas, *The Gospel of Thomas* (also known as the Coptic Gospel of Thomas), which showed that the world would end in May AD 482, did nothing to lighten the gloom. For example, 'four plagues of sword, famine, pestilence, and wild beasts raging everywhere throughout the world, the annunciations foretold by the Lord through his prophets came to fulfilment'. We also hear of 'starving mothers eating their children', bishops battling heresies, barbarian incursions; the instability of the western Roman Empire is indicated by the 'revolving door of emperors'. The sudden termination of *The Chronicle* in AD 468 is simply accounted for by Hydatius' death, not by any apocalypse.

The Byzantine Empire, Europe, Middle East, Asia and Africa

Plague reared its deadly head at the dystopian siege of Amida (in modern south east Turkey) by the Persians in AD 505 during the Anastasian War and prosecuted by troops of the Sasanian Empire under Kavadh I. The siege and its consequences were particularly repellent: it lasted 73 days and 80,000 inhabitants died in the ensuing reprisals. The Persians tied up all the men and incarcerated them in the local amphitheatre; many died of starvation or of its effects. The women, meanwhile, were famished as well and took to eating stone, the soles of old boots 'and other horrible things from the streets and squares'. Prostitution was a way out for many who exchanged sex for food but when the food began to run out the Persians deserted the women and left them to starve. According to our reporter, Pseudo-Joshua, what happened next was quite unbelievable: the women got together and planned acts of cannibalism where they would go out and overpower the vulnerable: other women, children and the old and infirm. Once boiled or roasted these victims would be eaten. The 'odour of the roasting' told the Persians what was going on; they tried to stop it through torture or execution.

The aftermath was no less horrific. The wildlife there got so used to feeding off the numerous corpses scattered around that, at the end of the war when the corpses had rotted away they began attacking the inhabitants in order to satisfy their taste for human flesh. The beasts would run off with children and devour them; farmers and solitary travellers were also attacked and eaten to death.

If all of this happened it illustrates well the depths to which besiegers and the besieged will sink to win or to survive. At the same time, though, it may be an example of a Christian writer using fictitious stories of such depravity to illustrate the dystopian world we all apparently live in and the repugnant things that go on which typify what may await us after judgement day. Early fake news?

True or not we learn that the very threat of siege had terrible consequences. In AD 560 rumours were put about in Amida that the Persians were on their way back. John of Ephesus recalls the reaction 'rage, madness and frenzy' this caused; it was the last straw for a town that in the last fifty years had endured the depredations of one siege, the loss of 30,000 more inhabitants during a three month plague and the collapse of its economy. Women and children were the main psychological sufferers of the madness and frenzy: 'barking like dogs, bleating like goats, meowing like cats, cock-a-doodle-dooing like cocks and imitating the sounds of all dumb animals'. More social anxiety set in with huddled groups 'confused, troubled, disturbed' staggering about at night, visiting the cemetery. They 'sang and raged and bit each other', their voices sounded like horns and trumpets; they swore 'as if from devils in person'. Involuntary gales of laughter, 'immodest talk and evil blasphemy' rang out. They leapt about and jumped off walls 'hanging themselves upside down, falling and rolling around in the nude'. None of them knew whether he or she were really alive.

Biological warfare in the ancient world

We have to go back to Hittite texts of 1500–1200 BC for the earliest documented use biological weapons. This records how victims of tularemia were herded into enemy territory, sparking an epidemic. Tularemia is an infectious disease, also known as rabbit fever or deer fly fever which typically attacks the skin, eyes, lymph nodes and lungs; it is caused by the bacterium *Francisella tularensis*. Some scholars believe that the Assyrians poisoned enemy wells with ergot, a parasitic fungus of rye which produces ergotism when the alkaloids produced by the *Claviceps purpurea* fungus are ingested.

During the First Sacred War or Cirraean War, in about 590 BC, Athens and the Amphictionic League poisoned the water supply of the besieged town of Kirrha near Delphi with toxic hellebore, so weak were the defenders with diarrhoea that Kirrha fell. According to Herodotus, during the 4th century BC Scythian archers dipped their arrow tips into decomposing cadavers of humans and snakes or in blood mixed with manure, with the intention of contaminating their enemy with lethal bacterial agents like *Clostridium perfringens* and *Clostridium tetani*, and snake venom.

In a naval battle against King Eumenes of Pergamon in 184 BC, Hannibal filled pots with venomous snakes and instructed his sailors to throw them onto the decks of enemy ships. The Roman commander Manius Aquillius poisoned the wells of besieged enemy cities in about 130 BC. In about AD 198, the Parthian city of Hatra (near Mosul, Iraq) repulsed the Roman army led by Septimius Severus by hurling pots filled with live scorpions at them. Like the Scythian archers, Roman soldiers dipped their swords into excrement and cadavers so that victims were infected by tetanus as result.

Elton, Hugh, 2018. *The Roman Empire in Late Antiquity: A Political and Military History*. Cambridge

Greatrex, Geoffrey, 2002, *The Roman Eastern Frontier and the Persian Wars (Part II, 363–630 AD)*. London

Mayor, Andrienne, 2003. *Greek Fire, Poison Arrows and Scorpion Bombs: Biological and Chemical Warfare in the Ancient World*. Woodstock, NY

Chapter 6

The Plague of Justinian: AD 541–AD 549

The beginning of the first Plague Pandemic

'During these times there was a pestilence by which the whole human race came near to being annihilated.'

– Procopius

The Plague of Justinian or Justinianic Plague was the first episode in the First Plague Pandemic, the first Old World pandemic of plague, that highly contagious disease caused by the bacterium *Yersinia pestis*. The disease remorselessly ravaged the whole Mediterranean basin, Europe, the Arabian peninsula and the Near East, with catastrophic effects on the Sassanian and Roman Empires, and not least on Constantinople.

Procopius was exaggerating to some degree but the mortality rate was certainly very high in Constantinople. He reports 5,000 deaths per day, so up to 12,000 over the four months the plague was ravaging, in a population estimated at half a million. We know, though, that often classical writers use such nice round figures as code for 'lots' or 'a big number'. The Roman empire had been split in two in AD 395 creating western and eastern empires, the latter with its capital at Constantinople. The Byzantine Empire was in effect the eastern half of the Roman Empire, and it survived over a thousand years after the western half fell in around 410. The plague ebbed and flowed but never really went away for another 200 years, spiking periodically afterward as the Roman plague of 590 (Byzantine Empire); the plague of Sheroe 627–628 (Mesopotamia); the plague of 664–689 (British Isles); the plague of 698–701 (Mesopotamia, Byzantine Empire, Syria and West Asia); and the plague of 746–747 (Byzantine Empire, West Asia, Africa). Some estimates suggest that up to 10 per cent of the world's population died. By the time the plague had run its course – c. AD 750 – the mortality was in the region of 50 million. The First Plague Pandemic generally and the Justinian Plague in particular are highly significant as Justinian's was the first recorded plague to ravage the world wreaking death, economic, political and social destruction.

It was not until 2013 that researchers were able to confirm earlier speculation that the cause of the Plague of Justinian was in fact *Yersinia pestis*. Ancient and modern *Yersinia pestis* strains closely related to the ancestor of the Justinian plague strain have been found in Tian Shan on the borders of Kyrgyzstan, Kazakhstan and China, suggesting that the Justinian plague originated in or near that region, some 300 years before Pelusium, as reported by Procopius.

As noted, the Plague of Justinian is generally regarded as the first historically recorded epidemic of *Yersinia pestis* based on literary descriptions of the clinical manifestations of the disease, mainly from the historian Procopius (AD 500 – AD 565), and on the discovery of *Y. pestis* DNA from human remains at ancient grave sites of that period.

Genetic studies published in *Nature Genetics*[1] and *The Lancet*[2] indicate that 'the origin of the Justinian plague was in Central Asia. The most basal or root level existing strains of the *Yersinia pestis* as a whole species are found in Qinghai, China. After samples of DNA from *Yersinia pestis* were isolated from skeletons of Justinian plague victims in Germany, it was found that modern strains currently found in the Tian Shan mountain range system are the most basal known in comparison with the Justinian plague strain.'

'This finding suggests that the expansion of nomadic peoples who moved across the Eurasian steppe, such as the Xiongnu and the later Huns, had a role in spreading plague to West Eurasia from an origin in Central Asia'.[3]

Earlier samples of *Yersinia pestis* DNA have been found in skeletons dating from 3,000 – 800 BC, across West and East Eurasia.[4]

The Byzantine Emperor Justinian (r. AD 527–565) has the unfortunate privilege of having the plague named after him. He himself contracted the disease in 542 but survived; his empire, though, was diminished soon after the plague struck. Coins of that era show him with a swollen face as a result, presumably, of plague buboes.

As noted, Procopius of Caesarea gives us our best evidence and detail regarding the Justinian Plague in his systematic *Histories of the Wars* – eight books on the wars conducted by Justinian based on a Thucydidian model of historiography. Procopius intentionally leans heavily on Thucydides to lend his account the authority and kudos which comes with Thucydidian history writing. Procopius, in his vituperative *Secret History* (*Anecdota*), in common with other Christian writers, blames Justinian for the pestilence, arguing that he had angered God by his 'unjust and capricious actions' and by his dependence on his notoriously licentious and cruel wife, Theodora. Procopius rose to become the legal secretary of the general Belisarius, and travelled with him throughout Justinian's campaigns in Italy, the Balkans and in Africa. In 542, he was witness to the plague in Constantinople. Christian writers and Christians generally saw themselves as qualified to make such a judgment as they now regarded themselves as the chosen people, a role which they believed the Jews had singularly failed to make a success.

Other sources include Syriac church historian John of Ephesus, (c. AD 507 – c. AD 588) a leader of the early Syriac Orthodox Church, in his fragmentary, passionate *Historia Ecclesiastica*, composed while travelling around the empire. It covered more than 600 years, from the time of Julius Caesar to AD 588. He was despatched by Justinian

---

1. Morelli, 2010
2. Wagner, 2014
3. Damgaard, *Nature*, 2028
4. Rasmussen, *Cell*, 2015

to convert such wayward pagans as remained in Asia Minor in 542, and informs us that he baptized 70,000. He also built a large monastery at Tralles, and more than 100 other monasteries and churches, mostly on top of demolished pagan temples. In 546 he collaborated with Justinian during a persecution of pagans in and around Constantinople. He performed this task meticulously, torturing all suspected of the 'wicked heathenish error', as John himself calls it, and unearthing much worship of the ancestral gods amongst the Empire's aristocracy.

Evagrius Scholasticus, who was a child in Antioch at the time and later became a church historian, was himself afflicted with the buboes symptomatic of the disease in 542 but survived; nevertheless, later spikes carried off his first wife, several children, a grandchild and many servants.[5] He had become a lawyer and honorary prefect living in Antioch and wrote his six volume *Historia Ecclesiastica* covering the years 431–594 at the end of the sixth century. Then there is the *Historia* of Agathias – a lawyer and poet who continued the history of Procopius focusing on the plague's second outbreak in Constantinople in 558.

The Byzantines had little or no idea how to mitigate the plague's infectivity: quarantine, social distancing, lockdown of a sort were tried in desperation:

> '…later on they were unwilling even to acknowledge their friends when they called on them and they shut themselves up in their rooms and pretended that they did not hear, although their doors were being beaten down, fearing, obviously, that he who was calling was one of those demons. But for some … they saw a vision in a dream and seemed to suffer the very same thing at the hands of the creature who stood over them, or else to hear a voice foretelling to them that they were written down in the number of those who were to die.'
> – adapted from Procopius, *Histories of the Wars* 2, 22, translated by
> H.B. Dewing, Loeb Library Collection, 1914

But all they could do was perform religious rituals, helplessly hoping and praying for salvation. To the peoples of the empire the plague was simply caused by supernatural forces visited on them by an angry God.

Procopius describes the supernatural element of the contagion:

> 'Apparitions of supernatural beings in human guise of every description were seen by many people, and those who encountered them thought that they were struck by the man they had met in this or that part of the body, and as soon as they saw this apparition they were seized also by the disease. Now at first those who met these creatures tried to turn them aside by uttering the holiest of names and exorcising them in other ways as well as each one could, but they accomplished absolutely nothing.'

---

5. 4, 29

It did not escape Procopius that even when the plague was raging through the land, Justinian I demanded tax assessment and collection be continued, charging survivors extortionate rates to compensate for the lost revenues of those who had died and for the dislocation of agriculture and trade.[6]

> 'When pestilence swept through the whole known world and notably the Roman Empire, wiping out most of the farming community and of necessity leaving a trail of desolation in its wake, Justinian showed no mercy towards the ruined freeholders. Even then, he did not refrain from demanding the annual tax, not only the amount at which he assessed each individual, but also the amount for which his deceased neighbours were liable.'

The price of grain rose in Constantinople. Justinian had spent huge amounts of money to finance wars against the Vandals around Carthage and the Ostrogoths' kingdom in Italy. He had spent heavily building magnificent churches, such as Hagia Sophia. He also enacted legislation to deal more efficiently with the glut of inheritance suits being brought as a result of victims dying intestate.[7] All the while very little was being spent on public health initiatives to provide for the sick, dying and dead.

Where did this plague come from? Africa is a popular candidate: according to Jacob of Edessa (d. 708), the 'great plague (mawtānā rabbā) began in the region of Kush (Nubia), south of Egypt, in the year AD 541–42'. Evagrius Scholasticus (d. 594) believed that the plague originated in Axum (modern day Ethiopia and eastern Sudan), possibly due to a traditional prejudice of the time that diseases came from hotter regions. Michael the Syrian, relying on the lost chronicle of John of Ephesus, has it that it began in Kush on the border of Egypt and in Himyar (Yemen). An inscription dated to 543 records how Abraha, the Ethiopian ruler of Himyar, repaired the Ma'rib dam after sickness and death had struck the local community; plague? *The Chronicle of Seert* records that Aksum (al-Habasha) was hit by the pandemic. Early Arabic sources record that plague was endemic in Nubia and Abyssinia. According to Peter Sarris, the 'geopolitical context of the early sixth century,' with an Aksumite–Roman alliance against Himyar and Persia, 'was arguably the crucial prerequisite for the transmission of the plague from Africa to Byzantium.'[8]

Procopius tells that the plague originated in the East, spreading to Pelusium near Suez in Egypt before reaching Constantinople from where it spread further throughout the empire. This is consistent with a route from the Red Sea region, possible via ship-borne rats if the Canal of the Pharaohs was still operating. The plague could have originated in commercial links with India or in growing Roman religious links with Nubia and Aksum.

---

6. *Anecdota* 23, 20
7. *Edict* 9, 3
8. Sarris (2007), Bubonic Plague in Byzantium

The plague later surfaced in Italy in 543, and reached Syria and Palestine in the same year. There, the contagion migrated to Persia, where it infected the Persian army and King Khusro himself, causing them to retreat east of the Tigris to the plague-free highlands of Luristan.[9] Gregory of Tours tells how St. Gall saved the people of Clermont-Ferrand in Gaul from the disease in 543;[10] Bede, recorded the devastation of Britain and Ireland by the plague in 664.[11] Some speculate that the plague may have spread to Ireland as early as 544. Agathias reports a second outbreak in Constantinople in 558.

Procopius says that the disease and the death it brought were inescapable and everywhere:

'During these times there was a pestilence by which the whole human race came near to being annihilated. Now in the case of all other scourges sent from heaven some explanation of a cause might be given by daring men... It started from the Egyptians who dwell in Pelusium. Then it split and moved in one direction towards Alexandria and the rest of Egypt, and in the other direction it came to Palestine on the borders of Egypt; and from there it spread over the whole world, always moving forward and travelling at times favorable to it. It seemed to move by fixed arrangement and to stay for a specified time in each country blighting all, in either direction right out to the ends of the world, as if fearing lest some corner of the earth might escape it. For it left neither island nor cave nor mountain ridge untouched wherever there was life; and if it had passed by any land it came back later.'

Procopius describes the symptoms: victims are struck by a sudden fever, although there was little or no physical manifestation such as the change of colour or body temperature one might expect in a febrile patient; there was no inflammation and a physician might be excused for believing that his patients had nothing to worry about, and would certainly not die. But there was quite a lot to worry about because very soon a bubonic swelling developed – black pustules about as large as a lentil – either in the groin, inside the armpit, and in some cases beside the ears and at different points on the thighs.[12] Buboes appear near the lymphatic nodes closest to where the individual was first infected with the disease; hence, the groin is a common site for buboes since fleas would see legs as an easy target. In short, the lymph nodes were being assailed. Vomiting of blood ensued without any visible cause; fatigue was followed by dehydration, delirium or coma and then, very often death. Contemporary medical science and the medical profession were at a total loss in terms of therapy and prognosis. What treatment there was showed different inconclusive results with different patients. Where there was a recovery it was due to nothing a doctor had done.

---

9. Procopius 2, 24, 8–12
10. *History of the Franks* 4, 5
11. *Ecclesiastical History of the English People* 3, 27
12. *Wars*, 2, 22, 17

This would be the paradigm that defined later outbreaks of the plague in the Near East. Procopius tells us that, when it left Constantinople, it moved on to Persia where it killed many more than it had in the Byzantine Empire.

He goes on to describe the coma and delirium which afflicted some of the victims[13] while at the same time, with commendable perspicacity, paying respect to the exhausted carers struggling to look after their dying loved ones who, indirectly, were just as much victims of the disease as the patients themselves. The comatose recognised no one they used to know and slept constantly; they would eat while asleep; some also were neglected and these would die through lack of sustenance. Those seized with delirium suffered from insomnia and were subject to paranoia, suspecting that 'men' were coming to get them; they would get excited and rush off, crying out at the top of their voices. Everybody pitied the carers no less than the sufferers for when the patients fell out of their beds and lay rolling upon the floor, they had to keep putting them back into bed, and when they rushed out of their houses, they would have to force them back with shoving and screaming.

We learn of the widespread deliberate smashing of pottery in Syria: this may be intended as a display of low level civil disobedience (a common feature of pandemics); a manifestation of people experiencing collective traumatic shock or it may even have been a desperate attempt to disturb and clear the air.

Evagrius described facial swelling, followed by a sore throat, as an early symptom, while some victims also suffered from diarrhoea.[14] Once the buboes appeared the disease progressed rapidly with infected individuals usually dying within two to three days.[15] The victim then often lapsed into a semi-conscious, lethargic state, refusing food and drink. This is when the delirium came in. Many people died in great pain when their buboes gangrened while some patients developed black blisters all over their bodies and soon died; others died vomiting blood.[16]

When the buboes grew to a great size they ruptured and suppurated[17] as the body evacuated the disease, in which case the patient usually recovered, although he or she would often suffer afterwards from muscular tremors. Doctors, therefore, sometimes lanced such buboes to discover that carbuncles had formed.[18] Those individuals who did survive were left with withered thighs and tongues, classic after-effects of the plague.

Pregnant women were particularly at risk. Some died through miscarriage, but others succumbed during childbirth along with their infants. However, Procopius reports exceptions: three women in confinement survived though their children died, and one woman died during the birth although the baby was born and survived. Agathias

---

13. *Wars*, 2, 22, 10, and John of Ephesus, fragment 11, E.

14. 4, 29

15. Agathias, 5, 10, 3; Evagrius, 4, 29; Gregory of Tours, 4, 31

16. *Wars*, 2, 22, 19–28; John of Ephesus, fragment 11, G

17. *Wars*, 2, 22, 37

18. *Wars*, 2, 22, 29; Evagrius,4, 29

tells us that young males suffered the heaviest toll overall.[19] Humans were not the only victims of this contagion: animals, including dogs, mice and snakes, contracted the disease. There is no mention in the sources, however, of the plague spreading to livestock which, if it had happened, would certainly have added to the turmoil and chaos.

John of Ephesus provides the most vivid and grotesque description of the plague, its effects on Palestine and in Constantinople. It must be conceded however that his apocalyptic writing, as a Christian, is informed by the sure belief that what he was witnessing was nothing less than the end of the world.[20] To him, the plague was simply a manifestation of divine wrath and a demand for repentance. He describes episodes of chaos in which men collapsed in agony in public. The fear of being left unburied, or of falling prey to scavengers, led many to wear identification tags, and when possible to avoid leaving their homes at all in self imposed lockdown. He described a house which men avoided because of the foul stench emanating from it. When the door was finally broken down over twenty corpses were found rotting away. Many also saw terrifying visions both before and after the disease produced symptoms in them. In typical apocalyptic style, John of Ephesus did not see these as hallucinations; to him they offered an insight into life on the other side, the afterlife. John also reported that ghost ships would could be seen floating rudderless at sea, eventually washing up on shore with all of their crew dead from plague. He also told of sailors reporting sightings of a spectral bronze ship with headless oarsmen and monsters in the sea off the coast of Palestine.

Plague itself presents in three forms: bubonic, pneumonic or pulmonary, and septicaemic. The bubonic variety must exist before the other two strains can become active; it is not directly contagious unless the patient hosts fleas. We can infer from Procopius that the bubonic form was most virulent in the Justinian plague. Pneumonic plague occurs when the disease bacilli, *Yersinia pestis*, invade the lungs; it is highly contagious and is spread by airborne droplets. Because Procopius observes that the plague was not directly contagious, and major symptoms of pneumonic plague, namely shallow breathing and tightness in the chest, were absent, this form was probably not very active. Septicaemia occurs when the infection enters the bloodstream, when death is imminent usually before buboes can form. Agathias, however, reported some victims dying as if by an attack of apoplexy[21] which would suggest that the septicaemic form did exist during the sixth century outbreak. Bubonic plague results in death in roughly 70 per cent of cases; pneumonic plague has over a 90 per cent mortality rate. Septicaemic plague shows no clemency. Although all three forms probably were present during the Justinian plague, the bubonic form clearly predominated.

The proper observance of funerary rites was of huge importance in the ancient world under pagan and Christian religions. As a preface to the wholesale abandonment of funerary ritual, Procopius gives us some interesting epidemiology:

---

19. *Wars*, 5, 10
20. Fragments 11E and G; also Michael the Syrian, 9, 28
21. 5, 10, 3

'Now the disease in Byzantium ran a course of four months, and its greatest virulence lasted about three. And at first the deaths were a little more than the normal, then the mortality rose still higher, and afterwards the death toll reached 5,000 each day, and again it even came to 10,000 and still more than that.'

At first everyone looked after the burial of the dead of his own house but this soon degenerated into throwing one's corpses into the tombs of others, either by stealth or by using violence. Soon confusion and anarchy was total and some people, even the notable men of the city, remained unburied for days.

'When all the tombs were filled with the dead, the people dug up all the places about the city one after the other, laid the dead there, and left; but later on those who were digging these trenches, no longer able to keep up with the number of the dying, scaled the towers of the fortifications in Sycae, tore off the roofs and threw the bodies in there in complete disarray; and they piled them up and almost filled all the towers with corpses, and then covered them up and put the roofs back on. As a result a vile stench pervaded the city and caused more distress for the inhabitants.'

– Procopius, *Wars*, 2, 23

All the customary rites of burial were now overlooked. The dead were not carried out escorted by a procession, while the usual chants remained unsung. Instead it was acceptable to carry a corpse on your shoulders to the seaside parts of the city and fling it down on skiffs in a heap, to be conveyed wherever it might go. Better news came with the observation that members of the factions (the Greens and the Blues) laid aside their mutual enmity and helped others whom they did not know, whatever their allegiance. Indeed 'those who in times past used to take delight in devoting themselves to pursuits both shameful and base, shook off the unrighteousness of their daily lives and practised the duties of religion with diligence…not due to some new found enlightenment but because they were so terrified by what was going on.' Sadly, Procopius tells us that this was no lasting Damascene transformation for as soon as the contagion had passed, those who survived reverted to their old irreligious ways.

Justinian, despite his preoccupation with tax revenues, his own illness and the alleged treason of Belisarius, nevertheless attempted to mitigate the disaster.[22] He ordered Theodora, his formidable wife, and the palace guard to help dispose of the corpses. Theodora was a government official, one of the *referendarii*, or legal secretaries, who handled and dispatched all of the emperor's correspondence.[23] She reacted to the mayhem by having huge pits dug across the Golden Horn in Sycae (Galata) and then hiring men to collect the dead. Although these pits reportedly held 70,000 corpses each, they all too soon overflowed.

There was of course catastrophic social and economic disruption: the urban poor were the first to suffer, but the pestilence soon crept into the wealthier districts.

---

22. *Wars*, 2, 23, 20
23. *Wars*, 2, 23

Bread became scarce and starvation loomed over a city once noted for its plenty; some victims may actually have died of starvation, rather than disease.[24] Many houses became tombs, as whole families died from the plague without anyone from the outside world knowing. Streets were deserted, and all trades were abandoned.[25] Inflation soared. In 544, Justinian's price controls were partly successful, but as the taxation base shrank, financial pressure on the cities soared. In an effort to economize, salaries for teachers and physicians were frozen and budgets for that all important public entertainment were slashed.[26] Bread and circuses were in short supply. Slaves found themselves without masters; masters without slaves; most work stopped including capital projects and infrastructure. When the plague finally passed crops stood rotting in the fields, inflation soared, and, as noted, Justinian I continued to scramble to collect the taxes which he diverted from civic construction projects to a programme of church building, a policy which he probably believed would please God who would then desist from visiting another pestilence on his empire.

Rural areas were afflicted less but those areas infected were laid waste. This, in turn, impacted the urban areas which relied on a good harvest to avoid food shortages. In Syria and Palestine, the plague reached the farmlands after the planting, and the crops ripened with no one to harvest them. The crisis was exacerbated when a disease, possibly anthrax, attacked cattle in 551, causing fields to be left unploughed due to lack of oxen.[27] Michael the Syrian says that when possible some work was done with mules or horses.[28]

The plague afflicted the army and the monasteries particularly badly. Philostorgius, (AD 368 – c. AD 439) an Anomoean Church historian describes the destruction of the military wreaked by the plague.[29] So many deaths naturally caused recruitment problems in the army so that the empire was increasingly defended by barbarian mercenaries.[30] 'So while he (Justinian) was emperor, the whole earth ran red with the blood of nearly all the Romans and the barbarians. Such were the results of the wars throughout the whole Empire during this time.' In Justinian's final years, there were virtually no men either to volunteer or to be pressed into the army. Fortunately for the Romans, the plague had also attacked and weakened the Persian empire to a similar degree. However, the effects were felt over a wide expanse of empire: in Italy, the Ostrogoths resumed the war, and new revolts broke out in the African provinces. Renewed threats from the eastern barbarian tribes escalated while what was left of the Asiatic Avars, whom Bayan I had reunited, massed on the imperial frontiers; Bayan I led the Avars along with some Bulgars into Pannonia where they established their khaganate from 568. The Kotrigur Khan attacked the Balkan territories.

---

24. *Wars*, 2, 23
25. John of Ephesus, frgs. II, E and G; Procopius, *Wars*, 2, 23
26. *Wars*, 2, 26
27. John of Ephesus, fragment 11, E
28. 9, 29
29. *Church History*, 11, 7
30. *Secret History*, 18

As mentioned, the monasteries suffered too. In Constantinople, records list over 80 monasteries before 542 but, after the plague, most of them had gone. As with soldiers in the close confinement of barracks, monks were always prey to highly infectious contagious diseases like the bubonic plague.

John of Ephesus disturbingly notes that officials in Constantinople were aware of the plague for two years before it reached the city but did nothing in the way of public health planning to prepare the city for its dystopian arrival. Whenever it invaded a city or village, John of Ephesus writes, it fell furiously and swiftly on it and on its suburbs as far out as three miles. It remained until it had run its course in one place and after becoming firmly rooted, it moved along, but only slowly. This, of course, allowed news of the plague to precede its arrival and to be reliably anticipated. The people of Constantinople had received such news regarding the looming advance of the plague over a period of one to two years.

Unfortunately for the Byzantines, bubonic plague and its resurgences were not the only terrible disasters the people of Constantinople and of the wider empire had to endure. In the *Secret History*, Procopius tells of natural catastrophes, including floods and earthquakes, as well as barbarian invasions, that had wrought havoc in the empire during Justinian's reign. He asserted that at least half of the survivors of these previous calamities went on to fall to the plague.[31] To Procopius the reason for such damnation was that God had turned away from the empire because it was ruled by a monster of an emperor. If proof were needed for this, the spectacular collapse of the original dome of Hagia Sophia following an earthquake provided it.

Procopius, of course, was not alone. Christian writers generally concurred that the plague was a punishment sent by God because of human sinfulness and adopted as their literary plague model the 'Book of Revelation'. 'It was known,' wrote Zachariah of Mytilene, 'that it was a scourge from Satan, who was ordered by God to destroy men.'[32]

Near Antioch, St. Symeon the Younger tearfully prayed to Christ, and received the following reply: 'The sins of this people are many, so why do you bother yourself about their diseases? For you love them no more than I.' God nevertheless granted Symeon the power to heal the believers. In this way, many who were infected with the disease visited St. Symeon and were cured.[33] We have noted how Gregory of Tours tells us how St. Gall saved his flock from the plague.[34] The message clearly is that you will pay for your sin but you may escape the ravages of plague through your belief in God.

The plague eventually took leave of Constantinople and turned its attention to 'the land of the Persians' – and destroyed the population there until AD 749 before

---

31. *Secret History* 18, 44
32. *The Syriac Chronicle*, 10, 9
33. *Vie de S. Symeon*, 69–70
34. 4, 5

abating and flaring up again in the Black Death which devastated the East from AD 1346–1360 and Europe from AD 1347–1352.

As with earlier pandemics, Justinian's Plague caused widespread anxiety, panic and disruption, wrecking the economy, depleting the military, and destabilizing all other aspects of life in the Byzantine Empire and beyond. However, while the pestilence exerted a powerful and influential impact on Justinian's empire it was but one of a number of influences, such as war, climate change and religious unrest which also affected the empire.

Bragg, Melvin, 21 January 2021, In Our Time: The Justiniac Plague, BBC Radio 4

Damgaard, Peter de B.; et al. 2018. '137 ancient human genomes from across the Eurasian steppes'. Nature. 557 (7705): 369–374.

Harbeck, Michaela '*Yersinia pestis* DNA from Skeletal Remains from the 6th Century AD Reveals Insights into Justinianic Plague'. *PLOS Pathogens.* 9 (5)

Little, L. K., 2008, *Plague and the End of Antiquity: The Pandemic of 541–750.* Cambridge

Morelli, Giovanna; et al. 2010. 'Yersinia pestis genome sequencing identifies patterns of global phylogenetic diversity'. *Nature Genetics.* 42 (12): 1140–1143.

Osen, William, 2008, Justinian's Flea: Plague, Empire and the Birth of Europe

Rasmussen, Simon; et al. 2015. 'Early Divergent Strains of Yersinia pestis in Eurasia 5,000 Years Ago'. Cell. 163 (3): 571–582.

Wagner, David M.; et al. 2014 'Yersinia pestis and the Plague of Justinian 541–543 AD: a genomic analysis'. *The Lancet.* 14 (4): 319–326

Plague in the Middle and Near East and in southern and north west Europe

Plague then was a key factor at the crossroads between the demise of the classical world and the beginning of the Middle Ages. Eight hundred years before the Black Death, this pandemic of plague had engulfed the lands in the Mediterranean basin, stretching as far east as Persia and as far north as the British Isles and Ireland. It persisted sporadically from 541 to 750 at the same time as the Byzantine Empire was developing with the prominence of the Roman papacy and of monasticism, the rise of Islam, the rapid expansion of the Arabic Empire, and the Carolingian dynasty in Frankish Gaul.

We must now take account of the plagues of the Near and Middle East, southern and north-western Europe which claimed millions of lives between AD 562 and AD 1346 throughout modern day Iran, Iraq, Syria, Turkey, Lebanon, Israel, Saudi Arabia and Egypt, among other places. These plagues may have been a resurgence of Justinian's Plague or another strain imported into the region through trade or the return of troops from various theatres of war. The Middle East outbreaks have received comparatively scant mention in the history books for a number of reasons which include: a reluctance of Near and Middle Eastern writers of primary sources to accept and address the issue; confusion in terminology between plague and cholera; the tendency of scribes to ignore affected regions beyond their own, imbuing outbreaks with religious interpretations which ignored or obscured the facts; a lack of translations of primary sources into Western languages; and the reliance of Western historians on earlier Western historians and travel writers instead of taking into account primary source material from further east.

The Chronicle of Zuqnin gives us details about the carnage in Syria in AD 743–745 noting that the plague 'was still capable of burying 500 people a day'. It was a chronicle written in Syriac concerning the events from Creation to c.AD 775. This gives a flavour of what is a vital work:

> 'At that time, God sent on us these most cruel and terrible plagues: the sword, captivity, famine and pestilence, because of our sins and the misdeeds that our hands had engaged in. I will send four plagues upon them, says the Lord: the sword to kill, the dogs to eat, the birds and beasts of the earth to devour and tear in pieces, and I will deliver them over to the earthquake... This is the carnage that the armies of Arabs have made between them. They have drowned the earth in their blood; the birds, the beasts and even the dogs are filled with their flesh. Men pillage one another. The plague ravages them, so that if someone goes outside the sword stops him; if he stays at home, plague and famine take him. One hears on all sides only sadness and bitterness.'

The Chronicle goes on to describe in graphic detail the suspension of all burial rites and bodies rotting in the street 'like litter'.

So profound was the impact of the Justinian Plague on the region that the Dark Ages seems relatively free of infectious disease – but not for any virological reasons – rather, the pandemic had taken so many to the grave that its reliance on feeding on crowds was seriously compromised. Spring fever (lencten adl) – tertian malaria – was common.

In the damp and gloomy lands further west and north we have evidence of jaundice, pleurisy and pneumonia attacking the Anglo Saxons, as well as the mystyerious sounding 'seo healfdeade adl' – the haldead disease which was possibly hemiplegia, the partial paralysis caused by stroke. Damp, dingy, dirty and smokey living conditions can only have depressed resistance to infectious diseases.

Cameron, M.L., 2008, *Anglo Saxon Medicine*, Cambridge

Pearse, Roger, 2010, The plague and famine under Hisham – from the Chronicle of Zuqnin. Posted on 4 August, 2010; https://www.roger-pearse.com/weblog/2010/08/04/the-plague-and-famine-under-hisham-from-the-chronicle-of-zuqnin/

By now the medical works of Hippocrates, Pliny the Elder, Soranus, Celsus and Galen were supplemented by others which include the *De Medicamentis* of Marcellus Empiricus (fl. AD 400); the *Etymologies* of Isidore of Seville (AD 636) and the work of Oribasius (c.320–400), Vindicianus (fl. 364–375), Cassius Felix of Numidia (fl. c.450) and Alexander of Tralles (c.525–605).

There were, of course, original sources of medical information, notably the leechbooks which provided a blend of the empirical, apocryphal and the magical. The most popular were *Bald's Leechbook* and the *Lacnunga* ('Remedies'). Diseases in the former are separated out into those which manifest externally (Book I) and those internally (Book II). *Lacnunga* provides 200 or so remedies including one for dweorh, a fever with delirium. Bede (d. AD 735) appreciated the importance of infection control when he advocated the segregation of the ill from the community.

Plagues in Francia (AD 541–590)

Francia or the Kingdom of the Franks was the largest post-Roman barbarian kingdom in Western Europe. It was ruled by the Franks during late antiquity and the Early Middle Ages. It is the forerunner of the modern states of France, Belgium, The Netherlands, Luxembourg and Germany.

Gregory of Tours records that there were numerous epidemics of plague in the Kingdom of the Franks after the Justinian Plague struck Arelate (Arles) and the surrounding region in the late 540s. Various portents were reported and to expiate them the inhabitants resorted to processions, prayers and vigils.

Gregory also reports an epidemic in 571 in the Auvergne and in the cities of Divio (Dijon), Avaricum (Bourges), Cabillonum (Chalon-sur-Saône), and Lugdunum (Lyon). He describes the plague causing wounds in the armpit or groin similar to snakebite and of patients dying delirious within two or three days – symptoms which would suggest bubonic plague. In 582 Gregory further reports an epidemic in Narbo Martius (Narbonne). According to him, the majority of the townsfolk at Albi in 584 died of an outbreak of plague.

Massilia (Marseille) was struck by plague in 588; there the king, Guntram, prescribed a strict diet of barley bread and water to allay it. Gregory blames a ship arriving from Hispania as the source of the contagion; the epidemic recurred several times. In 590 he records another plague epidemic at Vivarium (Viviers) and at Avenio (Avignon) at the same time as the plague broke out in Rome under Pope Pelagius II. Some historians and epidemiologists think that plague killed up to 50 million over two centuries of recurring outbreaks. With troop numbers depleted, it was only a matter of time before Francia's borders fell to the Goths and Vandals invading from the East.

The Plague of Mohill, Ireland AD 544

The plague of Mohill, a small town in County Leitrim, is the first recorded Irish plague; a resurgence of the Justinian Plague, it struck Mohill in 535 and 536 and ravaged the local population. The arrival of plague in Ireland seems to correspond with the westward trajectory of the Justinianic plague which had reached Gaul by 543. Another epidemic in AD 550, named the croin Chonaill (redness of Chonaill), or the buidhe Chonail (yellowness of C.), was focused on the Shannon area.

Manchán of Mohill, (fl. AD 464–538) was a Christian saint credited with founding many early Christian churches in Ireland; Manchán probably died as a result of famine caused by the extreme weather events of 535–536. The Gaelic Irish annals recorded the following: 'a failure of bread in the year 536 AD' – the *Annals of Ulster*; and 'a failure of bread from the years 536–539 AD' – the *Annals of Inisfallen*. There were also three huge volcanic eruptions in 536, 540 and 547. The extreme weather events were the most severe and protracted short-term episodes of cooling in the Northern Hemisphere in the previous 2,000 years caused by an extensive atmospheric dust veil from a huge volcanic eruption in the tropics or in Iceland; this led to unseasonable weather, crop failures and famines worldwide.

Mohill or Maothail Manachain is named after St. Manachan, who founded the monastery of Mohill-Manchan here. We find evidence for the Justinian plague from three contiguous townlands, south-west of the present town, all named in ancient times after Tamlachta: the word tam-lacht signifies a mass plague burial place. Confirmed bubonic plague mass burial sites at Maothaill-Manchan are Tamlagh More, Tamlaght Beg and Tamlaghavally.

Noel MacLochlainn in *Manchán of Mohill* explains that 'Tamlaghavally means the plague burial ground of the town or roadway. Taibhleacht is derived from tamh or taimh, an unnatural death as from a plague, and leacht signifies a bed or grave. It was a place where people who died from a plague were buried, generally in a common grave. People who passed the way were accustomed to raise a 'cairn' of stones over the spot by placing single stones over the grave. Tamlaght Beg and Tamlagh More are of the same origin. Some great plague or pestilence has left its name on those three townlands.' He goes on to add that 'The huge dying off in the 6th century,' suggested by the number of tamlachta sites would certainly have created fear if not widespread panic. This was a pandemic in which some people dropped dead in less than one day, some fell ill but recovered, and some remained unaffected. Such seemingly random infectivity and mortality was probably interpreted by the populace, even preached by the clerics, as evidence of divine selection.

Mohill and nearby Airgíalla suffered badly; this led to an upsurge in ring fort-building as the populace craved security and reassurance in the wake of all those mysterious and random deaths which were followed by cattle-raids and enslavement. The terror and and panic probably boosted conversions to Christianity and the veneration of Manchán as reflected in the many monasteries which sprang up across Ireland. Manchán was henceforth venerated for protection from plague.

More evidence of the climate events comes from in AD 536 when Procopius recorded in his chronicle on the wars with the Vandals, 'during this year a most dread portent took place. For the sun gave forth its light without brightness ... and it seemed exceedingly like the sun in eclipse, for the beams it shed were not clear'.

Dooley, Ann, 2007 (ed.). *The Plague and Its Consequences in Ireland. Plague and the End of Antiquity: The Pandemic of 541–750.* Cambridge, 215–230.

Haley, Gene C., 2002. 'Tamlachta: The Map of Plague Burials and Some Implications for Early Irish History'. 22, *Proceedings of the Harvard Celtic Colloquium.* 96–140.

The Djazirah Outbreak of AD 562, 'Mesopotamia'

As noted, the Byzantines of Constantinople took the view that the encroaching plague was not their problem and only realised their cataclysmic error when it was too late. On leaving Constantinople, it travelled East following the course described by Procopius – and struck at Mesopotamia, although precisely where is unknown. The later Arab writers describe this as the Plague of Djazirah (also known as Jazeera, 'island') which was their name for Mesopotamia ('the land between two rivers'). In 562 it killed 30,000 people in Amida (present-day Diyarbakir in southeastern Turkey) and struck again in AD 599.

Ahmad Fazlinejad, 2018, 'The Black Death in Iran According to Iranian Historical Accounts from the 14th through 15th Centuries.' *Journal of Persianate Studies* 11; 56–71.

Christensen, P., 2016, *The Decline of Iranshahr.* I.B. Tauris.

Ehsan Mostafavi, 2020. 'Plague in Iran: Past and Current Situation.' *Department of Epidemiology, Pasteur Institute of Iran, Tehran, Iran,* 1–22.

Farrokh, K., 2009, *Shadows in the Desert.* Osprey Publishing.

The Roman Plague of AD 590 was a perfect example of religion triumphing over public health. It was a continuation of the Plague of Justinian but was centred on Rome. It presented as a combination of bubonic, septicaemic and pneumonic plague with the bubonic strain most prevalent. As with earlier contagions it was officially seen as a punishment from God: Pope Gregory the Great (AD 540–604) decreed that it could only be stemmed by penitential processions through the city, begging for mercy through the intercession of the Virgin Mary. Obviously, and lethally, such processions had the deadly effect of bringing a large number of people into contact with each other, so spreading the infection in what was an abject lack of social distancing. There were even reports of people collapsing and dying as they processed through the streets of Rome. Notwithstanding, the processions continued in a perfect example of religion triumphing over public health, at whatever cost. Astonishingly, when the plague abated the processions were credited with appeasing God's wrath and ending the contagion.

Plague of Sheroe AD 627–628 CE, Sassanian Empire, Persia

The Plague of Sheroe takes its name from the Sassanian king Kavad II (r. AD 628) whose birth name was Sheroe or Shiroe. Kavad II came to power following the disastrous wars of his father Kosrau II (r. AD 590 – AD 628) who drained Sassanian treasuries in his efforts to destroy the Byzantine Empire. The Sassanian nobility finally overthrew Kosrau II and crowned the prince Sheroe as Kavad II in his place.

Kavad II was ruthless: he had all his brothers, half-brothers and stepbrothers killed to prevent them challenging his claim to the throne, and then initiated peace talks with the Byzantines leading to the planned reconstruction of the many cities damaged or ruined during Kosrau II's wars. But the plague had other plans and intervened ensuring that Sheroe did not have the time to complete any of his plans; the disease took his life in the autumn of AD 628, only a few short months into his reign. Since all the legitimate male heirs who could have then assumed the throne had been executed, he was succeeded by his 7-year-old son Ardashir III (r. AD 628–629) whose reign was overseen by the vizier Mah-Adur Gushnasp as regent. He was soon overthrown and both he and the young emperor assassinated.

The death of Kavad II destabilized the Sassanian Empire which was still struggling to recover from the losses incurred by Kosrau II's wars and the plague. When the Arab Muslims invaded during the reign of Yazdegerd III (AD 632–652), the Sassanian Empire was too weak to repel them: the plague galvanised the instability which contributed to the collapse of the Sassanian Empire.

The Plague of Amwas (عمواس طاعون, ṭā‘ūn ‘Amwās) or Emmaus, Syria AD 638–639

Amwas was a bubonic plague epidemic that afflicted Islamic Syria toward the end of the Muslim conquest of the region, most probably another resurgence of the Plague of Justinian. It was the second recorded plague of the Islamic era, which began in the 620s, and the first to directly afflict the Muslims. Amwas was the Arabic name for Emmaus-Nicopolis, a Roman army headquarters in the 1st century AD, which had grown into a small city by the early 3rd century. Called after Amwas in Palestine, the plague first struck the Muslim Arab troops encamped there before spreading across Syria–Palestine and affecting Egypt and Iraq; it finally subsided during Shawwal, 18 October 639. The plague killed up to 25,000 soldiers and their families, including the cream of the army's high command, and caused huge loss of life and displacement among the indigenous Christians of Syria as well as triggering inflation and hoarding. By 639, 4,000 Muslim troops were left out of some 24,000 in 637. The plague first struck during a nine-month drought in Syria called the 'Year of the Ashes' by the Arabs. This led to famine in Syria and Palestine which would have facilitated the plague due to weakened immune resistance and the stockpiling of food reserves in towns and villages which attracted plague-infected rodents.

The appointment of Mu'awiya ibn Abi Sufyan to the governorship of Syria in the wake of the commanders' deaths paved the way for his establishment of the Umayyad Caliphate in 661, while recurrences of the disease may have contributed to the dynasty's downfall in 750. Depopulation in the Syrian countryside probably led to the resettlement of the land by the Arabs.

Interestingly and importantly, the Muslims ensured that they learnt lessons from the plague in respect of their reactions to it: traditional narratives by Caliph Umar and his senior commander Abu Ubayda ibn al-Jarrah informed subsequent medieval Muslim theological responses to epidemics, including the Black Death. Principles derived from the narratives were cited in debates about predestination and free will, prohibitions on fleeing or entering plague-affected lands and contagion.

There were recurrences of the plague in Syria–Palestine nearly every decade between 688–89 and 744–45; in AD 688–689 Basra alone lost 200,000 people in three days. In AD 704–705 it re-emerged in north western Mesopotamia. This trend continued throughout the century until the Great Outbreak of AD 746–749 when bubonic plague killed upwards of 200,000 in Constantinople, Greece and Italy. As noted, the recurrences will have stunted population growth in Syria–Palestine, the centre of the Umayyad Caliphate, and weakened Umayyad power resulting in the rise of the Abbasid Movement there, which ultimately toppled the Umayyads in 750. In the following year the disease seemed to evaporate but it is now believed that it only lay surreptitiously dormant before returning yet again as the pernicious Black Death in the Middle Ages.

To many Muslims death by plague was regarded as a martyrdom, as exemplified by this poem recorded by the Damascene historian Ibn Asakir (d. 1175):

> How many brave horsemen and how many beautiful, chaste women were killed in the valley of 'Amwas/They had encountered the Lord, but He was not unjust to them/When they died, they were among the non-aggrieved people in Paradise./ We endure the plague as the Lord knows, and we were consoled in the hour of death.

The Plague of Amwas was used in the debate regarding predestination to argue that if a person fled or remained in a plague-affected area their death had already been decreed by God. In the Iraqi garrison city of Kufa, the prominent statesman and scholar Abu Musa al-Ash'ari (d. 662) turned away visitors to his home because someone in his household had the plague. Not only is this an early example of lockdown and self-isolation but it also reveals an early knowledge of contagion and infection.

Dols, M. W., 1974. 'Plague in Early Islamic History'. *Journal of the American Oriental Society.* 94, 371–383.

Sourdel-Thomine, J., 1960. 'Amwas'. In Gibb, H. A. R. (ed.). The Encyclopaedia of Islam, New Edition, Volume I: A–B. Leiden, 460–461.

The British Plague AD 664 and the Great Mortality in Ireland

Anglo Saxon records reveal that there were 49 British epidemics between 526 and 1087. In the mid 6th century, the island of Britain could be described as predominantly British: a Welsh-speaking land of belligerent Celtic princes who terrorised and plundered the produce of subsistence farmers. After the Romans left in 410 Britain had been unable to maintain an urban civilisation, but the Britons were nevertheless successful at keeping the Angles and Saxons (i.e. the colonist English, initially under Hengest and Horsa) confined to Anglia and Kent. There was little or no trade or social exchange between the Christian British and the pagan Angles and Saxons, once they had fought each other to a stalemate under King Arthur. The British carried on some trade with the lands of the Mediterranean basin, whereas the English were self sufficient and lived on what they could grow. One of the less welcome imports received by the British was plague which, like other cargoes, reached Britain in boats from mainland Europe; it killed up to half of the native British population but left the English colonists largely unscathed. St Augustine's mission to Christianise Britain in 547 may also have encouraged the spread of contagion.

This British plague also goes by the name of the Plague of Cadwallader's Time, for the King of Gwynedd (r. AD 655 to 682) who died of the disease in a 682 recurrence.

Recognising a depleted population, the English soon began to launch probing raids into British territory only to find that there was little opposition. This they communicated to their kinsfolk in Schleswig-Holstein and the Danish peninsula (whence they had come); the Angles west of what is now Hamburg knew a land grab opportunity when they saw one and invaded en masse. The English systematically extended their colonies in a plague-ravaged Britain from the borders of Wales to the middle of Scotland. The plague, then, changed the course of British history, allowing an influx of the Angles into what was hitherto British territory.

The plague of 664 was the first recorded epidemic in English history, notable for its long duration and because it coincided with a solar eclipse. It followed a period of turbulence in Britain with invasion and internecine strife. As a consequence of the astronomical event it was later referred to as 'The Yellow Plague of 664'. The epidemic is said to have lasted for 20 or 25 years, causing widespread mortality, social and economic dislocation and the abandonment of religious faith. The disease responsible was probably plague – part of the First Plague Pandemic – or else smallpox. Bede said of it that in Northumbria 'it brought low in grievous ruin an infinite number of men'. (*Historical Works* I, 485).

In 829 the monks at Christchurch, Canterbury were all but wiped out (five survived). This was followed in 897 by 'a great mortality of man and beast after the Danish invasion which Alfred at length repelled'. St Elphege, Archbishop of Canterbury, quelled the plague that was caused by the stench of rotting bodies by doling out consecrated bread – an early reference to miasma theory and the spread of disease. The plague in Annan in the Solway peninsula described by William of Newburgh (1136–1198) owed its orgin to the body of a revenant; the corpse was exhumed and cremated, after which the plague vanished.

How diverse was *Yersinia pestis* during the first plague pandemic (541–750 AD)? This intriguing question was partly answered when an international team of researchers led by the Max Planck Institute for the Science of Human History screened 183 samples of human remains from 21 archaeological sites to learn more about the bacterium's spread, diversity and genetic history over the course of the Justinian pandemic.

In a study published in *Proceedings of the National Academy of Sciences*[35] the researchers describe how they uncovered a previously unknown level of diversity in *Y. pestis* strains. Among other ground-breaking findings the researchers were able to 'offer genetic evidence for the presence of the Justinianic Plague in the British Isles, previously only hypothesized from ambiguous documentary accounts'.

So, the team found the earliest genetic evidence of plague yet found in Britain, from the Anglo-Saxon site of Edix Hill. By using a combination of archaeological dating and the position of this strain of *Y. pestis* in its evolutionary tree, the researchers concluded that the genome is likely related to an ambiguously described pestilence in the British Isles in AD 544.

According to the *Irish Annals of Ulster and Tigernach*, the plague was preceded by a solar eclipse on 1 May 664 – 'Darkness on the 1st of May' (*Tenebrae in Kl. Maii*) – a total eclipse indeed did occur on 1 May 664 over North America near Long Island, and a partial eclipse may have been visible from Ireland. Was this a portent of disaster? The same annalist closed his entry for the year with the statement that 'the plague first raged in the Plain of Ith of the Fothairt' (present-day Carlow-Kildare) and was soon being described as *mortalitas magna* ('the great mortality'). The *Anglo Saxon Chronicle* references it briefly. Bede also mentions the eclipse and the plague in his *Ecclesiastical History of the English People* (AD 731); Bede, however, got it wrong when he erroneously dated the eclipse to 3 May. Later records that refer to the plague year derive from Bede's history. From a regal standpoint Britain got off lightly because when King Eorcenberht (r. 640–664) died he was successfully succeeded by his father, Eadbald. After the death of Honorius, Archbishop of Canterbury, Eorcenberht had appointed the first Saxon archbishop, Deusdedit, in 655. The plague had profound repercussions in the church when Archbishop Deusdedit of Canterbury (r. 655–664) died in July 664.

The *Annals of Ulster* claimed that there was also an earthquake in Britain (*terremotus in Brittania*).

According to Adomnan, Abbot of Iona and biographer of Columba, the plague afflicted all of the British Isles except for much of what is modern Scotland. To Adomnan, as with others, the plague was divine punishment for mortal sins; he believed that the Picts and Irish who lived in northern Great Britain were spared from the plague due to the intercession of Saint Columba who had founded monasteries there. Adomnan walked among victims of the pestilence and claimed that neither he nor his companions fell ill. Writing in 697 he described the plague as 'the Great Mortality which twice in our time has ravaged a large part of the world'.

The 'Great Mortality' may well have been a resurgence of the Buide Conaill which had swept through Ireland in the 6th century. The pestilence continued into 665 and broke out with renewed vigour in 667–668. It then quietened down for about fifteen years but flared up again in 683–684 when it was described as the *mortalitas puerorum* (death of boys). Children seem to have been more susceptible then because

---

35. Marcel Keller et al, *PNAS* June 18, 2019 116 (25) 12363–1237

they had little immune resistance. The *Annals of the Four Masters* tells us that 'There died very many ecclesiastics and laics in Ireland of this mortality.'

In AD 700, the *Annals* report an outbreak of famine and pestilence and cannibalism (*fama et pestilentia*) in Ireland which lasted for three years, 'so that man ate man' (*ut homo comederet hominem*). As if this was not enough there was also an outbreak of something resembling foot-and-mouth disease (*bovina mortalitas*).

Kohn, George C., 2007. '*Yellow Plague of 664*'. *Encyclopedia of Plague and Pestilence: From Ancient Times to the Present*. Infobase Publishing

Maddicott, J.R., 1997. Plague in Seventh-Century England, *Past & Present*, Volume 156, Issue 1, 7–54

Shrewsbury, J.F.D., 1997. The Yellow Plague, *Journal of the History of Medicine and Allied Sciences*, 4, 5–47

Plague in Constantinople, AD 698–701

We know of an outbreak of bubonic plague in Constantinople, Syria and Mesopotamia from Theophanes the Confessor. He tells us that the contagion went on for four months and caused a large number of deaths in Constantinople. Emperor Leontios (r. AD 695 to AD 698) dealt with it decisively, ordering a market in the Neorion cargo port of Constantinople to be destroyed and the harbour dredged; animals were being sold here and it was suspected to be a reservoir for the plague and the source of infected animals imported from Syria. As a result of the plague the Arab army was forced to suspend its military operations. According to Syrian sources, the plague in Syria lasted for another two years.

The Plagues of AD 745–748, Sicily and Calabria

In the late 8th and early 9th century two historical works, the *Short History of Nikephoros* (*Breviarium*) *of Constantinople* (d. 828), and the *Chronicle of Theophanes the Confessor*, tell us about the bubonic plague which appeared in Sicily and Calabria in 745–6 spreading to Monembasia to the east and to the Greek mainland and the islands, before it erupted in Constantinople in 747–8 during the reign of Emperor Constantine V. It may have killed up to 30 per cent of the population in Asia Minor before it swept through the Peloponnese. Monemb(v)asia is a town in modern Laconia on a small island off the east coast of the Peloponnese. The island is linked to the mainland by a short causeway

Earlier plagues had found their guests in relatively good health; the plagues of 747 to 748, however, were visited on a Constantinople that was laid low by an earthquake (740), civil war and famine in 743–744; famine, as we have seen, promoted hoarding and storage which in turn attracted, in this case, plague-carrying fleas on vermin. Resistance to disease was generally low and immune systems were below par – ideal conditions for disease transmission. The political situation was complicated because Rome was now a protectorate of the Franks and Ravenna had fallen to the Lombards, while many were questioning whether the plague and earthquake were 'divine retribution for missteps in doctrinal policy'. St Nikephoros, St Theophanes the Chronographer and St Theodore the Studite are our sources. We have already met Nikephoros and Theophanes, Theodore (759–826) was a Byzantine Greek monk and abbot of the great St John of Stoudios Monastery in Constantinople; Theodore's plague account features in a funeral oration for his uncle, Plato, whose parents, Sergios and Euphemia, died in the plague. All three were important players in the iconophile resistance to iconoclasm ('iconophile apologists') so it comes as little surprise that Nikephoros blamed the plague on Constantine V and others who incurred God's displeasure by 'raising their hands against the icons'.

Theophanes[36] describes it as 'the pestilent illness of the bubo' with death occurring so swiftly that mourners planning to attend funerals had sometimes died before the funeral had taken place; Nikepheros[37] speaks of 'mortality' and 'pestilent death'. The following summer (747) regenerated the disease which thrived in the city heat and humidity of Constantinople.[38] All the familiar symptoms were there, psychological and physical: mental instability with victims greeting strangers and ignoring friends; motiveless murders; hallucinations; wandering around aimlessly zombie-like; the ramblings of the crazy were interpreted, just as crazily, as prophecies with hidden meaning – some had actually come true[39]; there were not enough living to bury the dead the Christian way and corpses were unceremoniously dumped in vineyards, water cisterns, fields and gardens. Towns became ghost towns,[40] 'populous cities in two months became an almost uninhabited wasteland'. Nikephoros[41] reports that the plague went away in the autumn almost as quickly as it had descended: more proof that 'God had dealt a crushing blow against his people.'

While Constantinople undoubtedly suffered most, we also hear in a letter from Pope Zacharias in 748 to St Boniface that Rome was deserted while Isamic sources tell us of areas of devastation. Bizarrely, our sources mention that the plague, or God, gave notice of his deadly retribution when he marked with an olive coloured cross the clothing of the people, the vestments of the clergy, church hangings, doors and lintels: those associated with such a cipher should be in no doubt that death was imminent. Nikepheros[42] says that this 'gave rise to great sadness and apathy'. Many would have been reminded of the plague in Exodus 12, 21–23 where the Israelites were ordered by God to daub their doors with blood of a ram to avert the angel of death. The Israelites had been helped by God; not so the people of Constantinople.

---

36. 1, 422–3
37. *Breviarium* 63
38. Theophilus 1, 423
39. Theophilus 1, 423, 15–16
40. Theodore, *Laudatio* col. 85
41. *Breviarum* 64
42. (*Breviarium* 62–43)

The effects of the plague obviously extended much further in the region with profound impacts on the social, economic and political fabric of Justinian's wider empire – just as it had done since AD 542 when it all began. It weakened the empire with its usual accompaniments: mass depopulation, diminished manpower, productivity and consumption, agricultural and agronomical catastrophe, social upheaval, serious shortfalls in the military, religious turbulence and cultural bankruptcy.

Creighton, Charles, 1891. *A History of Epidemics in Britain (Volume I of II) from A.D. 664 to the Extinction of Plague*, Cambridge.
Turner, David The Politics of Despair: The Plague of 746–747 and Iconoclasm in the Byzantine Empire *The Annual of the British School at Athens* Vol. 85 (1990), pp. 419–434

In the 9th century, when the plague had finally gone, scholars in Basra composed brief summaries of the history of the disease. Later Muslim historians considered these 'Books of Plague' highly authoritative but for us they are vitiated by being selective and incomplete.

The Plague of Justinian and the plagues in the region which followed clearly left the empire exposed and vulnerable to further socio-political and military crises. The plague's long-term effects on European, Near Eastern and Christian history were huge. As the disease spread to port cities around the Mediterranean and then to their hinterlands, the Goths were reinvigorated and their conflict with Constantinople reached a higher level. Just before, Justinian had recaptured North Africa from the Vandals and much of Italy from the Ostrogoths. Prospects for restoring the whole Roman Empire in its entirety looked good and much of the west might welcome his armies. However, the plague weakened the Byzantine Empire at a critical juncture just when Justinian's armies were on the verge of retaking all of Italy and the western Mediterranean coast; had it proceeded the campaign would have reunited the Western Roman Empire with the Eastern Roman Empire. Although the conquest did actually happen in 554, the reunification was short-lived. In 568, the Lombards invaded Northern Italy, defeated the small Byzantine army that had been left behind and established the Kingdom of the Lombards. Gaul suffered, as presumably did Britain.

Society and culture were radically and irretrievably changed. High mortality reduced the population sizes of the cities; the clergy was decimated as were the more literate groups in society. Deaths and depression and loss of population drained the recruiting pool for the legions so the Byzantine Empire had to downsize its field armies. Not only was the offensive in the West abandoned after 565, but the southern defences were so weakened that Islam, in the next century, was able to detach Egypt and Syria for itself leading to a significant opportunity for the development and spread of Islam in the region. Greek, Arab, and German dominance lasted for centuries.

Some scholars estimate that by AD 600 the plague may have reduced the population of the Mediterranean region to 60 per cent of its total a century earlier. Such a huge mortality rate would naturally result in social and economic ruin.

Chapter 7

The Japanese Smallpox epidemic AD 735–737

'Japan was particularly alert to the consequences of epidemics to the extent that they, with uncommon vigilance still not equalled by some developed nations in the 21st century, had adopted the Chinese policy of reporting disease outbreaks amongst the population at large.'

Smallpox: a global history

Smallpox is spread by an inhaled virus, which causes fever, vomiting and a rash which soon covers the body with pus-filled blisters. These turn into scabs which leave scars. Fatal in approximately one-third of cases, another third of those afflicted with the disease typically go blind. Smallpox existed in ancient times invading, among other places, Egypt, India and China. Although the origin of smallpox remains unknown, it is thought to date back to Egypt around the 3rd century BC based on a smallpox-like rash found on three mummies. The earliest written description of a disease clearly resembling smallpox emerged in China in the 4th century AD. We also have early written accounts from India in the 7th century and in Asia Minor in the 10th century.

As with other pandemics the global spread of smallpox goes hand in hand with the growth and spread of crowded civilizations, exploration and expanding trade routes and colonisation over the centuries: smallpox came to Europe during the Crusades of the 11th century. When Europeans began to explore and colonize other parts of the world, smallpox went with them. Smallpox has had a major impact on world history, particularly on indigenous populations where smallpox was non-native, such as the Americas and Australia; these peoples were rapidly weakened by smallpox along with other imported diseases during periods of early foreign contact.

Smallpox may have been implicated in the Plague of Athens (430 BC) and certainly was in the Plague of Cyprian when it hastened the decline and fall of the empire. Around 400 AD Indian medical literature recorded a disease marked by pustules and boils, saying 'the pustules are red, yellow, and white and they are accompanied by burning pain … the skin seems studded with grains of rice.' As so often when it comes to finding a rationale for the death and destruction, the Indian epidemic was thought to be punishment from a god: the survivors invented a goddess, Sitala, as the anthropomorphic personification of the disease. In Hinduism the goddess Sitala both causes and cures high fever, rashes, hot flashes and pustules – all symptoms of smallpox.

In 340, Chinese alchemist Ko Hung described the difference between smallpox and measles; a Christian priest, Ahrun, did likewise in Egypt in the 7th century. In AD 710 smallpox was re-introduced into Europe by the Umayyad or Muslim conquest of Spain. The clearest description of smallpox was given in the 9th century by the Persian physician, Muhammad ibn Zakariya ar-Razi, known in the West as 'Rhazes', who was the first to differentiate smallpox from measles and chickenpox in his *Kitab fi al-jadari wa-al-hasbah (The Book of Smallpox and Measles)*.

At the end of the 15th century Christopher Columbus led the way when he shipped in to the Americas a raft of deadly diseases for which the indigenous populations had no natural immunity: measles, smallpox, whooping cough, chickenpox, bubonic plague, typhus and malaria all had a role to play as efficient killers in the New World. Worldwide, smallpox was a leading cause of death in the 18th century killing an estimated 400,000 Europeans each year including five reigning European monarchs. Then every seventh child born in Russia died from smallpox. Most people were infected at some point during their lifetime, and about 30 per cent of people died from the disease. In the west, one in ten people died of smallpox, half of which were children. Smallpox was responsible for a third of all cases of blindness. Between 20 and 60 per cent of all those infected – and over 80 per cent of infected children – died from the disease.

In northern Japan, the Ainu population decreased drastically in the 19th century, due in large part to infectious diseases like smallpox introduced by Japanese settlers pouring into Hokkaido.

The Franco-Prussian War triggered a smallpox pandemic of 1870–1875 that claimed 500,000 lives; while vaccination was mandatory in the Prussian army, many French soldiers went un-vaccinated. Smallpox outbreaks among French prisoners of war spread to the German civilian population and other parts of Europe. Ultimately, this public health disaster inspired stricter legislation in Germany and England, though not in France.

In 1849 nearly 13 per cent of all Calcutta deaths were due to smallpox. Between 1868 and 1907, there were approximately 4.7 million deaths from smallpox in India. Between 1926 and 1930, there were 979,738 cases of smallpox with a mortality of 42.3 per cent.

Smallpox is exogenous to Africa. One of the oldest records of what may have been an episode of smallpox in Africa is associated with the Elephant War ca. AD 568, when, after fighting a siege in Mecca, Ethiopian troops contracted the disease which they took with them back to Ethiopia.

It seems likely that smallpox in Angola was introduced soon after the Portuguese settlement of the area in 1484. The 1864 epidemic killed 25,000 inhabitants, one third of the total population in that area. In 1713, an outbreak occurred in South Africa after a ship from India docked at Cape Town, bringing infected laundry ashore. Many of the settler European population suffered, and whole clans of the Khoisan people were wiped out as far as the Kalahari desert. A second outbreak occurred in 1755, again affecting both the white population and the Khoisan. A third outbreak in 1767 similarly affected the Khoisan and Bantu peoples.

Continued enslavement brought smallpox to Cape Town again in 1840, taking the lives of 2,500 people, and then to Uganda in the 1840s. It is estimated that up to 80 per cent of the Griqua tribe was exterminated by smallpox in 1831, and whole tribes were being wiped out in Kenya up until 1899. Along the Zaire river basin were areas where no one survived the epidemics, leaving the land completely depopulated. In Ethiopia and the Sudan, six epidemics are recorded for the 19th century: 1811–1813, 1838–1839, 1865–1866, 1878–1879, 1885–1887 and 1889–1890.

In Central and South America the effects of smallpox on Tahuantinsuyu, or the Inca empire, were even more devastating than on the Aztecs (see below). Beginning in Colombia, smallpox spread rapidly even before the Spanish invaders first arrived. The spread was probably facilitated by the efficient Inca road system. Within months, the disease had killed the Inca Emperor Huayna Capac, his successor and most of the other leaders. Within a few years smallpox claimed between 60 per cent and 90 per cent of the Inca population, with other waves of European disease weakening them further.

North American indigenous populations did not escape. The epidemics afflicting them are dealt with below. The first recorded outbreak in Australia, in 1789, devastated the aboriginal population, perhaps slaying about 50 per cent of Aboriginal populations on the east coast. It came in by either the first fleet of British settlers to arrive in the Colony of New South Wales, or by other visitors to Australia, such as Makassan mariners visiting Arnhem Land and Kimberley. Smallpox ravaged many indigenous Polynesians; Alfred Crosby, in his major work, *Ecological Imperialism: The Biological Expansion of Europe, 900–1900* (1986) showed that in 1840 a ship carrying smallpox was successfully quarantined, preventing an epidemic amongst the Māori of New Zealand. The only major outbreak in New Zealand was a 1913 epidemic, which affected Māori in northern New Zealand and nearly wiped out the Rapa Nui of Easter Island as reported in 1914.

In the 20th century, smallpox was probably responsible for a staggering 300–500 million deaths worldwide. In the early 1950s an estimated 50 million cases of smallpox occurred in the world each year. In 1967, the World Health Organization estimated that 15 million people contracted the disease and that 2 million died in that year. After successful vaccination campaigns during the 19th and 20th centuries, the WHO certified the global eradication of smallpox in December 1979.

Variolation

One of the earliest methods for controlling the spread of smallpox was the use of variolation. Variolation involved infecting a person via a cut in the skin with exudate from a patient with a relatively mild case of smallpox (variola), to bring about a manageable and recoverable infection that would provide later immunity. With variolation, people usually went on to develop the symptoms associated with smallpox, such as fever and a rash. However, fewer people died from variolation than if they had acquired smallpox naturally.

This practice of smallpox inoculation (as opposed to the later practice of vaccination) was developed possibly in 8th-century India or 10th-century China spreading into 17th-century Turkey. By the beginning of the 18th century, the Royal Society in England was discussing the practice of inoculation, and the smallpox epidemic in 1713 spurred further interest. It was not until 1721, however, that England recorded its first case of inoculation.

Crosby, Alfred, 1989, *Ecological Imperialism AD 900-1900*, London.
Hopkins D.R., 2002. *The Greatest Killer: Smallpox in History*. University of Chicago Press.
    Originally published as *Princes and Peasants: Smallpox in History* (1983)
Nicholas, R., 1981. 'The goddess Sitala and epidemic smallpox in Bengal, India'. *J Asian Stud*. 41 (1): 21–45
Whipps, Heather, 2008, 'How Smallpox Changed the World', *LiveScience*, June 23, 2008

Japan

We are fortunate that the quantity of information on disease, especially epidemic afflictions, is better for Japan than for most other civilizations, including western Europe. This is because the Japanese had the foresight to adopt the Chinese practice of reporting diseases in the community from around AD 700. Many of these reports were included in court chronicles. The quality of the reports, though, is somewhat wanting as communications between the provinces and the capital declined after 900, and many outbreaks of pestilence undoubtedly went unreported by the official recorders. What is more, even when the reporting system was operating well, the sources often do not provide crucial facts such as the nature of the disease, the regions afflicted, or levels of mortality. In addition, local records that would enhance our knowledge of diseases that prevailed are largely absent before 1100. But what we have is far better than nothing, which is the norm in early disease reporting.

The description, diagnosis, and treatment of disease in early Japan is heavily influenced by Chinese texts while Buddhist scriptures from India also determined how disease and medicine were perceived. Nevertheless, the native Japanese view of disease was also influential and it was widely believed that it was demonic possession to be exorcised by shamans and witch doctors. Geography plays an important part in epidemiology: Japan provides a good example of what is termed 'island epidemiology'; its comparative isolation meant that Japan remained relatively free of epidemic outbreaks as long as communication with the continent was kept to a minimum and remained sporadic. However, once an infectious disease was introduced to the country, by virtue of virgin soil immunity it was able to tear through those dense populations that had had virtually no opportunity to develop resistance to it. Thus, immunities were built up only very slowly over centuries. Additionally, Japan's topography and communications, its mountainous terrain, meant that an epidemic reached different regions at different times.

We can divide the history of epidemics in Japan until 1600 (when Japan banned travel and trade with most countries) into four periods: from earliest times to 700, when little is known about disease; 700–1050, an age of severe epidemics; 1050–1260, a transitional period when some historical lethal diseases became endemic in the population; and 1260–1600, a time of less disease despite the introduction of some new pestilence from the West. There is little or no evidence of infectious disease to be found in skeletons before about AD 550. After that date, though, hard evidence of disease starts to emerge: *The Chronicles of Japan*, the court histories, record that in

552 many people were hit with disease, contemporaneous with the time when gifts of a statue of the Buddha along with sutras (scriptures) arrived at the Japanese court from Korea: disease came too. The court blamed the outbreak on the introduction of a foreign religion and destroyed the gifts. In 585, the court blamed and banned Buddha again when the *Chronicles* recorded that many people were afflicted with sores 'as if they were burnt', indicating a fever. This is seen as the first outbreak of smallpox in Japanese history, although others believe that this 585 epidemic was measles.

The period between 585 and the end of the seventh century is a black hole when it comes to reports of contagion: either there was little or nothing to report or else the epidemics that did occur have gone unrecorded; the latter seems more likely as we know that during this time Japan sent eleven envoys to China, received seven from China, and had about 80 diplomatic exchanges with Korea. From AD 698, though, things really started to take off: there are 34 epidemics recorded for the 8th century, 35 for the 9th century, 26 for the 10th century (despite that decline in the availability of records), and 24 for the 11th century, 16 of which occur between 1000 and 1052. The diseases were clearly imported from the Asian mainland as the Japanese travelled to China and Korea to acquaint themselves with superior continental political and cultural systems, and to trade.

Disease had a pronounced impact on Japanese society, restraining economic development and influencing taxation systems, local government, land tenure, labour, technology, religion, literature, education, and all other aspects of life. On the positive side, by enduring so much disease trauma so early in their history, the Japanese were able to build immunities early on and escaped the worst of the diseases that beset the Incas, Aztecs and others with Western contact in the sixteenth century.

We can only identify five of the Japanese diseases: smallpox, measles, influenza, mumps and dysentery. Plague may be added to the list in 808 at a time when it was rampaging through the Mediterranean and the Middle East: Arab merchants and sailors often frequented Chinese, Korean and Japanese ports; they also made their way along the Silk Route.

The most deadly of the five or six diseases was smallpox (mogasa, 'funeral pox'). We know of serial epidemics for 735–7, 790, 812–14, 853, 915, 947, 974, 993–5, 1020, and 1036. Smallpox was especially lethal to adults here; it may have become endemic in the population by 1100 or even earlier.

The 735–37 Japanese smallpox epidemic (天平の疫病大流行) is 'the earliest well-reported smallpox epidemic in world history'[1]; it also goes by the name 'Epidemic of the Tenpyō era' and was a significant epidemic that prostrated much of Japan, killing approximately 30 per cent of the Japanese population. It was to have major nationwide economic and religious repercussions. As we have seen Japan was particularly alert to the consequences of epidemics to the extent that they, with uncommon vigilance still not equalled by some developed nations in the 21st century, had adopted the Chinese policy of reporting disease outbreaks amongst the population at large. Such recording

1. Farris 1985

proved to be very helpful in the the identification of the epidemic as smallpox in the years 735–37.

According to the *Shoku Nihongi* the smallpox epidemic made its first appearance in August 735 in the international port of Dazaifu, Fukuoka in northern Kyushu, western Japan where blame for the infection was laid at the door of a Japanese fisherman; he had contracted the disease when stranded on the Korean peninsula. The disease spread rapidly throughout northern Kyushu that year and into the next when tenant farmers were either dying or deserting their crops; this inevitably led to an immediate depletion of agricultural yields and ultimately famine. One record balefully reads that 'in recent times, there has been nothing like this'.

The *Shoku Nihongi* (続日本紀) is an imperially-commissioned Japanese history text. Completed in AD 797, it is the second of the *Six National Histories*, following the *Nihon Shoki* and followed by *Nihon Kōki*. It is one of the most important primary historical sources on Japan's Nara period. The work covers the 95-year period from the beginning of Emperor Monmu's reign in 697 until the tenth year of Emperor Kanmu's reign in 791, spanning nine imperial reigns.

Two other records describe the symptoms and treatment of smallpox. The disease initially presented as a fever, with the patient suffering in bed from three to six days. After the fever waned and the blotches started to disappear, diarrhoea was common. Patients also suffered from coughs, vomiting, nosebleeds and the regurgitation of blood. Remedies and treatments involved government doctors trained in Chinese, Indian and native Japanese medicine who advocated a variety of palliatives, including wrapping the patient in warm covers, drinking rice gruel, eating boiled scallions to stop the diarrhoea and force-feeding patients with no appetite. Medicines were seen as of little or no use. Survivors were advised not to avoid raw fish or fresh fruit or vegetables, to drink water, take a bath, have sex or walk in the wind or rain. Doctors also advocated mixing flour from red beans and the white of an egg, and applying the mixture to the skin to eliminate the pox. Other suggestions included bathing in a woman's menstrual blood or wrapping a baby in a menstrual cloth to wipe out the blotches; applying honey, powdered silkworm cocoons, white lead, or powdered falcon feathers and lard were also suggested.

Just when things seemed to be abating, a party of Japanese government officials made the mistake of passing through northern Kyushu at the same time as the epidemic was gathering its lethal pace there. Watching colleagues die around them, in 737 the diminished group decided not to proceed with their intended trip to the Korean peninsula and returned to Nara with the smallpox and, unwittingly spread it throughout eastern Japan and Nara. From there the pestilence continued to ravage Japan. One immediate effect was fiscal rather than public health orientated: by August 737, a tax exemption had been extended to all of Japan.

Tax records offer a glimpse of the mortality rates: in the year 737 alone, the province of Izumi near the capital lost 44 per cent of its adult population, while Bungo in northern Kyushu and Suruga in eastern Japan sustained death rates of about 30 per cent. The average mortality for all known areas was about 25 per cent. Population depletion for the three years probably amounted to between 25 and 35 per cent, making the epidemic comparable in its mortality to the European Black Death of the fourteenth century. All levels of society were of course affected. Many court nobles perished due to smallpox. The epidemic caused considerable dislocation, migration and imbalance of the labour markets throughout Japan with particular damage done to construction and farming, especially rice cultivation.

Smallpox led to population stagnation; it has been estimated that the population of Japan was 6 million in the eighth century; this had changed very little by 1050. Plagues led to the desertion of villages: an entire layer of village administration was abolished. The pestilence damaged agriculture as fields could not be cultivated. In 743, after the 735–37 outbreak, the aristocracy attempted to stimulate farming by enacting a policy giving permanent private tenure to anyone who would work the land. However, the pestilence had boosted migration and led to a shortage of labourers. The courts enacted legislation to tie peasants to their land in the 8th and 9th centuries, but to little effect. These labour shortages put an end to temple construction or rice planting, and by the year 800 construction projects and conscription to the army had been abandoned.

The repeated outbreaks of pestilence also had a profound influence on Japanese religion. The ground breaking introduction of Buddhism came about amidst a plague of smallpox. As a transcendental religion, Buddhism was perfectly adapted for an environment in which disease outbreaks were common. Early adherents reached out to Buddhism because of the promise it offered of protection from illness. After the epidemic of 735–37, the Emperor Shômu increased state support of the religion by ordering the construction of the great state temple Tôdaiji and its Daibutsu – a huge statue of Buddha – along with branch temples and statues throughout the land. The cost of casting the Daibutsu alone has been said to have nearly bankrupted an already financially weakened country.

The Gion Festival, today celebrated from 17 to 24 July, began as an attempt to rid Heian of epidemics. The festival was first conducted by Gion Shrine (later Yasaka Shrine) in eastern Heian (modern Kyoto), in 869, just after an epidemic. Sixty-six spears, one for each province in Japan, were placed on end and marched through the city to banish the disease. In 970 the festival became an annual affair, reflecting the frequency and prevalence of disease in the capital.

In 993, a festival to drive away disease gods was held in the Kitano section of the capital. Two palanquins (litters) were built by the state, Buddhist monks chanted a sutra, and music played. Several thousand citizens gathered and offered prayers to the gods. The palanquins, bearing the gods of the epidemic, were then borne by the crowds several miles to the ocean to wash away the smallpox.

Destructive waves of smallpox epidemics continued to wash over Japan: in 790 it returned via Chinese ports, predominantly afflicting those aged 30 or younger; the epidemic of 812–14 entered Japan via northern Kyushu and to swarm over the archipelago to the east. According to the records, 'almost half' of the population died. In 853, the disease focused on the capital, Heian before it spread to the countryside. The disease, however, mainly attacked adults this time. In 925, the Emperor Daigo caught it at the age of 41. The smallpox outbreak of 993–35 was particularly severe. In 993, the Emperor Ichijo became a victim at the age of 15. The disease was so virulent in the capital that 70 officials of the fifth court rank or higher died; the roads were strewn with corpses providing food for hungry dogs and vultures. In 1020 smallpox visited Kyushu again, possibly courtesy of continental invaders the previous year. A diary entry states that those aged 28 and under were particularly vulnerable. After AD 1000 or so the disease had become endemic in the Japanese population and thus less devastating during outbreaks.

The frequency, ubiquity and prevalence of smallpox caused the disease to become entrenched in Japanese mythology, in the form of the Smallpox demon (疱瘡神, Hōsōshin) or smallpox devil; this is a demon whose responsibility in Japanese life was to promulgate smallpox. People attempted to appease the smallpox demon by assuaging his anger, or they tried to attack the demon since they had no other effective treatment for smallpox. In those days, smallpox was considered to be the result of *onryō*, which was a mythological spirit who is able to return to the physical world in order to seek vengeance. Smallpox-related *kamis* (deities) include *Sumiyoshi sanjin*. In a book published in the Kansei years (1789–1801), we read that smallpox devils were enshrined in infected families in order to recover from smallpox.

Smallpox devils were afraid of red things and also of dogs so, people naturally showed off various dolls that were red. In Okinawa, they tried to praise and comfort devils with *sanshin*, an Okinawan musical instrument and lion dances before a patient clad in red clothes. They offered flowers and burned incense in order to please the smallpox demon. Also in Okinawa we find smallpox poetry composed in Ryukyuan; the purpose of smallpox poetry in the Ryukyu language is the glorification of the smallpox demon, or recovery from lethal infection of smallpox. Traditional smallpox folk dances have been seen even in today's Japan, including Ibaraki Prefecture and Kagoshima Prefecture, for the avoidance of smallpox devils.

The 'red treatment' caught on in a big way. In European countries it was practised from the 12th century onwards; when he caught smallpox, King Charles V of France dressed in a red shirt, red stockings and a red veil. Queen Elizabeth I of England was wrapped in a red blanket and placed by a burning fire when she fell ill with smallpox in 1562, and similar treatments were applied to other European monarchs. Many Japanese textbooks on dermatology held that red light was able to diminish the symptoms of smallpox and emulated in China, India, Turkey and Georgia. In western Africa, the Yoruba god of smallpox, Sopona, was associated with the colour red.

The 'red treatment' was given scientific authority by Nobel laureate Niels Ryberg Finsen, who claimed that the treatment of smallpox patients with red light reduced the severity of scarring and later developed rules governing erythrotherapy. This survived into the 1930s when scientists declared it to be bogus.

Measles

Measles (*akamogasa*, 'red pox') assailed Japan in 998 and 1025; *A Tale of Flowering Fortunes*, a chronicle of the tenth and eleventh centuries, states that the disease presented with a 'heavy rash of bright red spots'. The pestilence began in the early summer in the capital, where the wives of high ranking officials were first to be affected. Foreigners did not die from the disease which lends credence to Japan's island epidemiology.

In 1025 measles came back savaging people of all classes who had not caught it in the 998 epidemic. The capital seems to have suffered most although one source states that 'all under heaven' caught the disease.

Influenza

Flu was *gai byo* or *gaigyaku byo*, 'coughing sickness', which struck in 862–4, 872, 920, 923, 993 and 1015. Unlike smallpox and measles, which were most prevalent between late spring and autumn influenza usually struck in the late winter and early spring. The epidemics of 862–4 and 872 were particularly severe, killing many in and around the capital although mortality was less than from smallpox or measles.

Mumps

Records tell us that mumps (*fukurai byo*, 'swelling sickness') flourished in 959 and 1029, mainly in Heian. In both epidemics, historians have indicated that the disease was marked by the characteristic swelling of the neck.

Dysentery

Dysentery (*sekiri*, 'red diarrhea') was epidemic in 861, 915, and 947 in late summer and autumn. Often dysentery occurs with other infections as in the smallpox epidemic of 735–37. The dysentery epidemic of 861 was followed by influenza in 862 and 864. In 915 and 947, smallpox came with it. The measles epidemic of 1025 was also probably related to dysentery infections among the Heian nobility. Their diaries record that when patients caught dysentery they quickly lost their appetites and suffered from fever.

Malaria

Malaria (*warawayami*, *furuiyami*, or *okori*, 'the chills') was something of a mystery: doctors were still unaware that the disease could be carried by mosquitoes, although a court lady seemed to believe that butterflies were common where the disease broke out. Japan is a land characterised by swamps so malaria is likely to have had a marked effect on a peasantry trying to convert these low-lying lands into productive rice paddies.

Farris, William Wayne, 1985. *Population, Disease, and Land in Early Japan, 645–900*. Harvard University Asia Center. 51–52.

Jannetta, Ann Bowman, 2014. *Epidemics and Mortality in Early Modern Japan*. Princeton University Press.

Diseases of the Premodern Period in Japan https://www.mitchmedical.us/human-disease/diseases-of-the-premodern-period-in-japan.html

Table 3: 430 BC–AD 737: Disease impacts and mitigation efforts

NAME	DATE	DISEASE	IMPACT
THE PLAGUE OF ATHENS	430 BC	Typhus Fever?	A major contributory factor in Athens' defeat by Sparta: it weakened Athens' military power and diminished her hegemony and importance in ancient Greece for good.
THE ANTONINE PLAGUE	AD 165–180	Smallpox	Precipitated Rome's decline and fall due to weakening of army.
THE HAN DYNASTY EPIDEMIC	AD 200	Smallpox	Collapse of Han Dynasty and depopulation.
THE PLAGUE OF CYPRIAN	AD 250–271	Viral hemorrhagic fever, possibly Ebola?	Further weakened Rome and left her vulnerable to barbarian incursions in the Crisis of the 3rd Century. Significant military reform.
THE PLAGUE OF JUSTINIAN	AD 541–542	Bubonic plague	Seriously destabilised Byzantine empire.
THE PLAGUE OF SHEROE	AD 627–628	Bubonic plague	Weakened Sassanid Empire
PLAGUE OF AMWAS, SYRIA	AD 638–639	Bubonic plague	Incapacitated Umayyad Empire leading to its downfall
THE BRITISH PLAGUE	AD 664	Bubonic plague	Triggered invasions by Angles into traditional British territory; religious turmoil when Archbishop of Canterbury, Deusdedit, died of plague.
THE JAPANESE EPIDEMIC	AD 735–737	Smallpox	Total disruption of Japanese culture and traditions

THE MIDDLE AGES

Bubonic Plague: the Black Death: 1346–1353 (Start of the Second Plague Pandemic)

'First pray, then flee.'

– From Dr Alonso de Chirino's practical guide to the
plague for the layperson (c. 1431)

'The year of 1348 has left us alone and helpless. Where are our dear friends now? Where are the beloved faces? Where are the affectionate words? the relaxed and enjoyable conversations?'

– Francesco Petrarca, (b.1304), Petrarch

To the Florentine poet plague was a disease 'without equal for centuries'; it had 'trampled and destroyed the entire world'. It may well have all started in India, spreading through Asia, North Africa and then to Europe. Plague probably came to England courtesy of an infected rat or flea at Melcombe Regis (now Weymouth) at the end of July or beginning of August, 1348. It then spread through the south-west to Bristol and then eastwards to Oxford and London, which it had reached by the beginning of November travelling at the rate of about 1½ miles per day. In Europe, it is estimated around 50 million people died as a result of the Black Death, also known as the Great Mortality or the Great Pestilence. The population fell from some 80 million to 30 million. It killed at least 60 per cent of the population in rural and urban settings. It took the world population 200 years to recover to the level at which it stood in the early 1340s.

The 1347 pandemic plague was not referred to specifically as 'black' in the 14th or 15th centuries in any European language. In fact 'Black Death' was not used to describe the plague pandemic in English until 1755, when it translated the Danish: *den sorte død*, 'the black death'. As is usual, the poor were worst affected: they tended to live in single-storey thatched wattle-and-daub hovels. Rats burrowed under their earth floors and climbed the walls to build their nests in the roofs, from which blocked fleas could fall to infect the residents below. The houses of the better off often had an upper storey making them less attractive to rats and their fleas.

The Black Death in all its horror not only slew millions, it also was the trigger for mass hysteria, masochistic flagellent processions and persecution of the Jews. Jews were blamed and accused of a raft of crimes including contaminating food supplies through their concoctions 'of frogs and spiders mixed into oil and cheese to destroy Christendom'. The usual pogroms followed. The *Germania Judaica*, reports the annihilation of at least 235 Jewish communities around the time of the Black Death.

Flemish weavers and merchants in England also took a share of the blame and endured violent assaults as scapegoats.

Henry Knighton, a canon of St Mary's Abbey, Leicester and a plague witness, was one of the authors who have left us the wild, hysterical descriptions which allege to chronicle these darkest of dark days; their work was often a disturbing mixture of hysteria, fake news and conspiracy theory. Knighton claimed in his *Chronichon*, written between 1378 and 1396, that the earth had swallowed many cities in Corinth and Achaia; and in Cyprus, the mountains were levelled causing rivers to submerge the nearby cities. And, of course Knighton and everyone else all concurred that the Black Death was imposed by the wrath of God.

Here Knighton speaks of the appalling mortality rate and the economic toll, but he seems more concerned, and indignant, about more selfish and personal issues: the absolute need to secure death-bed payments of debts, the diminishing pool of hired help, and the preposterous demands of workers that they get a fair wage in the light of their new-found power in the employment market:

> 'Then the grievous plague penetrated the seacoasts from Southampton, and came to Bristol, and there almost the whole strength of the town died, struck as it were by sudden death. There died at Leicester in the small parish of St. Leonard more than 380, in the parish of Holy Cross more than 400; in the parish of S. Margaret of Leicester more than 700; and so in each parish a great number. Then the bishop of Lincoln gave general power to all and every priest to hear confessions, and absolve with full and entire authority except in matters of debt, in which case the dying man, if he could, should pay the debt while he lived, or others should certainly fulfill that duty from his property after his death.
>
> In the same year there was a great plague of sheep [anthrax?] everywhere in the realm so that in one place there died in one pasturage more than 5,000 sheep, and so rotted that neither beast nor bird would touch them...Sheep and cattle went wandering over fields and through crops, and there was no one to go and drive or gather them for there was such a lack of servants that no one knew what he ought to do. Wherefore many crops perished in the fields for want of someone to gather them...
>
> Meanwhile the king sent proclamation that reapers and other labourers should not take more than they had been accustomed to take [in pay]. But the labourers were so lifted up and obstinate that they would not listen to the king's command, but if anyone wished to have them he had to give them what they wanted, and either lose his fruit and crops, or satisfy the wishes of the workmen...there was such a want of servants in work of all kinds, that one would scarcely believe that in times past there had been such a lack. And so all necessities became so much dearer.'
>
> – From *History of England* by Henry Knighton,
> in *Source Book of English History*, by E.K. Kendall.

Indeed the Ordinance of Labourers, 1349 was a failed attempt by Edward III to freeze wages paid to labourers at their pre-plague levels; the ordinance is not only indicative of the labour shortage caused by the Black Death, it also adumbrates the beginnings of the redefinition of societal roles.

Across Europe people were frantic for an explanation: some attributed the pestilence to invisible particles blowing in the wind, others spoke of poisoned wells; many, as we have noted, predictably blamed the Jews. Some elected to face up to the plague by riotous living, others self-isolated and lived as recluses; others deserted their homes for the countryside; villages, towns, even whole cities were barred to sufferers. Everything failed. Corpses were slung out in the street or committed to crisis burials. The depravity of some plumbed uncharted depths: for example, themselves already infected, they broke into houses and threatened to contaminate all within unless paid to leave. Desperate times required desperate remedies: some recommended the burning of aromatic woods and herbs; others suggested special diets, courses of bleeding, new positions for sleeping. The rich experimented with medicines made of gold and pearls. Flight remained the best option, and if you could not flee, then all you had was resignation and prayer.

Boccaccio (1313–1375) gives us an unusual consequence of the plague in the *Decameron*:

> '...it came to pass – something, perhaps, never before heard of that no woman, however attractive, fair or well-born she might be, rejected, when stricken with the disease, the advances of a man, young or old, or refused to expose to him every part of her body, with no more shame than if he had been a woman, submitting of necessity to that which her illness required; as a result there was a distinct loss of modesty in those who, after time, recovered. Besides which many now succumbed [to the plague], who would, perhaps, have escaped death.'

But there was another way:

The Flagellants were religious zealots who demonstrated their zeal and sought atonement for their sins by public demonstrations of vigorous self-flagellation and masochistic displays of penance. In the early days self-flagellation was imposed as punishment and as a means of penance for wayward clergy and laity. When plague ravaged Italy in 1259, Raniero Fasani, the Hermit of Umbria, corralled processions of self-scourging flagellants. Adopted first in Perugia, the movement developed into flagellant brotherhoods comprising laypersons as well as clergy and spread into Poland, Germany and the Low Countries in the mid-13th century. In the mid-14th century, flagellants terrified of the Black Death sought to mitigate the divine judgment that they feared to be round the corner. In 1349 Pope Clement VI condemned flagellation, as did the Council of Constance (1414–18).

The Catholic Church's condemnation only strengthened the movement to the extent that it attained its greatest popularity during the Black Death. Dressed in white robes, many adherents roamed around Europe dragging crosses while literally whipping themselves into a religious frenzy. On arrival in a town the brethren would head straight for the church, where bells would toll to announce their arrival to the townsfolk. The Brethren would then move to an open space and form a circle, stripping to the waist and then walking around in their circle until called to stop by the Master. They would then fall to the ground, adopting a crucifix position, holding three fingers in the air (perjurors) or lying face down (adulterers).

Despite their popularity on the European mainland the Flagellants did not really catch on in Britain: a large contingent did cross the English Channel in 1349 and converged on London but innate British reserve, even in those early days, prevented such conspicuous displays. Heinrich von Herford was one of the many who witnessed their painful ritual:

'Each whip consisted of a stick with three knotted thongs hanging from the end. Two pieces of needle-sharp metal were run through the centre of the knots from both sides, forming a cross, the end of which extended beyond the knots for the length of a grain of wheat or less. Using these whips they beat and whipped their bare skin until their bodies were bruised and swollen and blood rained down, spattering the walls nearby. I have seen, when they whipped themselves, how sometimes those bits of metal penetrated the skin so deeply that it took more than two attempts to pull them out.'

– Heinrich von Herford (c. 1300–1370),
Chronicon Henrici de Hervordia

'Some foolish women had clothes ready to catch the blood and smear it on their eyes, saying it was miraculous blood.'

– Jean Froissart (c.1337–c.1405)

Flagellants had to avoid speaking, have no contact with the opposite sex, avoid shaving, bathing or changing their clothes, and sleep on straw. Ironically, some towns started to notice that sometimes flagellants brought plague to places where it had not yet emerged. As a consequence they were denied entry.

There were other equally unsuccessful remedies for banishing the plague; they included: eating mustard, mint sauce, apple sauce and horseradish to balance wet, dry, hot and cold in your diet; rubbing onions or snake on your buboes or cutting up a pigeon and rubbing it over an infected body; drinking vinegar, eating arsenic, mercury or ten-year-old treacle; sitting close to a fire or in a sewer to drive out the fever, or fumigating the house with herbs to purify the air. Doctors tested urine for colour and health. Some even tasted it in the test.

Chapter 9

Plague quarantine in
Ragusa (Dubrovnik), 1377

'Some medical historians consider Ragusa's quarantine edict one of the highest achievements of medieval medicine.'

– Zlata Blazina Tomic, 2015

Around 1348, plague overtook cities like Venice and Milan and city officials, with admirable good sense and perspicacity, put emergency public health measures in place that are the 700-year-old precursors of today's best practices relating to social distancing and surface disinfecting. They had a good idea that people had to be very careful with traded goods since the disease could be spread on objects and surfaces, and that everyone had to do what they could to limit person-to-person contact. Personal and individual responsibility was paramount.

When plague hit Ragusa in 1377 it prompted the first known example of mandatory quarantine. The good people of the port were the first to pass a law requiring the mandatory quarantine of all incoming ships and trade caravans in order to screen for infection. That law 'stipulates that those who come from plague-infested areas shall not enter [Ragusa] or its district unless they spend a month on the islet of Mrkan or in the town of Cavtat, for the purpose of disinfection.' Zlata Blazina Tomic (2015) explains that Mrkan was an uninhabited rocky island south of the city and Cavtat was situated at the end of the caravan road used by overland traders en route to Ragusa. Tomic adds:

> '...that some medical historians consider Ragusa's quarantine edict one of the highest achievements of medieval medicine. By ordering the isolation of healthy sailors and traders for 30 days, Ragusan officials showed a remarkable understanding of incubation periods. New arrivals might not have exhibited symptoms of the plague, but they would be held long enough to determine if they were in fact disease-free.'

Our word 'quarantine' is derived from *quarantino*, Italian for a 40-day period, a number freighted with symbolic and religious significance to medieval Christians. When God flooded the Earth, it rained for 40 days and 40 nights, and Jesus fasted in the wilderness for 40 days. This was carried over into health where, for example, after childbirth a new mother was advised to rest for 40 days.

Ragusa can also take the credit as the first city to open the first state funded *lazaretto* or temporary plague hospital, on another island called Mljet.

Jane Stevens Crawshaw (2016) explains that the name *lazaretto* is a corruption of the word Nazaretto, the nickname for the lagoon island upon which Venice built its first permanent plague hospital, Santa Maria di Nazareth. The *lazaretto* served both as a medical treatment centre and a quarantine facility. It was a way to care compassionately for new arrivals and local citizens who fell sick with the plague while keeping them isolated from the healthy. At a *lazaretto*, plague-infected patients would receive fresh food, clean bedding and other health-promoting treatments, all paid for by the state. They also acted as convalescent homes, had cemeteries and were depots for the disinfection or destruction of infected goods. During the 1625 outbreak, London just had 'cabins in the fields'.[1] while in Germany, even small towns such as Überlingen had pesthouses, and indeed separate houses for the sick and for contacts. During an outbreak, overcrowding was normal; in 1630, Florence's San Miniato had 82 beds for 412 females, and 93 beds for 312 males.

Stevens Crashaw with reference to Venice:

> 'They're quite a remarkable early public health structure into which the government has to invest huge sums of money. Regardless of whether there's a plague in Venice, these hospitals are permanently manned, ready and waiting for incoming ships that may be suspected of carrying an infectious disease.'

The plague hospitals also illustrate the way in which medical facilities in Venice intersected with those of piety and poor relief and provided a model for public health which was influential across Europe.

Tomic, Zlata Blazina, 2015. *Expelling the Plague: The Health Office and the Implementation of Quarantine in Dubrovnik, 1377–1533*. McGill-Queen's University Press
Stevens Crawshaw, Jane L., 2016. *Plague Hospitals Public Health for the City in Early Modern Venice*, London

The following two epidemics – dancing mania and The Great Sweat – are quite different from all the other diseases covered here; for a start the mad dancing mania is not an infectious diseases although it could be said to have an infectious quality in that some observers of the mass dances found themselves unable to resist the temptation to join in.

---

1. Byrne 208ff

Chapter 10

Dancing to death, 1374 (Aachen) and 1518 Strasbourg

'When one is in the hold of this ill-wished beast, one has a hundred different feelings at a time. One cries, dances, vomits, trembles, laughs, pales, cries, faints, and one will suffer great pain, and finally after a few days, if unaided, you die.'
— Francesco Girolamo Cancellieri (1817)

When Marvin Gaye, William 'Mickey' Stevenson and Ivy Jo Hunter wrote *Dancing in the Street* and Martha Reeves and the Vandellas recorded the hit version of the song in 1964; and when Mick Jagger and Davie Bowie gave the song to the world in their video version for Live Aid in 1985, it is unlikely that any of them knew that they were evoking and reviving the well established dance plague of the 14th and 17th centuries in Europe.

Likewise when Horace McCoy, a seasoned bouncer at dance marathons, wrote his 1935 novel *They Shoot Horses Don't They?* about a disparate group of individuals desperate to win a Depression-era dance marathon, and when Sydney Pollack directed the 1969 film based on the book, it seems unlikely that they too were aware of the backstory integral to prolonged bouts of random dancing. Nevertheless, medical history, of course, tells us that neither Marvin Gaye nor Horace McCoy got there first.

Dancing mania (also known as dancing plague, choreomania, St. John's Dance and St. Vitus's Dance) was a socio-medical phenomenon that occurred primarily in mainland Europe between the 14th and 17th centuries. It involved groups of people dancing in a state of abandon, sometimes thousands at a time, sometimes for weeks on end. The mania afflicted men, women and children who often danced until they dropped from exhaustion. One of the first major outbreaks was in Aachen in 1374 and it quickly spread throughout Europe; another particularly notable outbreak occurred in Strasbourg in 1518.

In terms of longevity and cases it competes with plague, smallpox and influenza. The dancing plague afflicted thousands of people over several centuries in many episodes. Not surprisingly, there was little clue regarding its aetiology so remedies, such as they were, were based on folk medicine, superstition, spirit possession and guesswork. Naturally, musicians would accompany the dancers in the expectation that musical acompaniment might cure the problem. It didn't, but what it did do, unhelpfully, was to encourage more people to join in. Today we are none the wiser about its cause.

Theories abounded: religious cults were the cause; or, people did it to relieve themselves of the stresses of 14th century medieval life, not least a recent outbreak of the plague, flooding and their own abject poverty – dancing after all was free. Others blamed a corrupt clergy. For some, tarantism was to blame caused by the bite of the wolf spider (*Lycosa tarantula*) or, more likely *Latrodectus tredecimguttatus* or Mediterranean black widow or steppe spider, although no link between such bites and tarantism has ever been proved. The tarantella dance apparently evolved from a therapy for tarantism. It was originally described in the 11th century and was common in southern Italy, especially around Taranto, during the 16th and 17th centuries. The thinking was that victims needed to engage in frenzied dancing to prevent death from tarantism: the only antidote known was to dance to particular music to separate the venom from the blood.

'The tarantulees, after having danced for a long time, meet together in the chapel of Saint Paul and communally attain the paroxysm of their trance, ... the general and desperate agitation was dominated by the stylised cry of the tarantulees, the 'crisis cry', an ahiii uttered with various modulations.' Some indulged in other activities, such as tying themselves up with vines and whipping each other (reminiscent of Roman Bacchanalia), staging mock sword fights, drinking copious amounts of wine and jumping into the sea. Some died if deprived of music to accompany their dancing. Sufferers typically had symptoms similar to dancing mania, such as headaches, trembling, twitching and visions.

For others St. John the Baptist or St. Vitus (patron saint of dancers) were implicated because the condition was considered a curse sent by them or other saints; it therefore became known as 'St. Vitus' Dance' or 'St. John's Dance' and victims of dancing mania often ended their performance at places dedicated to that saint who was prayed to in an effort to end the dancing; outbreaks often occurred around the time of the feast of St. Vitus. At the other end of the religious spectrum others claimed to be possessed by demons, or Satan, leading to exorcisms on dancers.

In the 17th century dancing mania was diagnosed as Sydenham chorea, a disease of the nervous system which shares symptoms resembling those of dancing mania: a disorder characterized by rapid, uncoordinated jerking movements primarily affecting the face, hands and feet which results from childhood infection with Group A beta-haemolytic Streptococcus and occurs in 20–30 per cent of people with acute rheumatic fever.

Others proposed that it was a mass psychogenic illness (also called mass psychogenic disorder, epidemic hysteria, or mass hysteria, mass madness) defined as 'the rapid spread of illness signs and symptoms affecting members of a cohesive group, originating from a nervous system disturbance involving excitation, loss, or alteration of function, whereby physical complaints that are exhibited unconsciously have no corresponding organic aetiology'. Dancers seemed to be in a state of unconsciousness and unable to control themselves. Contemporary sources record that participants often did not dance where they lived but would travel from place to place while others would join them along the way. Bartholomew (2001) records that they brought customs and behaviour that were strange to the local people and how dancers wore 'strange, colorful attire' and 'held wooden sticks'. It was not all just good clean fun either: Bartholomew

notes that some 'paraded around naked' and made 'obscene gestures'. Some even had sex, while others behaved like animals, jumping, hopping and leaping about. The Swiss physician Paracelsus (1493–1541), christened the condition choreomania and put it down to three possible causes: an abnormal mental state, an unexplained physical illness, or lust.

Many were tireless for long periods: the abbot of a monastery near Trier recalled 'an amazing epidemic' in which a collection of hallucinating dancers hopped and leapt for as long as six months, some of them dying after breaking 'ribs or loins'. Dancers screamed, laughed or cried and some sang. Observers of dancing mania were sometimes shown violence if they declined to join in. Participants had a bizarre aversion to the colour red; in *A History of Madness in Sixteenth-Century Germany*, Midelfort notes they 'could not perceive the color red at all', and Bartholomew reports 'it was said that dancers could not stand... the color red, often becoming violent on seeing [it]'. Some asserted they were drowning in 'a red sea of blood'.

Dancers also exhibited a strange antipathy towards pointed shoes, while they enjoyed having their feet hit. Unsurprisingly, dancing maniacs suffered from a variety of ailments, including chest pains, convulsions, hallucinations, hyperventilation, epileptic fits, and visions.

In the later 18th century Francesco Girolamo Cancellieri (1751–1826) writer, librarian and bibliophile was a key opinion leader on the condition: he tells us that 'the sovereign and the only remedy is Music'.[1] Peasants it seems were particularly susceptible, especially on hot summer days when they would be overcome by lethargy and lassitude; the only way back to vitality was dancing to the accompaniment of a guitar:

> '...and we found the poor peasant oppressed with difficult breathing, and we observed also that the face and hands had started to become black. And 'cause his illness was known to all, a guitar was brought, whose harmony, immediately that he was understood, began first moving the feet, legs shortly afterwards. He stood on his knees. Soon after an interval he arose swaying. Finally, in the space of a quarter of an hour he was leaping, nearly three palms from the ground. Sighed, but with such great impetus, that it terrorised bystanders, and before an hour, the black was gone from his hands and face, and he regained his native colour.'
>
> – Cancellieri, (1817), p.11

Outbreaks reach back to the 7th century; one of the earliest-known incidents of this compulsive obsessive dancing occurred in 1021 in Kölbigk (in Saxony-Anhalt), where 18 peasants began singing and dancing around a church, disrupting a Christmas Eve service. The revellers ignored requests to cease and joined hands and danced a 'ring dance of sin', clapping, leaping and chanting in unison. The angry priest, recorded a local chronicler, cursed them to dance for an entire year as a punishment for their outrageous behaviour. It worked. Not until the following Christmas did the dancers

---

1. *Lettera sopra il Tarantismo, l'aria di Roma, e della sua campagna* (1817) p.6.

regain control of their bodies. Exhausted and repentant, they fell into a deep sleep. Some of them never woke up again.

One episode in 1237 involved a large group of children who travelled from Erfurt to Arnstadt (about 12 miles), jumping and dancing all the way, not that dissimilar from the legend of the Pied Piper of Hamelin which originated at around the same time. Another incident, in 1278, involved about 200 people dancing on a bridge over the River Meuse near Maastricht causing it to collapse drowning them all.

On 24 June 1374, one of the biggest outbreaks began in Aachen spreading to other German, Dutch and Belgian cities, and to Luxembourg and Italy with recurrences in 1375 and 1376, and an outbreak in Augsburg in 1381. In another incident in 1428 in Schaffhausen (northern Switzerland), a monk danced himself to death and, in the same year, a group of women in Zurich were reportedly seen cavorting in a dancing frenzy.

In July 1518, in Strasbourg, Frau Trauffea stepped outside her home and began dancing in the street. It was not a happy dance, more of a manic frenzy (similar presumably to the 'idiot dancing' of the 1960s and 70s). Despite the pleas of her husband she continued until night fell, when she collapsed from exhaustion. To everyone apart from Frau Trauffea that was thought to be the end of it but the next day – and the day after that – Frau Trauffea resumed her performance, soon to be joined by 400 or so other people, despite the physical pain she was in. At the end of the third day, her body bathed in sweat and her feet soaked in blood, she was bundled into a wagon and taken away to a 'healing' religious shrine up in the nearby mountains. Some of the 400 died. According to Michigan State University medical historian John Waller writing in *The Lancet*, 'One chronicle states that [the dancing] claimed, for a brief period at least, about fifteen lives a day as men, women, and children danced in the punishing summer heat.'

As with the 1374 outbreak the Strasbourg dancing may have been triggered by what was going on at the time: acute distress and anxiety would have been prevalent as the inhabitants of the region tried to come to terms with a succession of failed harvests, the highest grain (and therefore bread) prices for over a generation, the introduction of syphilis into the population and the re-emergence of leprosy and the plague. These were not good times for the people of Alsace: manic dancing was one way out.

Further incidents occurred in 1536 in Basel, involving a group of children; and in 1551 in Saxony Anhalt, involving just one man. In the 17th century, incidents of recurrent dancing were recorded by professor of medicine Gregor Horst, who reported:

'Several women who annually visit the chapel of St. Vitus in Drefelhausen [near Ulm]... dance madly all day and all night until they collapse in ecstasy. In this way they come to themselves again and feel little or nothing until the next May, when they are again... forced around St. Vitus' Day to betake themselves to that place... [o]ne of these women is said to have danced every year for the past twenty years, another for a full thirty-two.'

Ecstasy apart, the dancing had the additional benefit of banishing the physical ills the dancers had and keeping them fit and well for the rest of the year, until next time...

Many of the dancers were probably psychologically disturbed; others took part out of fear, or the need to fit in. Dancing mania remains one of the earliest-recorded forms of mass hysteria and is described as a 'psychic epidemic'. Waller concludes:

> '...there is no question that the 1374 and 1518 epidemics occurred. Dozens of reliable chronicles from several towns and cities describe the events of 1374. And the course of the 1518 epidemic can be minutely detailed with the help of municipal orders, sermons, and vivid descriptions left behind by the brilliant Renaissance physician, Paracelsus. These outbreaks represent a real and fascinating enigma.'

Europe's dancing plagues ended suddenly in the mid-1600s.

Mass psychogenic illness (MPI) is posited as a possible explanation [https://www.neuroscientificallychallenged.com/blog/dancing-mania-mass-psychogenic-illness]. 'MPI involves the appearance of symptoms that spread throughout a population, but don't have a clear physical origin. In other words, in MPI the brain is causing the patient to think they are afflicted by some ailment—even though the brain itself is the creator and orchestrator of the illness. This doesn't mean that the symptoms aren't real; there can be legitimate physical manifestations of MPI. But there's no evidence the symptoms are produced by something (like a poison or a germ) other than the nervous system.'

Bartholomew, Robert E., 2001. *Little green men, meowing nuns, and head-hunting panics.* McFarland. Jefferson NC.

Waller, J., 2009. 'A forgotten plague: making sense of dancing mania'. *Lancet.* 373 (9664): 624–5.

Waller, J., 2008. *A Time to Dance. A Time to Die: The Extraordinary Story of the Dancing Plague of 1518.* Cambridge.

Strasbourg 1518, BBC 2, 20 July 2020. Artangel project directed by Jonathan Glazer films lone performers around the world dancing till they drop.

Chapter 11

Sweating sickness 1485–1551

'Safer on the battlefield than in the city.'
– Thomas More reflecting on the dangers posed by 'the sweats' in a
letter to Erasmus 19 August 1517

*'There raged at that time, in London and other parts of the kingdom, a species of malady
unknown to any other age or nation, the 'sweating sickness', which occasioned the sudden
death of great multitudes though it seemed to be not propagated by any contagious
infection, but arose from the general disposition of the air and of the human body.
In less than twenty-four hours the patient commonly died, or recovered.'*
– Hume's History of England Vol II, page 384

Sweating sickness goes by many names including the Sweat, Sweats, English sweating sickness, English sweat, *sudor anglicus*, the Swat, hote iylls, hote sicknes, Stup-Gallant, Stoupe Knave and Know thy Master, Posting Sweat, and the New Acquainance. It was a terrifying contagious disease which is still very much shrouded in mystery; it afflicted England and later continental Europe in a series of epidemics beginning in 1485. The last outbreak occurred in 1551, after which the disease seems to have vanished. In between there were outbreaks in 1506, 1517 and in 1528. The 1551 outbreak struck on 7 July and lasted for twenty-three days in which time it killed nearly 1,000 people. The onset of symptoms was sudden, with death often occurring within hours. Its cause remains unknown, although there is speculation that an unknown species of hantavirus was responsible. Ague, rheumatic fever and influenza have also been proposed over the years. Ague is fever (such as from malaria) indicated by paroxysms of chills, fever and sweating recurring at regular intervals.

In 1517 London was thronged with foreign artisans while in 1528 Europe was preoccupied with the military operations of Francis I in Italy – both events obvious facilitators of disease transmission. Whatever the precise nature of the disease it would be contending with numerous other immune depressing contagions amongst the population of England: spotted fever, brain fever, epidemic flux, scurvy, diphtheria, smallpox, measles, scarlet fever, erysipelas to name but a few. In 1886 the journal *Science* concluded 'That England was not blotted out of existence by pestilential disease during this epoch is a marvel.'[1]

---

1. *Science* Vol. 8, No.186 (Aug. 27, 1886), p.190.

The disease broke in London on 19 September 1485 causing the postponement of the coronation of Henry VII until 30 October. One of the most alarming features of the disease was the speed with which it could claim its victims. There were numerous reports of people suddenly dropping dead in the street. Thomas Forrestier (or Le Forestier), a French physician living in London at the time, wrote of the disease:

'We saw two prestys standing togeder and speaking togeder, and we saw both of them dye sodenly. Also in die—proximi we se the wyf of a taylour taken and sodenly dyed. Another yonge man walking by the street fell down sodenly.'

Forrestier is our earliest source, writing in 1490; he notes the high mortality at 15,000 lives in London and more in Oxford, and the acute onset of:

'...sudden grete swetyng and stynkyng, with rednesse of the face and of all the body, and a contynual thurst, with a grete hete and hedache because of the fumes and venom...'

He added that some patients presented with black spots. It seems that the most dangerous stage of the disease was the first few hours; those who survived the first twenty-four hours would go on to make a full recovery.

Both Forrestier and Richard Grafton (in 1569) describe the plague as something 'new'; so it was probably not a recurrence of a previous epidemic. John Caius (or Keys) adds to the symptomatology. Caius, born in 1510, was physician to Edward VI, Mary I and Elizabeth I. He was a practising physician in Shrewsbury in 1551 when an outbreak occurred, and he described the symptoms and signs of the disease in *A Boke or Counseill Against the Disease Commonly Called the Sweate, or Sweatyng Sicknesse* (1552), which is still our main source of knowledge of the disease.

He opens his description with a sonorous 'this disease is not a sweat onely...but a feuer'. The disease had a sudden onset inducing anxiety, followed by cold shivers which sometimes were very violent, dizziness, headache 'and madness of the same', and severe pains in the back, shoulders and extremities accompanied by exhaustion, 'grief in the liver and nigh stomacke'. The cold stage might last from between half an hour to three hours, after which a feeling of hotness and sweating took over. The characteristic sweat broke out suddenly without any obvious cause. A sense of heat, headache, delirium, rapid pulse and intense thirst accompanied the sweat, palpitations and chest pain were frequent symptoms as well. No skin eruptions were noted by observers, including Caius. In the final stages, there was either general exhaustion ('marueilous heauinesse') and collapse, or an irresistible urge to sleep, which Caius thought was fatal if the patient submitted. Fluid and electrolyte imbalance may have been the actual cause of death.

One attack did not produce the consolation of immunity, and some people suffered several episodes before dying. The disease usually occured in summer and early autumn. The relatively affluent male adult population was most seriously afflicted, particularly the clergy. Unlike many other medieval diseases, it seemed to spare the very young and the very old. It was most prevalent in rural areas but also severely affected the nobility living in London and the student populations of Oxford and Cambridge. Caius, however, noted that the patients most at risk of the disease were 'either men of wealth, ease or welfare, or, not one to forego a stereotype – of the poorer sort, such as were idle persons, good ale drinkers and tavern haunters.'

In later outbreaks, Cardinal Wolsey would contract the disease twice, in 1517 and in 1528, and recover on both occasions although it claimed the lives of many of his household. The sweat may have been what afflicted Arthur, Prince of Wales (the elder brother of Henry VIII) and his wife Catherine of Aragon in March 1502; their illness was described as 'a malign vapour which proceeded from the air': other theories contend that it was tuberculosis, the Black Death and influenza. Catherine recovered, but Arthur died on 2 April 1502 at Ludlow Castle, age 15. Anne Boleyn contracted the disease but she too survived. Anne's brother-in-law William Carey did not. The disease's predilection for the young and wealthy led to it being dubbed the 'Stop Gallant' by the poorer classes because they observed how the posh boys of the day were disproportionately affected. Indeed, it resembled the 1918 Spanish flu pandemic in its choice of victim: healthy, fit, 25–35 year olds, men rather than women. We do, though, need to exercise caution regarding this demographic as such people would, by their nature, enjoy a high profile in society and were, therefore, more 'memorable' than victims of the lower classes.

The economic effects of the Sweat even invaded Tudor culture when in 1604 Shakespeare put the sweating sickness up there with the three great population shrinkers: war, executions and poverty in *Measure for Measure* (Act 1 Scene 2) when Mistress Overdone bemoans the loss of her trade:

> 'Thus, what with the war, what with the sweat, what with the gallows and what with poverty, I am custom-shrunk.'

A second outbreak occurred in 1507, followed by a third and much more severe epidemic later that year, which also spread to Calais where it remained mostly confined to the English ex-pat population.

This outbreak was frequently fatal; half the population died in some areas when it reached epidemic proportions in 1528 during its fourth outbreak. It erupted in London at the end of May causing panic and death and quickly spread over most of England, and although it did not infect Scotland, it did reach Ireland where Lord Chancellor Hugh Inge was the most prominent victim. It became known as 'The *English* Sweate' because it did not spread to Scotland and Wales. It also seemed to affect foreigners living in England less severely. In 1881 Arthur Bordier delivered a paper to the Anthropology Society of Paris entitled 'On the special susceptibility of the fair-haired races of Europe for contracting sweating Sickness'. In the paper, he presented an interesting, but unproven theory that Sweating Sickness did not solely affect Englishmen but instead had a tendency to infect those descended from the Anglo-Saxon and spared those descended from the Celts.

The disease would also affect the court of Henry VIII and, as noted, Anne Boleyn is said to have contracted it and survived. Chronicler Edward Hall commented on how it affected the king's court and nobility in London:

'Suddenly there came a plague of sickness called the sweating sickness that turned all his [the King's] purpose. This malody was so cruel that it killed some within two houres, some merry at dinner and dedde at supper. Many died in the Kinges courte. The Lorde Clinton, the Lorde Gray of Wilton, and many knightes, gentleman and officiers.'

A good number of Englishmen unsuccessfully tried to escape the disease by fleeing to Ireland, Scotland and France only to die there. John Caius wrote that 'It followed Englishmen like a shadow.' Because the mortality rate was so high in London Henry VIII suspended the court and left London, frequently changing his residence. In 1529 Thomas Cromwell, as mentioned above, lost his wife and two daughters to the disease.

The disease suddenly broke out in Hamburg, spreading so rapidly that more than a thousand people died in a few weeks. It swept through eastern Europe, arrived in Switzerland in December, then headed north to Scandinavia and east to Lithuania, Poland and Russia. There were no cases of the disease in Italy or France, except in the Pale of Calais which was controlled by England at the time following the Battle of Crécy in 1346. It also manifested in Flanders and the Netherlands, simultaneously in Antwerp and Amsterdam on the morning of 27 September. In each place, it prevailed for a short time, generally not more than two weeks. By the end of the year, it had entirely disappeared except in eastern Switzerland, where it lingered into the next year. After this, the disease did not recur on mainland Europe.

The last major outbreak of the disease occurred in England in 1551. John Caius wrote his 'eyewitness account' referred to above. Henry Machyn made this diary entry:

'...the vii day of July begane a nuw swet in London...the x day of July [1551] the Kynges grace removyd from Westmynster unto Hamtun courte, for ther [died] serten besyd the court, and caused the Kynges grase to be gone so sune, for ther ded in London mony marchants and grett ryche men and women, and yonge men and old, of the new swett...the xvi day of July ded of the swet the ii yonge dukes of Suffoke of the swet, both in one bed in Chambrydge-shyre...and ther ded from the vii day of July unto the xix ded of the swett in London of all dyssesus... [872] and no more in alle.'

–The Diary of Henry Machyn 1550–1563

There is a reference in the *Annals* of Halifax parish in 1551 to an outbreak there, resulting in 44 deaths while an outbreak of 'sweating sickness' occurred in Tiverton, Devon in 1644, recorded in Martin Dunsford's *Historical memoirs of the town and parish of Tiverton*, burying 443 people, 105 of them in the month of October.

Something similar kept breaking out in France between 1718 and finally in 1918 when a soldier presented in Picardy (one of two cases that year); it became known as the equally mysterious Picardy Sweat or *suette miliare* (miliary fever) with its 196 local epidemics. The poet John Churchill was a victim in 1764 at Boulogne and the outbreaks in 1840 and 1880 were particularly destructive.

Writing in the *British Medical Journal* Llywelyn Roberts noted 'a great similarity between the two diseases' although it was accompanied by a rash, which was not described as a feature of the English disease. However, Henry Tidy explains that away because John Caius' report applies to fulminant cases fatal within a few hours, in which no eruption may have developed. A 1906 outbreak of Picardy sweat struck 6,000 people around Charentes wiping out whole families in a few days; bacteriologist André Chantemesse led a commission which studied it, attributing the infection to the fleas of field mice. Henry Tidy found 'no substantial reason to doubt the identity of sudor anglicus and Picardy sweat'. Tidy describes the epidemics as 'explosive', noting that the attacks were short-lived, abating after two to three weeks, some patients had mild symptoms but in others mortality was between 30 and 40 per cent.

As for the rash, Tidy notes how it appears around day three or four with two characteristics: an erythema and 'glistening white miliaria', hence the name. The miliaria coalesce and form vesicles which spread across the whole of the body, but for one curious exception: the rash stops abruptly at the wrists and forms 'the miliary bracelet which persists after the eruptions have subsided elsewhere', as in the two 1918 cases. Tidy concludes by reminding us of Michael Foster's warning 'We should be unwise to regard it as necessarily a disease nearing extinction...(1919) 'Sweating Sickness in Modern Times').

What caused the Sweat? The aetiologic agent is still unknown but the most likely guilty suspect is sewage, poor sanitation and contaminated water supplies of the time providing reservoirs for the source of infection. The first confirmed outbreak was in August 1485 as the Wars of the Roses drew to a close; this has prompted the very English speculation that it may have been brought over from France by the French mercenaries whom Henry Tudor enlisted; there are no reports of it affecting the Tudor army. However, an earlier outbreak may have afflicted York in June 1485, before Henry and his army of mercenaries, disaffected Edwardian Yorkists and staunch Lancastrians, landed at Milford Haven on 7 August 1485. It is more likely that it entered England somewhere on the Yorkshire-Lincolnshire coast in cargoes or crews trading from Russia and Scandinavia.

The *Croyland Chronicle* reveals that Thomas Stanley, 1st Earl of Derby and a key ally of Richard III who contributed 30 per cent of the king's army, gave the sweating sickness as an excuse not to join with Richard III and travel from his home in Lancashire to Nottingham, after news of Henry Tudor's landing had broken and before Tudor's victory over Richard at the Battle of Bosworth.

Social and environmental issues may have been a factor. Erasmus, another lucky survivor who contracted the disease whilst in London in the summer of 1511, in a letter to Francis, physician to the Archbishop of York, explained how English houses were not built to make a through-draft possible and that their rush-strewn floors were totally unhygienic because sometimes they were not renewed for around twenty years and so they allowed 'spittle, vomit, dog's urine and men's too, dregs of beer and cast-off bits of fish, and other unspeakable kinds of filth' to fester. The streets were no better with all manner of refuse casually ejected from windows. Erasmus himself claims that 'if, even twenty years ago, I had entered into a chamber which had been uninhabited for some months, I was immediately seized with a fever'. Others blamed the damp, foggy English climate.

Relapsing Fever may have been the cause. This disease is spread by ticks and lice, and it occurs most often during the summer months, as did the original sweating sickness. Symptoms may include a sudden fever, chills, headaches, muscle or joint aches and nausea. A rash may also occur. These symptoms usually continue for two to nine days, then disappear. However, Relapsing Fever is marked by a prominent black scab at the site of the tick bite and a subsequent skin rash.

One of the most compelling arguments posited so far is shown by several researchers who have noticed that symptoms coincide with hantavirus pulmonary syndrome and have proposed an unknown hantavirus as the cause. Hantaviruses are spread by inhalation of rodent droppings and cause similar symptoms to sweating sickness before killing with bleeding and complications to the heart and lungs. In 1993, an outbreak of this disease struck the Navajo people in New Mexico. This outbreak, known as the Four Corners Outbreak after the region in which it was located, bore many resemblances to the Sweating Sickness, prompting investigators to suggest it as a potential cause.

Like Sweating Sickness, hantavirus is characterised by a sudden onset of a fever, joint pains, headache. This is followed by shortness of breath and rapidly evolving pulmonary oedema that usually requires mechanical ventilation and has a mortality rate of 35–40 per cent despite modern medical intervention. However, sweating sickness was transmitted from human to human, whereas hantavirus is usually not, although there is a report from 1997 that infection through human contact may have taken place in hantavirus outbreaks in Argentina.

In an article in *New Scientist* in 2004, microbiologist Edward McSweegan proposed that the disease may have been an outbreak of anthrax poisoning and that the victims could have been infected with anthrax spores present in raw wool or infected animal carcasses.

Evans, E., 1886, The Sweating Sickness. *Science*, 8 (186), 190.
Heyman, Paul, 2018. 'The English Sweating Sickness: Out of Sight, Out of Mind?' *Acta Medica Academica*. 47 (1): 102–11
Roberts, L., 1945. 'Sweating Sickness and Picardy Sweat'. *British Medical Journal*. 2 (4414): 196.
Thwaites, Guy, 1997. 'The English Sweating Sickness, 1485 to 1551'. *New England Journal of Medicine*. 336 (8): 580–2.

Chapter 12

The 1489 typhus epidemic, Granada, Spain

*'God punished the Egyptian with little things: with hailstones, and frogs, and grasshoppers;
and Pharaoh's conjurers, that counterfeited all Moses' greater works, failed in the least,
in the making of lice.'*

– John Donne (1572–1631), *Sermons*

Whenever and wherever large numbers of people are crowded together under less than sanitary conditions, then there is a potential for typhus to rear its head. It is inextricably associated with the social and health related upheavals caused by war, imprisonment and famine.

In 1489, when Spanish soldiers who fought the Turks in Cyprus came home to Spain they unwittingly brought typhus with them. During the Spanish siege of Baza against the Moors during the War of Granada (1482–92), 17,000 Spanish troops perished with typhus, more than five times the number killed by the Moors. Accounts mention fever, red spots over arms, back, and chest, attention deficit progressing to delirium and gangrenous sores and the associated stench of rotting flesh.

From Spain it spread to Italy, France and then northwards where it continued in a series of small outbreaks. The disease was described by several physicians such as Girolamo Fracastorius in 1546 in *De Contagione et Contagiosis Morbis*, referring to the Italian epidemics of 1505 and 1528 and distinguishing it from plague; Girolamo Cardano in his book *De Malo recentiorum medicorum Ursu Libellus* in 1536, and by Von Zavorziz in 1676 in *The Infection of Military Camps*.

Some contend that typhus was exported from Spain to the New World during the first half of the sixteenth century, but we now know that typhus fever existed among South American natives in pre-Columbian days and recognizable epidemics occurred in Mexico before the arrival of Cortez at Vera Cruz in 1519. At the end of the sixteenth century, typhus killed more than two million native Indians in the Mexico highlands.

The global roll call of typhus related deaths is truly staggering, with typhus a frequent bedfellow of large scale conflict:

1528	Naples, Italy: 21,000 French soldiers
1542	Hungary: 30,000 German and Italian soldiers
1552	Metz, France: 10,000 soldiers
1557–9:	10 per cent of the English population
1618–49	The Thirty Years War, France (1628). Half of the total population of Germany; 60,000 deaths in Lyon and 25,000 in Limoges

1756–63:   The Seven Years War: ? thousands
1812   Napoleon's invasion of Russia: 550,000 French; 61,964 Russian soldiers
1813–4:   Europe: 2 million people throughout Europe; 250,000 people in Germany
1816–19:   Ireland: 700,000 people
1847   Canada: 20,000 Irish immigrants
1854–56:   Crimean War: 134,000 soldiers
1914:   Austrian invasion of Serbia: 150,000 Serbs and 30,000–60,000 Austrian prisoners
1917–25:   First World War and Russian Revolution: 3 million Russians (from 30 million cases)

The disease has influenced the outcomes of wars and has led to epidemics in prison populations and in those who have survived natural disasters. Typhus fever tends to have a higher prevalence in colder months in those without adequate shelter or heating and who are crowding together for warmth.

The Irish epidemic was triggered during the famine caused by a worldwide reduction in temperature known as the Year Without a Summer. An estimated 70,000 people died. Typhus appeared again in the late 1830s, and yet another major typhus epidemic emerged during the Great Irish Famine of 1846 to 1849. The virulent Irish typhus spread to England, where it was called 'Irish fever'. It killed people of all social classes, as lice were ubiquitous and unconcerned with class, but as usual it hit the lower and vulnerable hardest.

A typhus epidemic erupted in Philadelphia in 1837 and killed the son of Franklin Pierce, 14th President of the United States, in 1843. Other epidemics occurred in Baltimore, Memphis and Washington DC, between 1865 and 1873. Typhus was also a significant killer during the US Civil War, although typhoid fever was the more prevalent cause of US Civil War 'camp fever'.

In Canada the typhus epidemic of 1847 killed more than 20,000 people from 1847 to 1848, mainly Irish immigrants cooped up in fever sheds and other forms of inhumane quarantine; they had contracted the disease aboard the crowded coffin ships in fleeing the Great Irish Famine. Public Health officials at the time obviously neither knew how to provide adequate sanitation nor understood how the disease spread.

The clipper *Ticonderoga* was infamous for her 'fever ship' voyage from Liverpool to Port Phillip in Victoria, Australia carrying 795 passengers in 1852. The overcrowded ship was insanitary and the ship's doctors were soon overwhelmed. During the voyage, 100 passengers died of typhus.

In 1922, the typhus epidemic reached its peak in Soviet territory, with some 25 to 30 million cases in Russia. Poland had been ravaged with some 4 million cases reported but by 1921 thanks largely to public health pioneers such as Hélène Sparrow (1891–1970) and Rudolf Weigl (1883–1957) things were getting under control. During the Russian civil war between the White and Red Armies (1917–1922), typhus killed 3 million people, mainly civilians. In 1937 and 1938 there was a typhus epidemic in Chile.

During the Second World War, many German PoWs after their massive defeat at Stalingrad died of typhus. Typhus epidemics killed those confined to PoW camps, ghettos and Nazi concentration camps who were held in ineffably disgusting conditions. Pictures of mass graves, including people who died from typhus, can be seen in footage shot at Bergen-Belsen concentration camp. Among the thousands of prisoners in concentration camps like Theresienstadt and Bergen-Belsen who died of typhus were Anne Frank, age 15, and her sister Margot, age 19.

Major epidemics in the post-war chaos were averted only by widespread use of the newly discovered DDT to kill the lice on millions of refugees and displaced persons. In 2018 a typhus outbreak spread through Los Angeles County mainly affecting homeless people. In 2019, city attorney Elizabeth Greenwood revealed that she, too, was infected with typhus as a result of a flea bite at her office in Los Angeles City Hall. As with many other diseases, typhus has not gone away.

A hundred years after the Thirty Years' War (1618–48), when epidemic typhus spread into Europe, Germany lost half to three quarters of her total population; Huxham, in 1739, made the first distinctions between typhus and typhoid; Boissier de Sauvages confirmed this in 18th century France and called it exantematic typhus.

Typhus is a group of infectious diseases that include epidemic typhus, also known as typhus fever, red louse fever, jail fever, sylvatic typhus, scrub typhus and murine (endemic) typhus. The diseases are caused by specific types of bacterial infection: epidemic typhus is due to *Rickettsia prowazekii* – as with other *Rickettsia spp.*, it is passed to humans from arthropod ectoparasites; the primary vector in the case of epidemic typhus is the human body louse (*Pediculus humanus corporis*). You might be forgiven for expecting the disease to be spread by the bite of an infected louse. Not so: the louse defecates shortly after taking your blood; you, the human host, naturally scratch the site because of a local inflammatory reaction from the bite, and in so doing auto-inoculate yourself with the organism from the faecal matter.

Incidents of transmission have been reported when aerosols of louse faecal dust are inhaled by physicians and laboratory personnel. *R. prowazekii* has been found to remain infective in louse faecal matter for over 100 days. The inhalational transmission capability in conjunction with the prolonged active phase makes it viable as an agent of bioterrorism.

Scrub typhus is due to *Orientia tsutsugamushi* spread by chiggers (a genus of harvest mites) on humans or rodents; murine typhus is due to *Rickettsia typhi* spread by fleas on animals such as cats and rats, most notably from the Norway rat, and is the least virulent.

In 1759 it was estimated that about 25 per cent of English prisoners died of the disease, thus earning the name 'jail' or 'gaol' fever. A year later it was being called typhus, a word deriving from the ancient Greek tûphos (τύφος) meaning 'smoky' or 'hazy', evoking the delirium, brain fog, sometimes developed in the infected. It was originally applied by Hippocrates to the confused states of mind frequently associated with high fevers.

Typhus often took hold when prisoners were crowded together into dark, dank, filthy, fetid cells in which lice could spread easily. Thus, 'imprisonment until the next term of court' was often tantamount to a death sentence. Prisoners brought before the courts sometimes infected members of the court. Following the assizes held at Oxford in 1577, later called the Black Assize, over 300 died from gaol fever. The Black Assize of Exeter in 1586 hosted another notable outbreak. During the Lent assizes court at Taunton in 1730, gaol fever led to the death of the Lord Chief Baron, as well as the High Sheriff, the sergeant and hundreds of others. Indeed, at this time more prisoners were dying from 'gaol fever' than were put to death by all the public executioners in Britain. In London, gaol fever often broke out among the prisoners of Newgate Prison and then migrated into the general population. In May 1750, the Lord Mayor of London, Sir Samuel Pennant, and many court officials were fatally infected in the courtroom of the Old Bailey which adjoined Newgate Prison.

There is an approximately 10–14 day incubation period before overt symptoms develop; earliest symptoms typically are severe headache and fever. The classic maculopapular, blanching rash that originates around the axilla and trunk within the first week of symptoms is actually present in between 25 and 80 per cent of cases depending on the population. This classical rash tends to spread to the entire body, with the exception of the face, palms and soles of the feet. A mild conjunctivitis and a brown furry tongue have also been seen. In severe cases, vasculitis may lead to vascular collapse and multi-organ damage such as cerebral ischemia or necrosis of the digits.

Most often the desperate search for therapies to combat pandemics is long, arduous and frequently elusive. Occasionally, though, the solution is disarmingly simple. In the early 20th century, French bacteriologist and Nobel Prize winner Charles Nicolle noticed that after receiving a hot bath and clean clothes a cohort of typhus patients was no longer infectious. By 1909 he correctly hypothesized the louse to be the vector for inter-human transmission of the disease. His discovery helped greatly on the Western Front saving countless lives during the First World War, when delousing stations were established. Unfortunately the Eastern Front had no such thing, leading to the death of 10 to 40 per cent of those infected. Nurses who treated the sick experienced an exceptionally high death rate. By the end of the war epidemic typhus had peaked with more than 3 million people, mostly civilians, dying in Russia alone. Countries such as Poland and Romania lost several million citizens as well. With no vaccine available, typhus was one of the most deadly aspects of the war along with combat mortality and injury and its atrocious sequel, the flu pandemic of 1918. When Germany invaded Poland and the Soviet Union in the Second World War, Nazi generals were not just preoccupied with strategy and the Red Army. As the war raged, typhus re-emerged in war-torn areas and in ghettos where crowded and insanitary conditions provided a perfect breeding ground for lice.

Rudolf Stefan Jan Weigl (1883–1957) was a Polish biologist and inventor of the first effective vaccine against epidemic typhus. In the First World War Weigl was drafted into the medical service of the Austro-Hungarian army and began research on typhus and its causes. He founded the Weigl Institute in Lwów (now Lviv), where he conducted vaccine research. Weigl came to the attention of the Nazi occupiers.

The Nazis ordered Dr. Weigl to produce a typhus vaccine. He created a technique that involved raising millions of infected lice in a laboratory and harvesting their guts to get the materials for a vaccine. Lice that had been infected with typhus bacteria would be encouraged to feed on human volunteers and then, after about five days, the lice would be dissected one by one. Scientists would pull out the 'louse gut', where the typhus bacteria grow and multiply, put it in a pot and simply mash it up with a chemical solution to make the vaccine.

Weigl's lab in Lviv sheltered Polish intellectuals, Jews and resistance fighters by employing them as lice feeders – they allowed thousands of lice – some infected with typhus, some not – to suck their blood. All intellectual life migrated to Weigl's laboratory. The lice were put in tiny cages that were attached to people's legs. To avoid catching the illness themselves, these volunteers had to be clean, have healthy skin and be able to resist scratching. His vaccines were smuggled into ghettos in Lviv and Warsaw, saving countless lives, until the Institute was shut down by the Soviet Union following their 1944 anti-German offensive. At the same time Weigl was sending weakened vaccines to the German army.

We return to the Spanish epidemic to outline the political situation which typhus did so much to influence when it ravaged the army of Ferdinand and Isabella in their failed attempt to eject the Moors from Spain. In 1489, a Spanish army of 25,000 had finally managed to blockade the Moors inside Granada and laid siege to the city, hoping that a successful campaign would finally end Moslem influence on the European continent. After louse-borne typhus struck the remnants of the Spanish army the survivors fled, and in so doing, introduced typhus to many other parts of Europe. In the event Granada held and it took a further 100 years of conflict before the Moors were expelled from Spain.

Allen, Arthur, 2015, *The Fantastic Laboratory of Dr. Weigl: How Two Brave Scientists Battled Typhus and Sabotaged the Nazis*, London

Baumslag, Naomi, 2005, *Murderous Medicine: Nazi Doctors, Human Experimentation, and Typhus*, Oxford

Olson, J.G., 1999, *Epidemic Typhus: A Forgotten but Lingering Threat in Emerging Infections*, Washington DC

Szybalski, Waclaw, 'The genius of Rudolf Stefan Weigl (1883–1957), a Lvovian microbe hunter and breeder'. In memoriam. McArdle Laboratory for Cancer Research, University of Wisconsin, Madison WI

Tansey, T., 2014, Typhus and Tyranny, *Nature* 511(7509), 291.

Vázquez-Espinosa, 2020. John Donne, Spanish Doctors and the epidemic typhus: fleas or lice? *Revista espanola de quimioterapia* 33, 87–93.

THE 16th – 19th CENTURIES

Chapter 13

The influenza pandemic: Asia, North Africa, Europe 1510

'Influenza has a long and sordid record of menacing humans.'
    – Amanda Yasgar, *Clinical Microbiology*, 3 January 2018

'On this day [July 13, 1510]…in Modena there appeared an illness that lasts three days with a great fever, and headache and then they rise…but there remains a terrible cough that lasts maybe eight days, and then little by little they recover and do not perish.'

We cannot help feeling anxious as we read these coldly clinical and disturbing early published description of what we now know as influenza. Its brevity and the description of its relative mildness are troubling because we know all about the carnage that was to ensue over the next 500 years. The account is by Tommasino De' Bianchi and describes the first recognised pandemic of influenza in 1510. He, along with a number of other observers, fascinatingly adumbrates what the western world knew about flu in the early 16th century; De' Bianchi (and the others) methodically describe what he believed the disease to be, its origin, the populations prone to it, complications, its morbidity and mortality and how it might be treated. What, of course, De' Bianchi and others could not know anything about were the bleak developments lurking round the corner.

De' Bianchi and his contemporaries knew something about contagion in the community but little or nothing about infection. The medical world still clung on to classical theories of humorism – a belief that too much or too little of any of four distinct body fluids in a person directly influenced their temperament and health. So doctors devoted much time and energy to eradicating the 'ill humors' which were believed to causing the disease they were treating. In order to do this various treatments were on hand, for example inducing diarrhoea or vomiting, or perspiration, or blistering, or, most dangerously, blood-letting. Paré claimed that 'neither bleeding nor purgation was otherwise of assistance in the rheumatism, but that all who adopted such agents for use were placed in mortal danger.'

As if to illustrate the uncertainty prevalent in the diagnosis of the respiratory diseases which confronted doctors and patients, various European languages adopted a whole range of names for it, whatever 'it' was; they include *cephalie catarrhale* (catarrhal headache), *coquelicot* (poppy because opiates were used to treat it), *tussis quinta* (fifth cough), and a lexicon of words describing 'hoods', such as *capuchon, cocoluccio, coqueluche, cuculionibus*, or *cucullo*, since those infected wore coverings over their heads. Coqueluche still survives in French today, but as pertussis (whooping cough), not influenza.

The year 1510 was a big one for the world: 1510 was the endpoint for a 20-year period of massive change on all sorts of fronts. Not least Columbus had discovered the New World in 1492 and in doing so had increased the size of and was mapping the new known world in a way thought unimaginable at the time. This New World was soon enduring wave after wave of European conquistadores intent on finding and exploiting El Dorado to the disadvantage of exotic native peoples; the Europeans settled and developed these lands, importing African slaves to do all the hard work, often dying in the act, to enable the invaders to establish lucrative new businesses. They took back to Europe not only fantastic descriptions of New World societies but also equally exotic emerging diseases such as syphilis.

It was a year of 'firsts' – the earliest description of a Christmas tree, the first successful slave revolt (on Hispaniola) and the advent of pocket watches. Florentine painter Allessandro Botticelli died that year, but Renaissance art flourished under da Vinci (1452–1519), Dürer (1471–1528), Michelangelo (1475–1564) and others. In 1510 medical literature and published medical research had not been discovered, but the printing press and moveable type were to change that: 'the most transformative technological product in centuries' in the words of David Morens and Anthony Fauci in their *Pandemic Influenza's 500th Anniversary* (2010). In 1510 flu struck.

Europe in 1510 was still trying to cope with the huge depopulation caused by the Black Death in the 1340s and was having to deal with the ravages of syphilis as well as pandemic or local epidemics of respiratory disease with fever, coughing and pneumonia. Worrying British and European epidemics of English sweating sickness had been recurring for 25 years, but influenza pandemics had never been seen before.

Tommasino de' Bianchi [de' Lancillotti] (1503–54) was an Italian chronicler who authored *Cronaca modenense* in the early 16th century, published in book form in 1862–64. He put the spread of flu in Modena down to the fact that '[i]t was so hot in August 1510 that the Christians [did] not live indoors but live[d] among the gardens and plants'. Turin professor Francisco Vallerioli (Valleriola) writes that the 1510 flu featured:

> '...constriction of breathing, and beginning with a hoarseness of the voice...[and] shivering. Valleriola added that 'not long after that there being a cooked humor which fills the lungs', followed by 'a great deal of clearing of the throat that is viscous, slow, not a little thin, and quite foamy. Following that there being sputum, coughing, and difficulty in breathing may return for several [days]...weakness of the body... and aversion to food...restlessness, weakness, wakefulness caused by a strong cough all press them...[and] from others a great deal of sweat flows.'

François Valleriola [né Variola] (1504–80) was a Montpellier physician, proto-epidemiologist, and contagion theorist who wrote *Loci medicinae communes, tribus libris digesti* (1562). Valleriola described flu as being more fatal to children and to those who had been extensively bled.

Polymath Jean Fernel (1497–1558) was physician to French King Henri III, physiologist, mathematician and astronomer who described the spinal canal and lunar craters. He wrote *De abditis rerum causis libri duo ad Henricum Granciae regem Christianissimum* (1548). Fernel rejected the orthodox and popular belief that it was a reflection of God's wrath; he claimed that the 'respiratory catarrh...with cardiac and pulmonary constriction, and coughing' was of unknown cause, and focused on describing what is now called its clinical and epidemiological characteristics.

Francesco Muralto, Italian lawyer and politician whose *Annalia Francisi Muralti* was written between 1492 and 1519 and published in 1861 described it as a 'precipitous illness...with coughing and a high fever', and noted that 'the disease killed ten people out of a thousand in one day', supporting a mortality rate of around 1 per cent.

The celebrated surgeon Ambroise Paré called it a 'rheumatic affliction of the head with...constriction of the heart and lungs'. Ambroise Paré (1510–90), anatomist and surgeon to French Kings Henri II, Francis II, Charles IX and Henri III invented surgical instruments and prostheses. The German edition of his collected works, *Wund Arztney, oder, Artzney Spiegell,* published posthumously in 1635, includes a full description of the pandemic.

Historian Jean Bouchet, (1476–1557) French barrister, poet and historian who wrote *Les annales Daquitaine* (1535) reported anorexia leading to 'extreme distaste for bread and wine', and Jacques Houllier [Hollerio] (1498–1562) French physician and surgeon who published *Magni Hippocratis Coaca Præsagia, Opus Plane Divinum, Et Veræ Medicinæ Tanquam Thesaurus, Cum interpretatione & commentariis* (1576) documented associated 'confusion and dizziness'.

So much for these informative first hand accounts; more detail comes from scholars born after 1510 who must have had access to primary sources. In the 17th century, Johannes Schenck von Grafenberg focused in his *De cephalgia seu catarrho epidemico* (1665) on 'respiratory constriction and hoarseness of voice, then soon shaking chills, fever, and robust coughing', while François-Eudes de Mézeray in his *Histoire de France, depuis Faramond jusqu'au règne de Louis le Juste* of 1685 described 'violent aching of the limbs...[with] delirium.' Taking a meteorological approach in *A General Chronological History of the Air, Weather, Seasons, Meteors, &c* of 1749, the physician Thomas Short described 'loss of strength...a terrible taring Cough... [and] Shortness of breath'. When Valleriola wrote that 'where it settled on the lungs...they were not able to expectorate it', von Grafenberg added that 'this might lead to suffocation', both apparently describing pneumonia.

There was disagreement about the extent of, and causes of, mortality. Houllier claimed high mortality, whereas Valleriola stated that the only victims were children although De' Bianchi had it that most people 'recover...and do not perish'. Jean Coytard de Thairé, writing in 1578, was sceptical, cautioning that '[i]t is now perilous or difficult to determine an estimate of the number that died...but of those who were seen with serious symptoms a sufficient number departed'. Both Schenck von Grafenberg and de Mézeray later rubbished such caution, concluding that there had been significant mortality. It is quite remarkable how the 16th-century chroniclers of this disease recorded how it caused moderate mortality in the very young, the elderly, in pregnant women and in the infirm, which are the basic features by which we know influenza today and how we would recognise it.

So, 1510 saw that acute respiratory disease emerge in Asia on its way through North Africa, the Middle East (Jerusalem and Mecca) and Europe. It probably originated in China: Gregor Horst in *Operum medicorum tombus primus* (1661) had a much wider view that it had started in the Orient, fanned out East to West along trade routes, had arrived in southern Europe from Africa via Malta, and had then advanced northward from Sicily into Italy and Spain, crossing the Alps and into all of Europe to reach the Baltic Sea. German medical writer Justus Hecker (1795–1850) suggested in his *History of Medicine, produced from the sources, from 2000 BC to the downfall of the Byzantine Empire in 1453*, that the 1510 influenza most likely came from Asia because of the historical nature of other influenzas to originate there in more recent pandemics. Hecker was a specialist in the history of disease, including plague, smallpox, infant mortality, dancing mania and the sweating sickness, and is said to be the father of the study of the history of disease. Medical historian Thomas Short believed that the 'island of Melite [Malta] in Africa' was flu's springboard into mainland Europe.

The first cases of influenza began to appear in Sicily around July on infected merchant ships from Malta. Influenza quickly spread out along the Mediterranean coasts of Italy and southern France via merchant shipping.

In Emilia-Romagna, Tommasino De' Bianchi, referred to above, witnessed Modena's first cases on 13 July 1510; in Bologna an 8-year-old named Ugo Bancopagni, who would later become Pope Gregory XIII, became very ill with flu but recovered. Pope Julius II attributed the outbreaks in Rome and the Holy See to God's wrath. Pope Gregory XIII would later blame the 1510 influenza in France on the resistance of King Louis XII to divine authority.

Flu spread over the Alps from Italy into Switzerland and the Holy Roman Empire. In Switzerland it was called *das Gruppie* by the Mellingen chronicler Anton Tegenfeld. A respiratory illness seemed to have menaced the Canton of Aargua in June, with the population falling ill with sniffling, coughing and fatigue. German physician Achilles Gasser records a deadly epidemic spreading over the Holy Roman Empire's upper kingdoms, branching into the cities and the 'whole mankind'.

André de Burgo's letters of 24 August 1510 reveal that Margaret of Austria had to intervene at a royal assembly between her father, Holy Roman Emperor Maximilian I, and Louis XII of France because the French king was too sick with 'coqueluche' to take part. The pestilence then spread out from the Holy Roman Empire into Northern Europe, the Baltic states and west towards France and England.

France received the pandemic courtesy of infected sailors arriving from Sicily through the ports of Marseille and Nice. As noted it was referred to as *cephalie catarrhal* by French physicians, then later *coqueluche*. Historian François Eudes de Mézeray gives us the etymology of *coqueluche*: in the 1410s victims would wear bonnets resembling *coqueluchons*, a kind of monk's cowl. Merchants, pilgrims, and other itinerants spread the virus throughout the western Mediterranean in July. By August it was in Tours and by September the whole country was afflicted. Poet and historian Jean Bouchet, in King Louis XII's Royal Court, wrote that the epidemic 'appeared in the entire Kingdom of France, as much in the towns as in the countryside'.

Coqueluche overran the hospitals in France. Louis XII's National Assembly of Bishops, Prelates, and university professors scheduled for September 1510 was postponed because of the ferocity of the flu in Paris. Jean Fernel later compared the 1557 influenza to the 1510 epidemic which attacked everyone with fever, a headache and violent coughing. Up to 1,000 Parisians per day were dying at the height of 'la 1510 peste'. Mézeray mentions that it disrupted judicial proceedings and colleges, and that the 1510 flu was more widespread and deadly in France than in other countries.

Fernel and Paré suggest that the 1510 influenza 'spread to almost all countries of the world', with the exception of the New World. An epidemiological study of past influenza pandemics reviewing previous medical historians has found England was affected in 1510 where there were reports of symptoms like 'gastrodynia' and noteworthy murrain among cattle.[1] The flu is also recorded to have reached Ireland.

In Spain and Portugal the trade and pilgrim routes connecting the Iberian peninsula with Italy provided a speedy highway for its transmission between the three countries. Spanish cities such as Barcelona, Cadiz, Cordova, Seville, Madrid and others were 'dispopulated' by the pandemic. Thomas Short describes some medicinal treatments for the 1510 flu including 'Bole Armoniac, oily lintus, pectoral troches, and decoctions'.

The 1510 pandemic is the first to be pathologically described, facilitated by advances in global communications brought about by the invention of the printing press and moveable type. This led to the publication of affordable books for the well off and a world-changing explosion of knowledge and its exchange around the world, up there with the wheel, the steam engine, penicillin and, most aptly, the internet. Infection rates were high, but fatality was low and said to be confined to weaker patients like children and those who had been bled. As with all its predecessors and successors the pandemic was responsible for major disruption in governments, church and society; 1510 saw infection rates close to universal infection and a mortality rate of around 1 per cent.

Put simply, influenza A is a zoonotic respiratory virus whose reservoir is in wild birds that affects birds, mammals and humans. On rare occasions these viruses are introduced into man and cause a flu pandemic. Influenza viruses are unique in their genetic instability, which frequently results in antigenic shift, a genetic process in which genes from multiple subtypes are reassorted to form a new virus; antigenic shifts are responsible for influenza epidemics. Influenza A pandemics have caused millions of deaths during the past several hundred years. So far the 1918–19 influenza pandemic is the worst in history in terms of mortality.

Influenza has left so many trails of destruction around the world for centuries that it has earned for itself a special place in infectious disease classification: two major conditions need now to be satisfied to classify an outbreak as a full-blown pandemic:

---

1. *The American Journal of Hygiene*: Monographic series. Johns Hopkins Press. 1921

a flu pandemic needs to be both an entirely new strain of influenza A, and must spread to multiple continents and countries.

What may have been influenza epidemics have been recorded in Babylon, or Babirus of the Persians in 722 BC and in Nineveh, during the reign of Sargon, King of Assyria in 591. We have described how Livy, the early 1st century AD Roman historian, refers to a pestilence resembling the flu in Book 4, 52, 3–5. The symptoms of human influenza are first described by Hippocrates around 410 BC in Book 1, 1 of the *Epidemics* as experienced in Northern Greece. The world has been seeing what it believes to be influenza-like illnesses, contagious upper respiratory tract infection, since the 7th century when monks tell of an epidemic ravaging Britain, its spread accelerated by delegates returning from a synod at Whitby Abbey in 664.[2]

In the time of Charlemagne (AD 748 – AD 814) the respiratory tract disease known as *febris Italica* (Italian fever) pursued his armies around Europe, incubating silently in the troops and infecting the baggage train and anyone who got in the way. There are thought to have been 31 known instances of flu pandemics since the first unanimously agreed outbreak in 1580. The 1173–74 pandemic, affecting England, France and Italy, is the first pandemic to be reported: 'In May, an inflammatory plague swept all over the Occident,' according to a French chronicle 'and all eyes wept following a cruel rhinorhea'. At the time many hard hitting epidemics were called a plague.

About the same time the clerics of Melrose Abbey reported 'an eveil and unheard-of-cough'. The term influenza is first used to describe a disease in 1357 when people called an epidemic in Florence *influenza di freddo*, which translates literally to 'cold influence'. A Montpellier doctor reported an upper respiratory tract infection that was 'so important that only one in ten of the population could escape the disease' which affected mainly the elderly. *Influenza di freddo* would be applied again to the epidemic in 1386–87 in Italy; this too specifically targeted elderly and vulnerable persons with underlying health conditions and gives us probably the first documentation of a key epidemiological feature of both pandemic and seasonal influenza.

Jacob von Königshofen states in the *Strasburg Chronicle*, 'A general pestilence invaded the whole country, attended with cough and fever; hardly one among ten were unaffected.' The 1410 epidemic of flu-like violent coughing disease is referred to as *le tac, le taq* or *horion* and is associated with spontaneous abortions in pregnant women. According to Pasquier of Paris writing in 1665 contagion in the air during convalescence also caused profuse haemorrhages from the mouth, nose and bowels. Four years later in 1414 Paris endured another outbreak of flu that affected up to 100,000 people right across society. Historians said it originated from *vent puant et tout plein de froidure*, or a 'malodorous and intensely cold wind'. Victims 'lost the eating and drinking unable to do anything other than rest. They had a very high fever with shivering and cough.' The 1427 epidemic – a true influenza pandemic – was possibly the first time the disease was referred to as *coqueluche;* it also went by the name *dando = dans le dos*, or *Ladendo*. Symptoms included cough, insomnia, renal pains, anorexia, constant

---

2. Creighton 1965

rigors. The modish greeting everywhere on meeting friends on the streets was '*Have you had Ladendo?*' The monks of St Albans report that 'it invaded the whole people, and so infected the aged as well as the younger and so conducted a great number to the grave'.

The 1557 influenza pandemic spread from Asia to the Ottoman Empire, then into Europe, the Americas and Africa and is the first to be reliably recorded as spreading worldwide by medical historians and epidemiologists; this is when flu received its first English names. The 1557 pandemic lasted for at least two years and unlike the 1510, this had highly mortality with deaths registered as due to 'pleurisy and fatal peripneumony'. High mortality in pregnant women is also recorded. Herman Thompson has it that symptoms are 'tightness and dreadful oppression over the chest, as if bound with red hot chains; the same sensations over the abdomen and stomach.' The 1580 influenza pandemic originated in Asia during the summer, spreading to Africa and then to Europe along two routes from Asia Minor and North-West Africa. Infection and illness rates were high with 8,000 deaths reported in Rome; populations in some Spanish cities were decimated; in the Americas, over 90 per cent of the population was apparently infected. Bleeding or bloodletting (venesection) was a first line and common treatment which consisted of bleeding those who were ill until they were weak, pale and occasionally unconscious. There is little doubt that this contributed to the overall mortality rate of this outbreak, as did another debilitating therapy, purgation. Anna, wife of Philip I of Spain, died of the disease.

In 1647 the Caribbean was ravaged with high morbidity; on each of the Islands of Barbados and St. Kitts there were 5,000 to 6,000 cases.

Influenza was back in 1729 when a pandemic emerged in Moscow; within six months it had spread westwards in ever expanding waves to infect all Europe with high death rates. Bizarrely Louis XV was infected and said that the disease spread like 'a foolish little girl', or *follette* in French.

An influenza pandemic originated in the Americas in the spring of 1761 and leapfrogged to Europe and around the globe in 1762. It is the first pandemic to enjoy concentrated study by multiple international scientists and physicians in learned societies and through medical journals and books. The clinical characterisation of influenza was enhanced at this time as physicians painstakingly and meticulously recorded observations on series of patients and attempted to understand what would later be called the pathophysiology of the disease.

In mid-1700 Britain, as elsewhere, it was thought that the influence of the cold (*influenza di freddo*), along with astrological influences or the conjunction of stars and planets (*influenza di stelle*), caused the disease. These supernatural causes included: 1411 – diabolical pollution of the air with pestilential vapours arising from the air and ground; these caused bleedings from the mouth, nose and bowels, and in women caused abortions; 1580 – bad conduct of Sirius the dog star, caused by anger; 1658 – blast from the stars according to Thomas Wills, MD of Oxford and 1742 – malign influence (Influenza) of the stars.

Doctors were still ill-equipped to handle the disease. Many believed the flu was caused by the synchronization of certain atmospheric factors. Medical journals show theories attempting to correlate phenomena like wind speed, temperature changes and barometric pressure with a wave of influenza.

In 1768 Voltaire was in St Petersburg when he describes in a letter a disease which he calls 'la grippe' (from the German *grippen*, to catch) that had swept in from Siberia and infected him. The word 'influenza' was by now the word of choice describing the URTI (upper respiratory tract infection). Lord Chesterfield wrote in a letter to his son describing an epidemic in London 'as a little fever which kills nobody but elderly people that is now called by a beautiful name, influenza'. Five years later a French doctor named Bachaumont describes the spread in France of 'an epidemic cold' which emanated from London; it was causing so much anxiety, he says, that British people were migrating in droves to southern France to escape it with the inevitable result that deaths were now reported in Marseille, Toulon and Paris – up to twelve deaths amongst the elderly were reported in the capital.

The 1780–82 global pandemic originated on the borders of China and India, spreading to Russia and the USA; it was given the name Russian Catarrh. Tens of millions of cases of infection were reported worldwide as the virus spread relentlessly and as quickly as contemporary transportation would allow. At its peak, the infection afflicted 30,000 people a day in St. Petersburg and affected half to two-thirds of the population in Rome. In the USA George Washington caught it. The British fleet sailed from Plymouth and Portsmouth on 6 May, 1782. No further contact was had with the land, yet, amazingly, on 27 May the flu broke out in the fleet. In 1788 the same thing happened to US sailors on board ships 100 miles from land.

This pandemic is probably the first in which the concept of influenza as a distinct entity with characteristic epidemiological features was first appreciated. Despite the high morbidity this pandemic had relatively low mortality rates.

The year 1803 saw another epidemic in France with much death amongst the 'vigorous people'. The German ambassador in Paris, Johann Freidriech Reichardt witnessed a large epidemic in which younger people were worst afflicted. There were other possible flu epidemics in 1817, 1830 and 1837. The 1830–33 influenza pandemic erupted in winter 1830 in China, spreading southwards to reach the Philippines, India and Indonesia and across Russia into Europe. By 1831, it had reached the Americas. Overall the attack rate is estimated at 20–25 per cent of the population, but the mortality rate was modest. In 1837 a French chronicler reported that 'half the population of Paris was in bed, transforming Paris into a giant hospital in which half the inhabitants were afflicted by influenza and the other half were taking care of the cases.'

In 1878 avian influenza was recorded for the first time, in Italy; before this it was known as Fowl Plague. The 1889–92 pandemic goes by the name the 'Russian pandemic' affecting 14 per cent of the world's population. Infections were reported from 14 European countries and in the United States: the pandemic would take only four months to circumnavigate the globe, arriving in the United States 70 days after the original outbreak in Saint Petersburg. In 1901 the causative organism of avian influenza was discovered to be a virus.

The notorious 1918–1920 Spanish flu (H1N1) pandemic was one of the most lethal natural disasters ever, infecting an estimated 500 million people across the globe and claiming between 50 and 100 million lives. To put its rapacity into some kind of context, if today's COVID-19 had killed at the same rate as the 1918 pandemic there would be more than 200 million deaths globally rather than just over 3 million as of mid-April 2021. This pandemic would be described as 'the greatest medical holocaust in history' and is estimated to have killed in a single year more people than the Black Death killed in four years from 1347 to 1351. The next big outbreak was a new, virulent influenza A virus subtype H2N2 which broke in Guizhou, China in 1957 and spread to the neighbouring Yunnan and Hunan provinces. This evolved into a pandemic (category 2) and killed between 1 and 4 million people.

In 1968–69 the Hong Kong flu (H3N2) pandemic broke out. In 1976 swine flu was identified at a US army base in Fort Dix, New Jersey. Four soldiers were infected resulting in one death. To prevent a major pandemic, the United States launched a vaccination campaign. The agent for the 1977 Russian flu (H1N1) epidemic was a new influenza strain isolated in northern China. A similar strain prevalent in 1947–57 meant that most adults had good immunity: most patients were children born after 1957. In 2009, a new flu virus (H1N1) pandemic, first recognized in the state of Veracruz, Mexico, spread rapidly across the United States and the world. Worldwide, nearly 1 billion doses of H1N1 vaccine were ordered while 74 countries were affected with 18,500 deaths.

Alibrandi, Rosamaria. 'When early modern Europe caught the flu. A scientific account of pandemic influenza in sixteenth century Sicily'. *Medicina Historica*. 2: 19–25.

Belshe, R.B. 2008 An introduction to influenza: lessons from the past in epidemiology, prevention, and treatment. *Managed Care*. 2008 Oct;17 (10 Suppl 10):2–7.

Fauci A.S. 2006. 'Pandemic influenza threat and preparedness'. *Emerging Infect. Dis.* 12 (1): 73–7.

Morens, David M. *Lancet*. 2010 Dec 4; 376(9756): 1894–1895. Eyewitness accounts of the 1510 influenza pandemic in Europe.

Chapter 14

1519–1520 smallpox epidemic, Mexico

'Sores erupted on our faces, our breasts, our bellies; we were covered with agonizing sores from head to foot. The illness was so dreadful that no one could could walk or move.'
— A native account

History has blamed an African slave, Francisco Eguía, for this contagion, but this seems unlikely – a white Spanish invader is a more probable culprit. Indeed others say, more credibly, that Eguía was on the ship carrying Pánfilo de Narváez and his army, which had been detailed to capture Hernán Cortés, 'Cortés the Killer', and take him back to Spain. Very few men can claim to have been responsible for so much death and destruction as Francisco Eguía, whatever his role. During the 16th-century, in the name of colonisation, 'many native records were destroyed by Christian authorities in campaigns to eradicate vestiges of indigenous religion'[1]. This would have included such primary sources as eye-witness reports, annals, chronicles and histories, some of which no doubt included early descriptions of smallpox and other epidemics.

Mexico, indeed all of the Americas, knew nothing about smallpox until the Europeans turned up. The Spanish did the Mexicans no favours at all when they introduced the deadly disease which left the ravaged and depopulated country in such a state of wretched desolation that the disease can be said to have played a significant role in the downfall of the Aztec Empire. Hernán Cortés left Cuba having helped acquire the island for the Spanish, and arrived in Mexico in 1519 on his mission to open trade talks on the Veracruz Coast only. However, Cortés was having none of this: so intent was he to despoil Mexico that he scuttled his fleet to preclude any possibility of an early withdrawal and then he ignored the Cuban governor and began to invade the interior with his 500 men. The whole Mexican empire of an estimated 16 million people was now under threat from Spain, an empire the Mexicans had built up through conquest and tribute radiating out some 80,000 square miles from the great island capital city of Tenochtitlán in Lake Texcoco. Tenochtitlán boasted a population of 200,000.

The aggrieved governor sent Pánfilo de Narváez after Cortés. Unfortunately, Narváez's forces were by now harbouring at least one infectious case of smallpox and when the Narváez expedition stopped at Cozumel and Veracruz in 1520, the disease gained a lethal foothold in the region.

---

1. McCaa 1994

In 1520 another group of Spanish landed in Mexico from Hispaniola, bringing with them the smallpox which had already been ravaging that island for two years. When Cortés heard about the other group, oblivious to the disease prevailing amongst them, he attacked and defeated them. Unfortunately, Cortés was not the only victor: one of Cortés's men contracted the disease and when Cortés returned to Tenochtitlán, he took the disease with him. The first recorded outbreak of smallpox in Hispaniola, previously a disease of the Eastern hemisphere, occurred in December 1518 among enslaved African miners. As in Mexico later the natives had no immunity to European diseases. By May 1519, as many as one-third of the remaining inhabitants had perished driving the population to near extinction by 1520. Hispaniola, an island now split between the Dominican Republic and Haiti, is the most populous island in the West Indies and the region's second largest after Cuba.

Soon, the Aztecs rebelled against Cortés and his men. Outnumbered, the Spanish were forced to flee. In the fighting, the Spanish soldier carrying smallpox died. This was the Noche Triste – 'The Night of Sorrows' (30 June 1520) – when Cortés, his army of conquistadors, and their native allies were driven out of Tenochtitlán. The name is derived from the sorrow that Cortés and his surviving followers felt and expressed at the loss of life, and booty, incurred during the flight from Tenochtitlán. Cortés did not return to the capital until August 1521 while all the while smallpox was laying waste the Aztec population. It killed most of the Aztec army and 25 per cent of the overall population at large. On Cortés' return, he found the Aztec army's chain of command in total disarray: the soldiers who were still alive were prostrated by the disease. Cortés, with his new found insidious ally, easily defeated the depleted Aztec army and entered Tenochtitlán. The Spaniards said later that they could not walk through the streets without stepping on the bodies of smallpox corpses.

From May to September 1519, smallpox spread inexorably 150 miles inland to Tepeaca and Tlaxcala, and to Tenochtitlán. It was well established by April or May 1520.

A native account describes the dreadful effects of smallpox upon the people of Tenochtitlán:

> 'It began to spread…striking everywhere in the city and killing a vast number of our people. Sores erupted on our faces, our breasts, our bellies; we were covered with agonizing sores from head to foot. The illness was so dreadful that no one could could walk or move. The sick were so utterly helpless that they could only lie on their beds like corpses, unable to move their limbs or even their heads. They could not lie face down or roll from one side to the other. If they did move their bodies, they screamed with pain. A great many died from this plague and many others died of hunger. They could not get up to search for food, and everyone else was too sick to care for them, so they starved to death in their beds.'

Cortés could also take advantage of the widespread local animosity toward the capital city and its ruler, establishing alliances with many disaffected locals. Though vastly outnumbered, he and a small force marched on Tenochtitlán, where Montezuma

(Motecuhzoma II) received them graciously. Cortés thanked him by taking him prisoner and laid siege.

The people were both starving and dying from smallpox. Bernal Diaz, Cortés' chronicler, described the scenes in the city:

> 'We could not walk without treading on the bodies and heads of dead Indians.
> I have read about the destruction of Jerusalem, but I do not think the mortality was
> greater there than here in Mexico. Indeed, the stench was so bad that no one could
> endure it…and even Cortés was ill from the odours which assailed his nostrils.'

After two years Cortés finally conquered the Aztec capital in August 1521. His victory had little to do with military might or ingenuity: his ally was the smallpox his army had brought with it. This had spread inland from the coast of Mexico and more than decimated the densely populated city of Tenochtitlán in 1520, reducing its population by 40 per cent in one year. Military and diplomatic strength were destroyed. Cortés only mentions one native leader who died of smallpox, Maxixcatzin, a Tlaxcalan loyal to Cortés; however, we know that Cuitláhuactzin, ruler of the Mexica (a Nahuatl-speaking indigenous people of the Valley of Mexico who were the rulers of the Aztec Empire), and other native rulers – friend and foe alike – also succumbed to 'the pustules'. Chimalpahin reports the death of some lords in Chalco from the disease as well – all part of the widespread epidemic which decimated the common population. Estimates of mortality range from one-quarter to one-half of the population of central Mexico.

With the sudden death of Cuitláhuactzin, Cortés was able to pick off Mexica towns one by one, often through diplomacy; Hassig[2] says 'with the fall of Tenochtitlán, the rest of Mesoamerica fell to Spanish domination with little or no struggle'.

The native people of the Americas, including the Aztecs, were particularly vulnerable to smallpox because they had never before experienced the virus and so possessed no natural immunity. For smallpox this was virgin territory. A Franciscan monk, Toribio Motolinia, who accompanied Cortés gave this description:

> 'As the Indians did not know the remedy of the disease, they died in heaps, like
> bedbugs. In many places it happened that everyone in a house died, and as it was
> impossible to bury the great number of dead, they pulled down the houses over
> them, so that their homes became their tombs.'

For plague, Alonso de Chorino, a Jewish doctor, recommended in his layperson's guide to the plague to first pray, and then flee. For smallpox he prescribed social distancing.

As with earlier epidemics there were serious life-changing ramifications: depopulation when it killed so many people, particularly infants and young children; the death toll amongst adults seriously depleted the workforce as did illness and the

---

2. 1992 p.164

fact that many adults became full time carers so that they were unable to work and earn; at the same time the morbidity amongst adults reduced the number of carers which had serious implications because it was well known that good nursing and caring reduced mortality.[3] The disease also badly affected the number of people able to make bread, leading to malnutrition and starvation in some communities. Others suffered depression or lost the will to resist the Spanish invader; this had an effect on the economy, not least productivity, notably in agriculture where land was neglected and crops failed, resulting in extensive famine which in turn compromised the immune systems of many leaving them prone to infection.

The Aztec Empire was effectively finished and New Spain was born. Although uncontrolled disease had a large part to play in the destruction and demise, the causes were multi-factorial: superior weaponry and more sophisticated military tactics brought to bear by the Spanish, the religious beliefs of the Aztecs, and the long history of ritual sacrifice and persecution of the other peoples living in Mexico all played essential roles. As McCaa (1994) says:

> 'But the role of disease cannot be understood without taking into account massive harsh treatment (forced migration, enslavement, abusive labor demands and exhorbitant tribute payments) and ecological devastation accompanying Spanish colonization. Killing associated with war and conquest was clearly a secondary factor.'

And it was not just the Aztecs who were nearly wiped off the globe. Other indigenous peoples suffered from the introduction of European diseases. In addition to North America's native American populations, the Mayan and Incan civilizations were also nearly exterminated by smallpox. Measles and mumps and other infectious agents took their substantial tolls – altogether reducing some indigenous populations in the New World by 90 per cent or more. It has been estimated that the population of Mexico fell from over 30 million people before the arrival of Cortés, to a mere 1.5–3 million by 1568. We will never know the exact numbers who perished in the New World generally but it is estimated that smallpox killed between 40 and 50 million of the native population. Some estimates are even higher and state that as many as 90 per cent of the population died.

Smallpox is particularly suited to deployment in biological warfare: in the 18th century, the British tried to infect native American populations with the agent at the Siege of Fort Pitt, Philadelphia in 1763 with items from a smallpox infirmary given as spurious gifts to Native American envoys. One general wrote, 'We gave them two blankets and a handkerchief out of the smallpox hospital. I hope it will have the desired effect.' Things don't get more atrocious and inhumane than that.

The Spanish-Aztec debacle is one more sobering reminder that defence budgets are not the only way of facilitating colonialisation and bankrolling ethnic cleansing: history has numerous examples where the course of events has been definitively

---

3. McCaa, p. 421–422

altered by outbreaks of disease, natural or otherwise, which vie with the masters and machinery of war to eradicate whole populations.

Acuna-Soto, R., Emerg Infect Dis. 2002 Apr; 8(4): 360–62. Megadrought and Megadeath in 16th Century Mexico

Acuna-Soto, R., Large epidemics of haemorrhagic fevers in Mexico 1545–1815. *Am J Trop Med Hyg*. 2002.

McCaa, R., 'Revisioning smallpox in Mexico City-Tenochtitlán, 1520–1950: What difference did charity, quarantine, inoculation and vaccination make?' 2000

McCaa, R., Spanish and Nahuatl Views on Smallpox and Demographic Catastrophe in the Conquest of Mexico: Robert McCaa *Journal of Interdisciplinary History*, 25:3 (1995), 397–431.

Chapter 15

The Cocoliztli epidemics:
1545–1548 and 1576–1580

*'The fevers were contagious, burning, and continuous, all of them pestilential, in most part
lethal. The tongue was dry and black. Enormous thirst. Urine of the colors of sea-green,
vegetal green, and black, sometimes passing from the greenish color to the pale. Pulse was
frequent, fast, small, and weak – sometimes even null. The eyes and the whole body were
yellow. This stage was followed by delirium and seizures.'*

– Francisco Hernández

T he cocoliztli epidemics is the name given to millions of deaths in New Spain
in present-day Mexico in the 16th century attributed to one or more illnesses
collectively called cocoliztli which ravaged the Mexican Highlands in epidemic
proportions near modern-day Puebla City. Given the death toll, this epidemic is often
referred to as the worst disease epidemic in the history of Mexico. Shortly after its
initial outbreak, however, it may have spread as far north as Sinaloa, and as far south as
Chiapas and Guatemala, where it was called *gucumatz*.

Mexico in 1545 was still reeling from the population collapse caused by the 1520
smallpox epidemic. The catastrophic epidemics that began in 1545 and 1576 subsequently
killed an additional 7 to 17 million people in the highlands of Mexico. The exact identity
of the cocolitzli continues to evade scientists, but epidemiologists suggest that the
events in the 1545 and 1576 epidemics, associated with a high death rate and referred
to as cocolitzli (Nahuatl for 'pest'), may have been due to indigenous haemorrhagic
fevers. Recent bacterial genomic studies have suggested that salmonella, specifically a
serotype of *Salmonella enterica* known as Paratyphi C, was at least partially responsible
for this initial outbreak.[1]

Cocoliztli epidemics usually occurred within two years of a major drought;
tree ring evidence, which reveals the levels of precipitation, indicates that the worst
drought to afflict North America in the past 500 years occurred in the mid-16th
century, when severe drought extended at times from Mexico and Venezuela to Canada.
These droughts interacted with ecologic and sociological conditions, magnifying the
impact of infectious disease in mid 16th-century Mexico. The correlation between
drought and the disease has been thought to be that population numbers of the vesper

---

1. (Vågene (2018), *Salmonella enterica genomes recovered from victims of a major 16th century
epidemic in Mexico).*

mouse, a carrier of viral haemorrhagic fever, increased during the rains that followed the drought, as conditions improved. Drought too would have lowered sanitary conditions and encouraged poor personal hygiene. Periodic rains would have increased the presence of New World rats and mice.

The epidemic of cocoliztli from 1545 to 1548 killed an estimated 5 million to 15 million people, or up to 80 per cent of the native population of Mexico – one of the worst demographic catastrophes in human history, approaching even the mortality of the Black Death.

Depopulation apart, the epidemics had significant impacts on Mexico. The death of so many Aztecs created a void in land ownership, with Spanish colonists desperate to exploit these newly vacant lands. The Spanish Emperor, Charles V, had been looking for a way to emasculate the *encomendero* class, and establish a more efficient and 'ethical' settlement system; this gave him his opportunity. These infections appear to have been stimulated by contemporary extreme climatic conditions and by the poor living conditions and harsh treatment of the native people under the *encomienda* system of New Spain. This was a labour system set up by the Spanish crown whereby a Spanish *encomendero* was granted a number of native labourers who would pay tribute to him in exchange for his protection – virtual slavery. They were poorly fed and inadequately clothed, and were hideously overworked as farm and mine labourers which left them particularly vulnerable to epidemic disease.

At the end of the 1549 outbreak, the *encomenderos*, laid low by the loss in profits, were compelled to comply with the new *tasaciones* (regulations), known as *Leyes Nuevas*. These aimed to limit the amount of tribute *encomenderos* could levy, while also prohibiting them from exercising absolute control over the labour force. At the same time non-*encomenderos* began claiming lands lost by the *encomenderos*, as well as the labour provided by the natives. This developed in to the implementation of the *repartimiento* system, which established a superior level of oversight within the Spanish colonies and maximized the overall tribute extracted for public and crown use. Rules regarding tribute itself were also changed in response to the epidemic of 1545, when fears over future food shortages ran rampant among the Spanish. By 1577, after years of debate and a second major outbreak of cocoliztli, maize and money were designated as the only forms of acceptable tribute.

The cocoliztli epidemic from 1576 to 1578 killed an additional 2 to 2.5 million people, or about 50 per cent of the remaining native population. We have long suspected that newly introduced European and African diseases such as smallpox, measles and typhus were the suspected cause of the population collapse in both 1545 and 1576 because both epidemics preferentially killed native people. But recent research related to the 1545 and 1576 epidemics now indicates that they were probably haemorrhagic fevers, caused by an indigenous virus and carried by a rodent host.

Friar Juan de Torquemada, a Franciscan historian writing in 1577, described cocolitzli in vivid detail:

> 'It was a thing of great bewilderment to see the people die. Many were dead and others almost dead, and nobody had the health or strength to help the diseased or

bury the dead. In the cities and large towns, big ditches were dug, and from morning to sunset the priests did nothing else but carry the dead bodies and throw them into the ditches. …It lasted for one and a half years, and with great excess in the number of deaths. After the murderous epidemic, the Viceroy Martin Enriquez wanted to know the number of missing people in New Spain. After searching in towns and neighborhoods it was found that the number of deaths was more than two million.'

Cocoliztli was a notoriously rapid spreading and highly lethal disease. Francisco Hernández de Toledo (1514–1587) the Proto-Medico of New Spain, one time personal physician of King Philip II and one of the highest qualified physicians of the day, witnessed the symptoms of the 1576 cocoliztli infections. He was among the first wave of Spanish Renaissance physicians practising according to the revived principles established by Hippocrates, Galen and Avicenna.

Philip despatched him to Mexico to see what he could find out about native medicines. Hernandez learned five Indian languages and wrote fifty volumes based on his own observations and interviews with hundreds of Indians, carrying out post-mortems on many of the victims of the 1576 epidemic. But the books arrived back in Spain just after Philip II's death. Philip III considered the project too expensive to publish, and the manuscript disappeared for 400 years; around 1950 it resurfaced in the Hacienda Library in Madrid. Six years later, Mexican physician German Somolinos d'Ardois published a version of that manuscript and was able to conclude that Hernandez considered the 1576 epidemic to be different from those that had come earlier.

Hernandez vividly described the atrocious cocoliztli symptoms with clinical precision:

'The fevers were contagious, burning, and continuous, all of them pestilential, in most part lethal. The tongue was dry and black. Enormous thirst. Urine of the colors of sea-green, vegetal green, and black, sometimes passing from the greenish color to the pale. Pulse was frequent, fast, small, and weak – sometimes even null. The eyes and the whole body were yellow. This stage was followed by delirium and seizures. Then, hard and painful nodules appeared behind one or both ears along with heartache, chest pain, abdominal pain, tremor, great anxiety and dysentery. The blood that flowed when cutting a vein had a green color or was very pale, dry, and without serosity. . .Blood flowed from the ears and in many cases blood truly gushed from the nose. This epidemic attacked mainly young people and seldom the elder ones.'

'This was certainly not smallpox,' Dr. Acuña-Soto, professor of epidemiology in the Faculty of Medicine at Universidad Nacional Autonoma de Mexico (2002) says. 'If they described something real, then it appeared to be a haemorrhagic fever.' Haemorrhagic fevers are viral diseases with dreaded names like Ebola, Marburg and Lassa. They strike with sudden intensity, rarely respond to treatment, kill at high rates, then vanish as mysteriously as they came. They are called haemorrhagic because victims bleed, haemorrhaging in their capillaries, beneath the skin, often from the mouth, nose, and ears.

This provoked two questions. First, were people prepared to absolve the Spanish of responsibility for one of the great evils of the colonial era? The destruction of ancient Mexico's culture by the Spanish invaders is an integral part of every Mexican's education relating to their country's history. The plague years were always one of the evils of colonialism. The second question was, if the Spanish were not responsible for the cocolitzli, what was?

The prevailing social and physical environment of colonial Mexico could not help but facilitate the spread of the 1545–1548 epidemic and attain the severity that it did. War and the fact that the Aztecs were forced into easily governable *reducciones* (congregations) that focused on agricultural production and conversion to Christianity, would have brought people in much closer contact to one another. Animals too may have been implicated be it rats, chickens, pigs, or cattle, or even animals imported from the Old World – all were potential disease vectors.

Spanish colonizers may have used exaggerated fears of the pestilence to spread and enforce Christianity; Gonzalo de Ortiz (an *encomendero*) says 'God sent down such sickness upon the Indians that three out of every four of them perished,' suggesting that the Spanish colonizers were less susceptible to this 'act of God'. Toribio de Benavente Motolinia, an early Spanish missionary, seems to contradict Ortiz by suggesting that 60 to 90 per cent of New Spain's total population decreased, regardless of ethnicity. Bernardino de Sahagún, another Spanish clergyman and author of the *Florentine Codex*, caught the disease himself and in 1576, Sahagún identified both African slaves and Spanish colonists as being preferred by the disease.

The geography of the 16th century cocoliztli epidemics supports the belief that they may have been indigenous fevers carried by rodents or other hosts native to the highlands of Mexico. Acuña-Soto (2002) adds:

'In 1545 the epidemic affected the northern and central high valleys of Mexico and ended in Chiapas and Guatemala. In both the 1545 and 1576 epidemics, the infections were largely absent from the warm, low-lying coastal plains on the Gulf of Mexico and Pacific coasts. This geography of disease is not consistent with the introduction of an Old World virus to Mexico, which should have affected both coastal and highland populations.'

Because the Aztec census records were so meticulous Acuña-Soto found he could track the movement of epidemics from village to village across the country.

Shortly after 1548, the Spanish started calling the disease *tabardillo* (typhus), recognized in Spain since the late 15th century. However, the symptoms were not identical to typhus, or spotted fever, as observed in the Old World then. In 1970 Germain Somolinos d'Ardois took a systematic look at all the suggestions at the time, including haemorrhagic influenza, leptospirosis, malaria, typhus, typhoid and yellow fever but none of these quite matched the 16th century accounts of cocoliztli, leading him to conclude the disease was a result of 'viral process of hemorrhagic influence'. In other words, cocoliztli was not the result of any imported Old World pathogen, but possibly a virus of either European or New World origins. The viral agent responsible for cocoloztli remains obscure; if it is not extinct, the microorganism that caused cocoliztli could reappear given favourable climatic conditions. Rodolfo Acuña-Soto, the Harvard-trained epidemiologist, warns that the fever may still be lurking in remote rural areas of Mexico.

Acuna-Soto R., 2002. Large epidemics of hemorrhagic fevers in Mexico 1545–1815. *Am J Trop Med Hyg.*

Callaway, Ewen, 2017. 'Collapse of Aztec society linked to catastrophic salmonella outbreak'. *Nature.* 542 (7642): 404.

Marr J.S., 2000. Was the Huey Cocoliztli a haemorrhagic fever? *Med Hist.* 44:341–62

Prem, Hanns, 1991. 'Disease Outbreaks in Central Mexico During the Sixteenth Century'. In Cook, Noble David; (ed.). 'Secret Judgments of God': Old World Disease in Colonial Spanish America. Norman:, OK. 20–48.

Chapter 16

1561–1562 Chile smallpox epidemic and the Balmis Expedition

The 'severest scourge known to humanity.'
– Edward Jenner on smallpox

In Europe, at the end of the 18th century, an average of 400,000 people died every year from smallpox. Jenner had discovered a means to prevent smallpox when he injected the exudates from a cowpox pustule into the arm of 8-year-old James Phipps on 14 May 1796. Jenner's vaccine was initially controversial, but his discovery was later accepted by the medical community. Soon after this breakthrough, King Charles IV of Spain vowed to help rid the world of smallpox using Jenner's method. Many members of the Bourbon royal family became infected with the smallpox virus: Gabriel, King Charles's brother, and his sister-in-law, the Portuguese queen Maria Ana Victoria, succumbed while the king's daughter, Queen Maria Luisa, and the Princess of Parma were all infected with the smallpox virus but survived. Urged by the queen, King Charles IV ordered that the unaffected members of the royal family should be variolated.

When Francisco de Villagra Velázquez (1511–1563), conquistador and four times governor of Chile between 1547 and 1563, disembarked at La Serena, northern Chile in 1561 to take up his post as Royal Governor he could have had no idea what he was bringing with him – unbeknown to Villagra he was hosting smallpox, the disease which Spanish soldiers had introduced into Chile for the first time in 1554; it struck again in 1561 and again in 1591. Before 1561 Chile had been isolated from Peru and protected by the Atacama Desert and Andes mountains, but at the end of 1561 and in early 1562 Francisco de Villagra put an end to all that natural protection.

Smallpox manifested in a destructive epidemic in Valparaiso and Santiago, but also assailed the native Mapuches with even greater severity. Contemporary chronicles and records have left us with no accurate data on mortality, but recent estimates say the Mapuches lost between 20 and 25 per cent of their population. Historian Ward Churchill[1] has claimed that the Mapuche population fell from half a million to 25,000 within a generation as result of the Spanish occupation and the famine and disease which came with it. One Spanish historian said that even the gold mines had to shut down when all their native Indian labour perished. Mapuche fighting Spain in Araucanía

---

1. *A Little Matter of Genocide*, p.109

viewed the epidemic as a magical attempt by Francisco de Villagra to exterminate them because he could not defeat them in the Arauco War.

Some 200 years later smallpox returned and scourged Central and South America, impacting mainly on the indigenous populations; 1790 saw a major epidemic that erupted in the Valley of Mexico, mainly affecting children, although more people recovered than died. For example, in Mexico City, of 5,400 cases admitted to hospital, 4,431 recovered and 1,331 died. This epidemic coincided with a rise in the price of corn, causing famine, and with a typhus epidemic.

Four years later another smallpox epidemic plagued Mexico via Guatemala with Oaxaca and Chiapas hit first; it then spread to Puebla, and then to Mexico City and Veracruz by 1797 reaching Saltillo and Zacatecas in the following year. This outbreak is significant because it marked the first time that public health and preventive campaigns were implemented in New Spain, including quarantines, inoculation, self-isolation and road closures. The 'Ayuntamiento' or city council, the Catholic Church and 'Real Tribunal del Protomedicato', which was an institution founded in 1630, managed all sanitary aspects of New Spain including the establishment of quarantines. A charity board was created, where the wealthier people of the city donated money to build hospitals and to help and cure the sick. This charity board was led by the Spanish archbishop Alonso Núñez de Haro y Peralta. It was not as philanthropic as it might at first seem, as the high death toll triggered economic problems and the depleted indigenous population caused a serious shortfall in tax revenues and labour.

Efforts to eradicate smallpox got off the ground in 1779 when José Ignacio Bartolache published his book on smallpox treatment entitled *Instrucción que puede servir para que se cure a los enfermos de las viruelas epidemicas que ahora se padecen en México (Instructions that may help to cure smallpox in Mexico)* in which he included an introduction describing the disease and how to treat it: methods included drinking warm water with salt and honey, gargling with water and vinegar, maintaining personal hygiene and finishing treatment by taking a purgative. He believed that smallpox was a remedy imposed by nature to lift low mood and that doctors should not accelerate the process of healing because it was contrary to nature. He wrote a letter to propose his measures in which he also included such recommendations as purifying air with gunpowder and scent, ventilating churches where bodies were buried and building cemeteries outside the city. This strategy was approved by city council in September 1779.

The church hospitals and cemeteries demanded that people bury their dead with lime outside the towns and cities. Isolation of sick people in hospitals or charities outside the cities was another important measure taken to stop the smallpox infection. These institutions took care of patients and provided them with food and medicine. During the 1797 and 1798 outbreak, they also provided inoculation and were called inoculation houses. Nevertheless, the miasma theory of contagion was still widely believed.

In 1796, *Gaceta de México* ran an article in which inoculation was promoted, giving examples of kings and other notable persons who had taken the jab. In January 1798, the eradication of the 1790s epidemic was declared. The government proposed that the measures taken in that epidemic be implemented as the official policy in the event of a recurrence and it was approved by the city council in April 1799. Viceroy

Miguel José de Azanza, ordered an article written on 14 November 1799 about the benefits resulting from the inoculation in the 1790s epidemic and distributed it to the population.

In 1803, Spanish doctor Francisco Javier de Balmis was appointed physician to King Charles IV; that same year Charles issued a royal command for a ground breaking vaccination expedition to Spain's colonies. King Charles appointed Balmis and Dr. Jose Salvany to lead this mission of mercy to propagate the recently discovered vaccine against smallpox which reduced the severity and mortality in the epidemics that followed. The Balmis Expedition (the Real Expedición Filantrópica de la Vacuna (Royal Philanthropic Vaccine Expedition)) sailed from La Coruña and travelled to Puerto Rico and Venezuela, vaccinating thousands of people along the way. When they got to Venezuela, they divided into two groups: Salvany went to various countries in South America but had become ill and later died of pulmonary tuberculosis, which manifested as episodes of massive haemoptysis. Balmis travelled to Puerto Rico, Puerto Cabello, Caracas, Havana, Mérida, Veracruz and Mexico City. The vaccine was carried as far as Texas in the north and New Granada in the south. In Mexico City, the challenge Balmis faced was to convince the viceroy, José de Iturrigaray, but he did so, and the viceroy had his son vaccinated.

His expedition is considered one of the most crucial events in the history of medicine and the vaccine programme was used until 1951 when smallpox was officially declared eradicated in Mexico. Military surgeon, Cristóval María Larrañaga, used this vaccine in the New Mexico province to inoculate thousands of people starting in 1804. It has inspired, for example, Dr. Carlos Canseco, President of Rotary International, to start the worldwide vaccination programme Polio Plus to eradicate polio.

On 5 February 1805, Balmis took twenty-five Mexican orphan children aged 4–6 with him on the perilous voyage from Acapulco to Manila, carrying the vaccine for smallpox. Because of the lengthy duration of the journey and the absence of any refrigeration the vaccine had to be kept alive by arm-to-arm vaccination from one child to another. Each child would be a repository for the vaccine for around ten days after which an extract from the child's lymphatic fluid was cut into next child, and so on. Balmis vaccinated two children at a time for insurance, just in case something happened to one of them: twenty-five children could carry the vaccine for a three to four month trip, all being well. Balmis reached Manila with his precious cargo on 15 April 1805. By 1806, a smallpox institute and vaccination board were established in Manila. Two years later, immunizations were already being administered in the provinces. Things don't get more magnanimous and humane than that.

Filipino historian Jose Bantug writes that the introduction of vaccination in the Philippines 'reads like an epic poem' worthy of universal pride and praise. Edward Jenner refers to the Balmis expedition as such: 'I don't imagine the annals of history furnish an example of philanthropy so noble, so extensive as this.' Macao and China followed while Napoleon, who was waging war with Britain, had all his French troops vaccinated and awarded Jenner a medal, and at the request of Jenner, he released two English prisoners of war and permitted their return home. Napoleon remarked he could not 'refuse anything to one of the greatest benefactors of mankind'.

There was another serious outbreak in 1814 Mexico which started in Veracruz and extended to Mexico City, Tlaxcala and Hidalgo. This epidemic caused Viceroy Félix Calleja to take mitigating measures such as fumigations and vaccination, which were successful. There were sporadic outbreaks until 1826 when smallpox re-emerged in Yucatán, Tabasco and Veracruz imported by North American ships. In 1828, there were reported cases in Hidalgo, Oaxaca, State of Mexico, Guerrero, Chiapas, Chihuahua and Mexico City.

Inoculation and vaccination

Edward Jenner, FRS FRCPE [1749–1823) pioneered the concept of vaccines including creating the smallpox vaccine, the world's first vaccine. The terms vaccine and vaccination are derived from *Variolae vaccinae* (smallpox of the cow), as devised by Jenner to denote cowpox. He used it in 1798 in his *Inquiry into the Variolae vaccinae known as the Cow Pox*, in which he described the protective effect of cowpox against smallpox. Jenner is often called 'the father of immunology', and his work is said to have 'saved more lives than the work of any other human'.

In 1768 English physician John Fewster had realised that prior infection with cowpox rendered a person immune to smallpox. In the years following 1770, at least five investigators in England and Germany successfully tested a cowpox vaccine against smallpox in humans. One, Dorset farmer Benjamin Jesty, successfully vaccinated and induced immunity with cowpox in his wife and two children during a smallpox epidemic in 1774; a similar observation was made in France by Jacques Antoine Rabaut-Pommier in 1780.

Observing that milkmaids were generally immune to smallpox, Jenner postulated that the pus in the blisters that milkmaids received from cowpox (a disease similar to smallpox, but much less virulent) protected them from smallpox.

Jenner's hypothesis was that the initial source of infection was a disease of horses, called 'the grease', which was transferred to cattle by farm workers, mutated, and then presented as cowpox. On 14 May 1796, Jenner tested his hypothesis by inoculating James Phipps, an 8-year-old boy who was the son of Jenner's gardener. He scraped pus from cowpox blisters on the hands of Sarah Nelmes, a milkmaid who had caught cowpox from a cow called Blossom whose hide now decorates the wall of the St. George's Medical School Library, Tooting. Phipps was the seventeenth case described in Jenner's first paper on vaccination.

Jenner inoculated Phipps in both arms that day, subsequently producing in the boy a fever and some anxiety, but no full-blown infection. Later, he injected Phipps with variolous material, the routine method of immunization at that time. No disease ensued.

The medical establishment deliberated at length over Jenner's findings before accepting them. Eventually, vaccination was given the OK and in 1840, the British government banned variolation – the use of smallpox to induce immunity – and provided vaccination using cowpox free of charge through the Vaccination Acts of 1840, 1853, 1867 and 1898.

Although the World Health Organization declared the disease eradicated in 1979, some pus samples still remain in laboratories in the Centers for Disease Control and Prevention in Atlanta, USA, and in the State Research Center of Virology and Biotechnology VECTOR in Koltsovo, Novosibirsk Oblast, Russia. Both are under WHO supervision. The US smallpox stockpile, which includes samples from Britain, Japan and the Netherlands, is stored in liquid nitrogen. *The Guardian* reported in 2014 that 'A government scientist cleaning out an old storage room at a research center near Washington made a startling discovery last week – decades-old vials of smallpox packed away and forgotten in a cardboard box.' The virus samples were found in a cold room connecting two laboratories at the National Institutes of Health in Bethesda, Maryland, that has been used by the Food and Drug Administration since 1972. The implications for possible bioterrorism if similar vials exist unrecorded are horrendous.

The Guardian goes on to explain how 'The six glass vials of freeze-dried virus were intact and sealed with melted glass, and the virus might have been dead, officials at the Centers for Disease Control and Prevention said Tuesday.' Smallpox can be lethal even after it is freeze-dried, but the virus usually has to be kept cold to remain alive and dangerous. Initially a CDC official said he believed the vials were stored for many years at room temperature, which would suggest the samples are dead. But FDA officials said later in the day that the smallpox was in cold storage for decades. For many years world health authorities have believed the only samples left were safely stored in secure laboratories in Atlanta and in Russia.

The Guardian adds that 'vials of smallpox were found at the bottom of a freezer in an Eastern European country in the 1990s, according to Dr. David Heymann, a former World Health Organization official ...[and] professor at the London School of Hygiene and Tropical Medicine'.

Should we be worried?

Durbach, Nadja, 2004. Bodily Matters: *The Anti-Vaccination Movement in England, 1853–1907*. Raleigh, NC.

Jenner, Edward. 'An Inquiry Into the Causes and Effects of the Variolæ Vaccinæ, Or Cow-Pox. 1798'. *The Harvard Classics, 1909–1914*.

Riedel, Stefan , 2005. 'Edward Jenner and the history of smallpox and vaccination'. *Proceedings of the Baylor University Medical Center*. 18 (1): 21–25.

van Oss, C.J., 2000. 'Inoculation against smallpox as the precursor to vaccination'. *Immunological Investigations*. 29 (4): 443–46.

Chapter 17

Plague in the 16th century

1563–1564, London Plague

'I met with wagons, cartes, and horses full loden with young barnes, for fear of the black Pestilence...'

– Physician William Bullein quotes a beggar who watched
the inevitable flight from London:

After more than a decade of plague free years Londoners, their memories short, had grown somewhat complacent, as had the officials running the city in the reign of Elizabeth I where sanitation, overcrowding and population growth were as critical as ever. Complacency turned to fear and panic in 1563 and memories were jolted when plague broke out in Derby and Leicester, quickly reaching London; so virulent was it that the pestilence spread to English troops garrisoned at Le Havre, forcing a surrender to French forces. The English were there because of the Wars of Religion when on 8 May 1562 the reformers took the city, looted churches and expelled Catholics. The English sent troops but the armies of Charles IX, commanded by Anne de Montmorency, attacked Le Havre and the plague-ridden English were finally expelled on 29 July 1563. Not only did they lose Le Havre but they also lost Calais: the latter was being held as a hostage for Le Havre.

In London weekly Bills of Mortality for 1563 show the first seventeen recorded plague deaths for the week ending 12 June; Elizabeth began coordinating a government response to the epidemic by strict preventative measures at the local level such as painting blue crosses on the houses of the infected and government orders to kill and bury all stray cats and dogs 'for the avoidance of plague', with special officers appointed for the job. The miasma theory of contagion was still prevalent, of course, so orders were given by Queen Elizabeth's Council on 9 July that, at 7pm all householders should light bonfires in the street to snuff out the corrupt air. In February 1564, the Lord Mayor of London prohibited the public performance of plays because of the plague. This happened to coincide roughly with the birth of Shakespeare whose home town of Stratford lost 25 per cent of its inhabitants to the pestilence. The 1602 plague saw theatres closed for a year or so which forced Shakespeare's company (The Lord Chamberlain's Men) out on to the road to tour their productions.

Inevitably, cases began to escalate: by the end of July the weekly death toll was in the hundreds. Physician William Bullein quotes a beggar who watched the inevitable flight from London: 'I met with wagons, cartes, and horses full loden with young barnes, for fear of the black Pestilence...' It was of course the urban poor who took the brunt of the disease with the worst afflicted areas being Saint Poulkar's parish with its fruit market and general filth which was so attractive to rats, Fleet Ditch's Turnagain Lane, Seacoal Lane and the overcrowded and insanitary areas around the River Fleet.

By the end of August Londoners were dying by the thousand every week while panic, like the plague, was out of control. An anxious Elizabeth set a poor example when she relocated the Royal Court to Windsor Castle and erected a gallows in the town square, threatening to hang anyone who followed them from London. She banned the transportation of goods into Windsor from London and wrote to the Archbishop of York to recommend universal prayer and fasting for hastening 'remedy and mitigation' of the plague.

Between 27 August and 1 October an average of 1,449 people were dying weekly, peaking at 1,828 plague deaths for the week ending 1 October. Elizabeth's government now ordered that all houses with infected individuals should have their doors and windows boarded up and that no person inside was to make contact with persons outside for forty days. This strict quarantine had the desired effect with plague deaths dropping over 30 per cent to 1,262 for the week ending 8 October. Winter came and went, and with it the plague.

We all know about the insidious transmission of *Yersinia pestis* with the rats and its fleas. But the process of infection is fascinating: the mouth of the rat flea is tailor made for passing on the plague, functioning rather like a combined syringe, needle and blood-culture bottle. When an infected rat is bitten, a bloody suspension of living plague bacilli is drawn up into the flea's stomach, where they multiply and block the gut. The flea soon gets hungry, but cannot feed until this blockage is cleared. It is at this point what occurs is termed a 'blocked flea'. When it bites its next victim, the flea injects its previous meal, now cultured into a teeming mass of living plague bacilli, into the bitten area. The flea defecates and the host, you or I, naturally scratches the fleabites to inoculate faecal plague bacilli. Within a few days the lymph nodes draining the bitten area form buboes, and a new case of plague is there for all to see.

Britain was spared the depradations of the first plague pandemic – Justinian's in the 6th century – because the rat had not arrived on the British Isles. Rats do not feature in a 10th-century list of pests from which parish priests were expected to protect the altar bread. The earliest certain reference to rats is in a doodle of two rats hanging a cat at the end of a thirteenth-century genealogical roll now in the British Museum. By the early fourteenth-century references to rats are proliferating: Chaucer (born around 1340) mentions shops that sold rat poison.

Cummins, Neil,. 'Living standards and plague in London, 1560–1665'. *The London School of Economics and Political Science*

The Plague of Tenerife (1582)

The list of epidemics at Santa Cruz is rather formidable, e.g. 1621 and 1628, peste
(plague); 1810 and 1862, yellow Jack; 1814, whooping cough, scarlatina, and measles;
1816–16, small-pox (2,000 victims); 1826, cough and scarlet fever; 1847, fatal dysentery;
and 1861–62, cholera (7,000 to 12,000 deaths).

– Richard F. Burton, *To the Gold Coast for Gold*

By 1582 the Canary Islands were no strangers to pestilence of one kind or another.
The first major outbreak of plague occurred in 1506, ten years after the end of the
Castilian conquest, when the disease spread freely in Spain. Tenerife did what it could
to defend itself but, inevitably, plague came by sea from Gran Canaria, Fuerteventura
and Lanzarote, which in turn, had been exposed by the ships which brought with
them the pathogens that already plagued the mainland. The ports on Tenerife
were closed but it was too late and the disease spread rapidly throughout the island.
This first outbreak lasted two years; worst affected was the recently founded Santa
Cruz de Tenerife and also La Laguna, where the sick were isolated in the Bufadero and
San Andrés valleys. The first *lazaretto* was built in 1512, in Puerto Caballo next to the
port. Anaga too was ravaged; many Guanches lived here and suffered terribly because
they did not have any immunity mechanism to protect them. The Guanches were the
aboriginal inhabitants of the Canary Islands, confirmed in 2017 to be genetically most
similar to ancient North African Berber peoples.

From 1513, anyone on a ship reaching the anchorage of Santa Cruz had to present a
health certificate before being allowed to go ashore – early border control and quarantine.

A young Charles Darwin was frustrated in his desire to visit Tenerife en route to
South America on the second survey expedition of *HMS Beagle* under captain Robert
FitzRoy. Having arrived at Santa Cruz in early January 1832, they were prevented from
going ashore due to a cholera outbreak in England that required them to be quarantined
for twelve days. Time was of the essence so the captain gave orders for the ship to
proceed to the Cape Verde Islands.

A shocking footnote in Richard F. Burton's *To the Gold Coast for Gold* reports
the onslaught of disease from the 17th century to the 19th:

'The list of epidemics at Santa Cruz is rather formidable, e.g. 1621 and 1628,
peste (plague); 1810 and 1862, yellow Jack; 1814, whooping cough, scarlatina, and
measles; 1816–16, small-pox (2,000 victims); 1826, cough and scarlet fever; 1847,
fatal dysentery; and 1861–62, cholera (7,000 to 12,000 deaths).'

The 1582 plague began in San Cristóbal de La Laguna, whence it spread over much
of the island: it is regarded as one of the world's most serious outbreaks in relation to
the number of inhabitants. Something as innocent as imported tapestries are to blame
when they brought the rat flea from Flanders (hence its alternative name 'the plague of
Flanders'). It began around the Corpus Christi Day of that year when the new governor
of the islands hung tapestries from the balconies triggering an outbreak which in a

couple of weeks had killed more than 2,000 people in La Laguna alone. The final toll was between 7,500 and 9,000 which represented more than half of the population of Santa Cruz and La Laguna.

The plague of 1601 was caused simply by the mindless disobedience of the crew of a ship from Seville: two boats arrived at Garachico from Seville; they were forbidden to enter, but one of them disobeyed. The disease soon spread through Los Realejos, Icod, Los Silos and Santa Cruz. From Tenerife, it spread to Gran Canaria and from there to Fuerteventura and Lanzarote.

The Plague of Malta (1592)

When the 1592–93 plague epidemic raged, Malta was ruled by the Order of St John. It came in three waves between June 1592 and September 1593 and resulted in approximately 3,000 deaths, about 11 per cent of the population. It arrived in Malta indirectly from Alexandria in Ottoman-ruled Egypt. Four galleys of the Grand Duchy of Tuscany or the Order of Saint Stephen had captured two vessels from Alexandria, and took their cargo and about 150 Turkish captives with them to Malta. On the way an outbreak of the plague killed 20 crew members.

The galleys arrived in Malta on 7 May 1592. The outbreak was initially misdiagnosed as a sexually transmitted infection. The Infermeria delle Schiavi of Birgu, a hospital for galley slaves which had previously housed the Sacra Infermeria before its transfer to Valletta in 1575, was converted into an isolation hospital. When things got really serious in March 1594, Grand Master Hugues Loubenx de Verdalle requested assistance from the Viceroy of Sicily, who sent Pietro Parisi from Trapani, a doctor with experience of contagious diseases. Parisi arrived on 15 May and took control. A temporary isolation hospital was established in Marsamxett Harbour known as the Isolotto (later Manoel Island); 900 suspected and confirmed cases were sent there and were kept separate from each other. The rest of the population was told to self-isolate in their own houses, with only one person per family being allowed to go out daily for essential errands. These measures were enforced with harsh penalties, including flogging and death.

Washing facilities near the sea were set up in Valletta, Birgu and Senglea allowing suspected cases to wash in an attempt to purify themselves and their clothes. Walls of houses with confirmed or suspected cases were washed with seawater and whitewashed with lime; similar measures were undertaken in burial grounds. In Valletta dogs were culled but cats were not, since they were seen as useful in controlling the rat population, even though at the time it was not known that rat fleas were the cause of the disease. Extramural plague cemeteries were set up for the first time in Malta.

The epidemic began to subside by June 1593 and attempts were made to purify the island to remove any traces of the disease which might have been left. However, plague struck again in 1623; it began in the household of the Port Chief Sanitary Officer, caused by handling refuse from the earlier epidemic. Two further outbreaks occurred in Hospitaller-ruled Malta, a limited outbreak in 1655 which killed 20 people and a massive epidemic in 1675–76 which killed some 11,300 people, the best part of the island's population. In the 17th century, a permanent *lazaretto* was built on the Isolotto, on the site of the temporary plague hospital of 1592–93.

Tully, James D. (1821). *The History of Plague… with Particulars of the Means Adopted for Its Eradication*. London

The Plague of London (1592–1593)

'…by the weekly certificates, it doth appear that the present infection within the city of London doth greatly increase, growing as well by the carelessness of the people as by the want of good order to see the sound severed from the sick'.
                    – 10 September 1592, from a letter the Privy Council
                    wrote to the Lord Mayor and Aldermen of
                    London emphasising general non-compliance.

The late 1580s and early 90s were to witness increasing signs of plague along England's southern and eastern coasts: an outbreak at Newcastle in 1589 took 1,727 residents while from 1590 to 1592 there were 997 plague deaths at Totnes and Tiverton. The pestilence eventually reached London in September 1592. First indications of a return of the plague to the capital came when first the Thames Fair was postponed, and then the induction of the new Lord Mayor of London. London was to lose about 18,000 people (with a further 4,900 in surrounding parishes) mainly, again, in the rat-infested slums around the Thames, while the Fleet Ditch area around Fleet Prison became the most heavily infected part of the city. Since the winter of 1592–93 was mild, the fleas only partially hibernated and the disease flared up again in the spring of 1593 before being extinguished by the cold winter of 1593–94. The 8.5 per cent mortality rate makes this a relatively minor outbreak by London standards.

On 7 September, soldiers marching from the north of England to embark on foreign campaigns were diverted around London due to concerns about infection, and by the 21st at least thirty-five parishes were 'infeckted' with plague. A group transporting the spoils of a Spanish carrack from Dartmouth was ordered to stop at Greenwich. London's theatres, temporarily closed since a riot in June, had their shutdown orders extended to 29 December.

On 10 September 1592, the Privy Council wrote to the Lord Mayor and Aldermen of London that 'by the weekly certificates, it doth appear that the present infection within the city of London doth greatly increase, *growing as well by the carelessness of the people* as by the want of good order to see the sound severed from the sick'. The reference to 'the carelessness of the people' is particularly resonant. James Balmford, the curate of St Olave's, Tooley Street, observed that some sufferers went mad, leaping out of windows or running into the Thames. He attributed much of the blame for the contagion on the 'bloody error' that many people made, in thinking that the 'Pestilence' was not contagious. He dedicated his *A Short Dialogue concerning the Plagues Infection of 1603* to his parishioners: a publication in which he 'set down all that I have publicly taught' and tried to disabuse them of this fatal misconception that led 'men, women and children with running sores' to 'go commonly abroad and thrust themselves into company'.

Although plague burials took place at dusk when there were fewer people around, to minimise the chance of the disease spreading, not everyone took heed. Balmford grieved to see how 'the poorer sort, yea women with young children, will flocke to burials, and (which is worse) stand (of purpose) over open graves, where sundry are buried together, that (forsooth) all the world may see that they feare not the Plague.'

Thomas Dekker beautifully likened the advent of plague to Death pitching his tents in the 'sinfully polluted suburbs', from where he commanded his army of 'Burning Fevers, Boils, Blaines, and Carbuncles'. These generals led his rank and file: 'a mingle-mangle' of 'dumpish Mourners, merry Sextons, hungry Coffin-sellers, scrubbing Bearers, and nastie Grave-makers'.

Meanwhile the rich and the aristocratic were busy fleeing the city: 'The plague is so sore that none of worth stay about these places' sniffed one of their number. In November, London's College of Physicians convened a meeting to discuss the 'insolent and illicit practice' of London's unlicensed medical physicians with the intention to 'summon them all' before the college for quackery. Elizabeth's royal court cancelled the annual Accession Day tilt celebrations for 17 November, also known as Queen's Day, due to the possibility of contagion at the royal court.

Some records of the plague as copied by John Stow showed around 2,000 Londoners died of plague between August 1592 and January 1593. Government orders forbidding performances at theatres were again extended into 1593. By August Queen Elizabeth's royal court had evacuated to Windsor Castle (again). The city's sugar refineries, for example, continued business as usual even though public houses remained closed on government orders in a bid to halt the spread of infection. There was consternation at Windsor caused by the death of Elizabeth's chambermaid Lady Scrope from plague on 21 August which almost put the royal court to flight a second time. But they all stayed at Windsor Castle where Elizabeth got to host her tilt celebrations.

The government had published advice against catching the plague in 1578. This offered (those who could read) a range of preventative measures and cures – potions and lotions made up of ingredients like vinegar or various herbs and spices, or what to burn to purge the air. If you could not afford the ingredients, no problem: 'The poor which can not get vinegar nor buy Cinnamon, may eat bread and Butter alone, for Butter is not only a preservative against the plague, but against all manner of poisons.'

There was plenty of unofficial medical advice if the official guidance failed to save you: various remedies were prescribed in the twenty-three books published on the subject between 1486 and 1604. Beer and ale had medicinal qualities, and alehouses were notably busier at times of plague. Simon Kellwaye's 1593 tract was amongst the more inventive; he suggested applying live plucked chickens to the plague sores to draw out the disease:

'Take a cock chicken & pull all the feathers of his tail very bare, then hold the bared part of the pullet close upon the sore & the chicken will gape and labour for life & will die; then do so with another pullet till it die, & so with another: till you find the last chicken will not die, cannot be killed by the infection being altogether extracted, for when all the venom is drawn out the last chicken will not be hurt by it & the patient will mend speedily: one Mr Whatts hath tried this on a child of his, & 8 chickens one after another died & the ninth lived, & the sore being hard & hot was made soft by the first chicken as papp, the 2nd drew it clean away.'

Infected houses were boarded up and daubed now with a red cross to warn others away. A shut up house was boarded up or padlocked by a constable, and marked as unclean and a one foot long red cross and the words 'Lord have mercy on us' were daubed on the door. The constable was supposed to check everyday that the warning signs were still in place.

Shakespeare describes how plague victims were quarantined in *Romeo and Juliet*:

'Here in this city visiting the sick, the searchers of the town, Suspecting that we both were in a house Where the infectious pestilence did reign, Seal'd up the doors, and would not let us forth so that my speed to Mantua there was stayed... I could not send it,... here it is again,...Nor get a messenger to bring it thee, So fearful were they of infection.'

– Act V Scene 2, Friar John to Friar Laurence.

James Balmford is a little more prosaic: 'think it an hell to be so long shut up from company and their business: the neglecting whereof is the decay of their state'. Commercial ruin wreaked by the plague was a very real concern for those of modest means. Balmford callously dismissed such concerns, remarking that those infected should be 'content to forbear a while, since in the Plague they usually mend or end in short time'.

Dogs were thought to be carriers of infection and were culled by the authorities. Clothes belonging to the deceased were also not to be trusted. In Kent, in 1610, a man sold a coat belonging to his lodger, who had recently died of the plague. Unfortunately, the man who bought it died soon afterwards, as the coat was 'not well aired or purified'.

Preventing crowds from gathering and maintaining social distancing was top of the agenda. Theatres, many of which were in Southwark, were closed on 23 June, and did not open again until August 1594. The Westminster law courts were unable to commence their new term in October, and by the end of the month it was decided to hold them in Hertford instead. The High Court of Admiralty, which usually met in Southwark, was relocated to Woolwich. On 11 October, the usual ceremonies held to inaugurate the new Lord Mayor of London were cancelled, and the Queen suggested the budget be spent on relieving 'those persons whose houses are infected' instead.

Xenophobia and discrimination were never far away; we have seen how the Jews were scapegoated. Some blamed immigrants in general for introducing the plague to London. Miranda Kaufmann (2020) takes up the unfortunate story:

'The 'filthy keeping' of foreigners' houses was identified by the city authorities as 'one of the greatest occasions of the plague'. This might have helped to trigger the anti-immigrant feeling expressed by London apprentices in the spring of 1593. The trouble began in April when they set up 'a lewd and vile ticket or placard' on a post in London threatening violence against 'the strangers'. A series of 'divers lewd and malicious libels…published by some disordered and factious persons' appeared in the following weeks. One castigated the 'beastly brutes, the Belgians, or rather drunken drones, and fainthearted Flemings: and you, fraudulent father, Frenchmen' and threatened that if they did not 'depart out of the realm' by 9 July, over 2,000 apprentices would rise up against them. The verse set upon the wall of the Dutch church at Austin Friars in the City of London in early May did 'exceed the rest in lewdness': 'Strangers that inhabit in this land!…Egypt's plagues, vexed not the Egyptians more/Than you do us; then death shall be your lot'. The threatened violence never actually erupted. Some of the culprits were rounded up and 'put into the stocks, carted and whipped, for a terror to other apprentices and servants'. The Privy Council encouraged the Lord Mayor to use torture if necessary to prevent these 'lewd persons' from their 'wicked purpose to attempt anything against strangers'. For 'out of such lewd beginnings, further mischief doth ensue'.

Benedictow, Ole, 2004. *The Black Death 1345–1353: The Complete History*. Woodbridge

Fowler, Catherine 2015. 'Moving the Plague: the Movement of People and the Spread of Bubonic Plague in Fourteenth Century through Eighteenth Century Europe'. *University of Mississippi*

Kaufmann, Miranda, 13.3.2020, The Plague of 1592–3-echoes of today? http://www.mirandakaufmann.com/blog/the-plague-of-1592-3-echoes-of-today

Scott, Susan, 2004. *Biology of Plagues: Evidence from Historical Populations*. Cambridge

Chapter 18

1600 – 1650 South America malaria epidemic

If you think you are too small to make a difference, try sleeping with a mosquito.

– Dalai Lama

Malaria is a dangerously lethal disease caused by parasites of the genus *Plasmodium*, which is transmitted to humans by a bite of an infected female mosquito of the species *Anopheles*. The parasite, in the form of sporozoite, after a bite by an infected female mosquito, enters the human blood and after half an hour of blood circulation, enters the hepatocytes. The most common species in the Americas and Europe are *P.vivax* and *P.malariae*, while in Africa it is *P.falciparum*. Malaria persists as the leading cause of mortality around the world – only early diagnosis and fast-acting treatment prevent even worse outcomes than already prevail. It is the most common disease in Africa and some countries of Asia, while in the developed world malaria occurs as imported from endemic areas. The sweet sagewort plant was used as early as the second century BC to treat malaria fever in China. Much later, quinine took on the role of an anti-malaria drug.

Malaria enjoys a unique ever-present place in our history. Over thousands of years its depradations have been endured by Neolithic dwellers, early Chinese, Greeks and Romans, the rich, privileged, the poor and the marginalised. Just in the 20th century, malaria claimed between 150 million and 300 million lives, accounting for 2 to 5 per cent of all deaths. Although its main sufferers today are the poor of sub-Saharan Africa, Asia, the Amazon basin, and other tropical regions, 40 per cent of the world's population still lives in areas where malaria is transmitted. This is despite more than a century of global effort and research aimed at improving the prevention, diagnosis and treatment of malaria. The malaria mortality rate globally ranges from 0.3 – 2.2 per cent, and in cases of severe forms of malaria in regions with tropical climate it jumps from 11 to 30 per cent. Various studies have shown that the prevalence of malaria parasite infection has increased since 2015 mainly due to budget constraints.

Ancient writings and artifacts testify to malaria's long reign. Clay tablets with cuneiform script from Mesopotamia mention deadly periodic fevers suggestive of malaria. Malaria antigen was recently detected in Egyptian remains dating from 3200 and 1304 BC.[1] Indian writings of the Vedic period (1500 to 800 BC) called malaria the 'king of diseases'. In 270 BC, the Chinese medical canon, the *Nei Chin*, linked tertian

---

1. Miller et al., 1994)

(every third day) and quartan (every fourth day) fevers with enlargement of the spleen (a common finding in malaria), and blamed malaria's headaches, chills and fevers on three demons – one carrying a hammer, another a pail of water, and the third a stove. Homer (c. 750 BC) mentions malaria in *The Iliad*, as does Aristophanes (445–385 BC) in *The Wasps*, and Aristotle (384–322 BC), Plato (428–347 BC), and Sophocles (496–406 BC). Like Homer, Hippocrates linked the appearance of Sirius the dog star (in late summer and autumn) with malarial fever and misery. The malaria epidemic of AD 79 devastated the fertile, marshy croplands surrounding Rome, causing local farmers to abandon their fields and villages. The Roman Campagna would remain sparsely settled until finally cleared of malaria in the late 1930s.

Cunha, C.B., 2008. Brief history of the clinical diagnosis of malaria: from Hippocrates to Osler. *J Vector Borne Dis.* 45: 194–199

Dobson, M.J., 1989. History of malaria in England. *J R Soc Med.*; 82: 3–7

Sallares, R., 2002. *Malaria and Rome: a history of malaria in ancient Italy.* New York

Schlagenhauf, P., 2004, Malaria: from prehistory to present. *Infect Dis Clin North Am.* 18: 189–205

So great is the fear inspired by *Anopheles* that people were prepared to die rather than expose themselves to the chance of getting a lethal bite. Take for example Lu Tsu Chang, 'an official of talent and reputation' in 627 who was ordered by his emperor T'sai-tsung to go as governor to Giaio Province in northern Vietnam, pacify and defend it. The emperor warned him against refusing the posting on the grounds that it was so far away; Lu Tsu Chang did decline to go, but not because of the distance but because he knew there was 'much malaria in the south' and he feared that he would never return. His malariaphobia was greater than his fear of imperial anger: the emperor was indeed angry and had Lu Tsu Chang beheaded.

Most malaria cases in South America occur in the Amazon basin. In 2015, the four countries accounted for 83 per cent of malaria cases in the Americas: Brazil (24 per cent), Venezuela (30 per cent), Colombia (10 per cent), and Peru (19 per cent). Malaria continued to plague the United States until the early 20th century. Hundreds of thousands of Civil War soldiers were debilitated; for example, in 1862, General McClellan's army en route to Yorktown was stopped in its tracks. During the early days of the Pacific campaign in the Second World War more soldiers fell to malaria than to enemy forces. With the Vietnam War, the American military discovered that drug-resistant malaria was already widespread in Southeast Asia.

But malaria has enjoyed its richest pickings in Africa and proved to be a major stumbling block to colonization. Portuguese traders in the late 1400s and early 1500s were the first foreigners to confront the killing fever. For the next three centuries, whenever European powers tried to establish outposts on the continent, they were repelled time and again by malaria, yellow fever and other tropical scourges. This was indeed 'the White Man's Grave'.

The Oxford team behind the development of the Oxford-AstraZeneca vaccine (the ChAdOx1 nCov-2019 coronavirus vaccine) has another significant claim to pharmaceutical fame: the Oxford based Jenner Institute announced in early December 2020 that it was 'due to enter the final stage of human trials' with its cheap and effective vaccine for malaria – a vaccine which will form a powerful weapon in the battle against malaria which kills half a million people every year, most of them children. Professor Adrian Hill, director of the Jenner Institute said that 'malaria is a public health emergency. A lot more people will die this year in Africa from malaria than will die from COVID…probably ten times more'. Malaria kills a child every two seconds in the poorest parts of the world. Over 100 years of research has not yielded a fully licenced vaccine for malaria; the most successful vaccine so far, by GSK, has only 30 per cent efficacy.

Bruce-Chwatt, L.J., 1988. History of malaria from prehistory to eradication. In: Wernsdorfer W, ed;. Malaria: *Principles and Practice of Microbiology*, Edinburgh

Hempelmann, E., Krafts, K., 2013. 'Bad air, amulets and mosquitoes: 2,000 years of changing perspectives on malaria', *Malar. J.* 12 (1): 213.

Loy, Dorothy E., 2017. 'Out of Africa: origins and evolution of the human malaria parasites Plasmodium falciparum and Plasmodium vivax'. *International Journal for Parasitology*. 47 (2–3): 87–97

Reiter, P., 2000, From Shakespeare to Defoe: Malaria in England in the Little Ice Age. *Emerging Infectious Diseases*. 6(1):1–11.

Chapter 19

1616–1620 New England
infections epidemic

Nine parts ten, yea 'tis said nineteen parts twenty, Indians perished.
                                       – Puritan minister Cotton Mather

Why did the native American Indians of Massachusetts not exterminate the hapless Pymouth colonists during that atrocious winter of 1620–1621? After all, there was no love lost between the two as evidenced by a number of hostile conflicts between 1605 and 1620 when the British showed their customary violence in atrocities towards the native populations leading to 'invetrate malice towards the English'. 'Halfe of their company dyed…of 100 and odd persons, scarce 50 remained.' Scurvy did for the fatalities, as indeed it did for half the crew of the *Mayflower*, rendering survivors prey to other opportunistic diseases.

Disease and its bedfellow, famine, provide the answer. The 1616–1620 contagion raging through New England felled much of the native manpower focusing the minds of the survivors on the exclusion of what must have seemed like yet another minor incursion. There have been various attempts at assessing the plague mortality rate: in 1675 John Jocelyn reported that three tribes in Massachusetts were reduced from 30,000 to 3,000 (99 per cent attrition); Captain John Smith asserted in 1631 that 'it is most certaine that there was a great plague among them for where I have seen two or three hundred, within three yeares after remained scarce thirty.' (90 per cent). General Daniel Gookin files the most conservative depopulation estimates but even his show nothing below an 80 per cent loss: the Pequots declined from 4,000 to 300 (93 per cent); the Narragansetts from 5,000 to 1,000 (80 per cent); the Pawtuckets from 3,000 to 250 (90 per cent); and the Massachusetts from 3,000 to 300 (90 per cent).

Such a comprehensive and universal demographic decline could only have helped the Pilgrim newcomers, especially as the native survivors would have been weakened further because there were now fewer of them to do the necessary hunting in what was 'the starving time'.

It seems likely that the disease, whatever it was, was introduced from Europe when Sir Ferdinando Gorges sent Richard Vines and a company of traders to Maine to winter with the Indians in 1616–17. Captain Thomas Dermer tells us: 'We might perceive the sores of some that had escaped, who described the spots of such as usually die.'[1] Daniel Gookin reported that:

> 'I have discoursed with some old Indians, who were then youths, who say that the bodies all over were exceedingly yellow, describing it by a yellow garment they showed me, both before they died and after.'
> – Gookin, *Historical Collections of the Indians in New England* 1, 148

Bratton, T., 1988. The Identity of the New England Indian Epidemic of 1616 *Bulletin of the History of Medicine*, 62(3), 351–383.

Crosby, Alfred W., 1976, Virgin Soils Epidemics as a factor in the aboriginal depopulation in America, *William & Mary Quarterly* 33, 289–299

Hornbeek, Billee, 1976, An investigation into the cause or causes of the epidemic which decimated the Indian population 1616–1619, *New Hampshire Archaeologist* 19, 35–46

Cook, Sherburne F., 1973, The Significance of disease in the extinction of the New England Indian, *Human Biology* 45, 485–508

---

1. Baxter, *ibid* 1, 219–220.

Chapter 20

Plague in the 17th century

The Great Castilian Plague of 1596–1601

'Where ships go, the plague goes'

No one thought anything of the ship which, in late 1596, sailed from the Netherlands and docked in Santander; no one knew that one of its cargoes was plague; why should they? ...plague was not listed on the ship's manifest. Plague reached Madrid by 1599 and Seville by 1600. Over five years the disease killed some 500,000 people in Castile, around 10 per cent of the population. Add to this the mortalities from the 1646–52 Great Plague of Seville and the plague of 1676–1685 and historians estimate that the cost in human lives throughout Spain, in 17th century, was nearly 1.25 million. Consequently, the population of Spain scarcely increased between 1596 and 1696.

Mackay, Ruth, 2019, *Life in a Time of Pestilence The Great Castilian Plague of 1596–1601*, 2019, Cambridge

1600: a very bad year all round

Fake news is not a product of modern times nor is it confined to the on-line world. Sensationalist and alarmist hyperbole have been with us ever since the publication of the first news sheets. This extract gives a taste of the sensational reporting of contrived information that was so prevalent in the early 17th century and the inextricable link that was made between natural phenomena, famine and pestilence.

'The year 1600 was remarkable for pestilence in almost every part of Europe. Spain, where the disease was fatal the year before, was this year almost depopulated. There raged throughout Europe, a pestilential, mortal cholic which destroyed the lives of all whom it seized, within four days. The patient, as soon as he was seized, became senseless – the hair fell from his head – a livid pustule arose on the nose, which consumed it – the extremities became cold and mortified.

In Florence a terrible earthquake destroyed many buildings. The winter of 1600 was very cold. In the summer of 1600 there was a severe drought of four or five months; and a violent dysentery followed, with double tertians and continual fevers.

The plague raged in Portugal, attended with black round worms. At Christmas, there was an earthquake in England. The same year there was an earthquake at Arequipa, in Peru, accompanied by an eruption of a volcano.

In Muscovy [Moscow] the famine raged for three years ...attended with the plague. Parents devoured their dying children; cats, rats and every unclean thing was used to sustain life. All the ties of nature and morality were disregarded; human flesh was exposed to sale in the open market. The more powerful seized their neighbors; fathers and mothers, their children; husbands, their wives, and offered them for sale. Multitudes of dead were found, with their mouths filled with straw, and the most filthy substances. Five hundred thousand persons were supposed to perish in Muscovy, by famin and pestilence. At the same time, the famin in Livonia [on the eastern coast of the Baltic Sea, north of Lithuania], and the cold winter of 1602, destroyed 30,000 lives. The dead bodies lay in the streets, for want of hands to bury them. At the same time, raged a most dreadful pestilence in Constantinople, which also followed a famin. In England, there was also a dearth, and in 1603 perished 36,000 in London, of the plague, which was said to be imported from Ostend.

...In August 1603 in Paris died 2000 persons weekly of the plague. This disease was attributed to the diet and filth accumulated, under a defective police... The period under consideration was remarkable for the universality of the action of subterranean fire. The earthquakes of 1600 and 1601 and the bursting of a volcano in South-America have been mentioned. In 1603 there was an explosion of Etna. In 1604 a second eruption in Peru, and a comet.'

Webster, Noah (1758–1843). *A brief history of epidemic and pestilential diseases; with the principal phenomena of the physical world, which precede and accompany them, and observations deduced from the facts stated.*

The London Plague 1603

Pregnant women were advised to shield themselves from plague by eating toast covered in vinegar, butter and cinnamon.

– one of the measures introduced by James I

Regular publication of the Bills of Mortality began in 1603 when 33,347 deaths were recorded from plague. Between then and 1665, only four years passed with no recorded cases; 1625 saw 41,313 dead, between 1640 and 1646 there were 11,000 deaths, spiking in 3,597 with 1647. The 1625 outbreak was called the 'Great Plague', until deaths from the plague of 1665 outstripped it. Bills of Mortality gave their readers a picture of how 'in the Plague time how the sickness increased or decreased, so that the rich might judge of the necessity of their removal, and Tradesmen might conjecture what doings they were likely to have'.

– John Graunt, *Natural and Political Observations Made Upon the Bills of Mortality*, London, 1662.

The year 1603 was another bad year all round for England. In March the death of Elizabeth I was announced; she was succeeded by James I (James VI of Scotland). Then the plague arrived; it would go on to claim around a quarter of London's population. One of James' first reactions was to issue a book of Orders outlining rules and procedures to be followed in an attempt to stop the spread of the disease and to help those suffering from it. Thomas Dekker published his pamphlet, a *Wonderfull Yeare*: an account of the death of Elizabeth, accession of James I, and the 1603 plague which attempted to chronicle the extraordinary events of that year ('wonderful' meaning astonishing). Two more plague pamphlets, *News From Gravesend* and *The Meeting of Gallants at an Ordinary* were published. *The Seven Deadly Sins of London* (1606) was another plague pamphlet in circulation.

For James, quarantine, self-isolation and hygiene were the orders of the day: houses were 'to be closed up' for six weeks if one of the inhabitants fell ill, and the sick were encouraged to be 'restrained from resorting into company of others' for fear of spreading infection. If they did leave the house, they were to mark their clothes so as to warn others that they were infected. The ruling was enforced by watchmen – breaking these orders was punished by time in the stocks. 'Clothes, bedding and other stuffe as hath been worne and occupied by the infected of this disease' were burnt. As we have seen, pregnant women were advised to shield themselves from plague by eating toast covered in vinegar, butter and cinnamon. Those who were already exhibiting sores could ease them with a warmed mixture of onions, butter and garlic, or if these were not to hand, you could try simply laying 'a load of bread to it [the sore] hot as it commeth out of the oven'. James also ensured the sick would not lose everything: he ordered that collections should be made in order to support those who were locked in their houses and to replace their possessions.

Early face coverings were all the rage: people were advised to carry herbs such as rosemary, juniper, bay leaves, frankincense, sage and lavender to repel the bad airs, or else breathe through a handkerchief dipped in vinegar. Dekker colourfully described London's streets strewn with dead herbs, lying alongside the sick and dying: 'where all the pauement should in stead of greene rushes, be strewed with blasted Rosemary: withered Hyacinthes, fatall Cipresse and Ewe, thickly mingled with heapes of dead mens bones'.

Local lockdown and government 'following the science' came later in 1625:

'Orders thought meet by His Maiestie, and his Privy Councell, to bee executed throughout the counties of this realm, in such townes, villages, and other places, as are, or may bee heerafter, infected with the plague, for the stay of further increase of the same. Also, an advice set downe by the best learned in Physick within this realme, containing sundry good rules and easie medicines ... as well for the preseruation of his good subjects from the plague ... as for the curing.'

– England and Wales. Sovereign (1603–1625: James I)

Wilson, F.P., 1925. *The Plague Pamphlets of Thomas Dekker*. Oxford.

The Italian Plague (the Great Plague of Milan) 1629–1631

Ferrara: successful integrated disease management, the Renaissance way.

The Italian Plague of 1629–31 was a series of outbreaks of bubonic plague that tore through northern and central Italy claiming up to one million lives, or about 25 per cent of the population. The plague may well have been a factor in the decline of Italy's economy relative to those of other Western European countries.

Once again war, and the associated troop movements, had a role to play. German and French troops brought the plague to Mantua in 1629 during the Thirty Years' War (1618–1648). Infected Venetian troops spread the infection further afield when they retreated into northern and central Italy. October 1629 saw it reach Milan; despite effective public health measures, including quarantine and limiting the access of German soldiers and trade goods, the plague smouldered. A major outbreak in March 1630 resulted from health measures being relaxed during the carnival season; a second wave came in the spring and summer of 1631. Overall, Milan suffered approximately 60,000 fatalities out of a population of 130,000.

The Republic of Venice was hit in 1630–31 with the city of Venice recording 46,000 casualties out of a population of 140,000. Some historians contend that the huge loss of life, and its impact on commerce, contributed to the downfall of Venice as a major commercial and political power. Bologna lost an estimated 15,000 citizens to the plague, with Modena and Parma also being badly affected. This outbreak of plague also spread into the Tyrol of western Austria and northern Italy.

But while the pestilence was devastating the greater part of northern Italy, one town, Ferrara, escaped with not one fatality. How did they do it? Simple: by strict adherence to rules relating to aggressive border controls, robust sanitary laws and rigorous personal hygiene – integrated disease management, the Renaissance way. In Ferrara (population 30,000), reaching the highest threat level meant closing all but two of the city gates and posting permanent surveillance guards made up of wealthy noblemen, city officials, physicians and apothecaries. Anyone arriving at the city gates could not enter without identification papers called Fedi ('proofs') to confirm they had arrived from a plague-free zone. Then they would be screened for any signs of disease. Within the city people suspected of infection were moved into one of two *lazaretti* or plague hospitals outside Ferrara's city walls. Similar plague hospitals in Florence treated over 10,000 patients during the Plague of 1630–31, all paid for by the state.

Ferrara could boast a viable municipal sewer system since 1425. During the plague streets were swept of rubbish and cleared of 'filthy' animals like dogs, cats and chickens. Lime powder was spread liberally on any surface that may have come in contact with an infected person. Residents tried a range of measures to disinfect objects and surfaces. Any damaged or cracked furniture was removed and burned, while valuable objects and money were heated close to a fire and perfumes were sprayed throughout the house for fifteen days. Clothing and other textiles were hung out in the sun, beaten and doused with perfumes.

The citizens of Ferrara set a lot of store by a medicinal oil called Composito. By law, a ready supply of Composito had to be stored in a locked box set into the wall of the municipal palace for distribution in times of plague. The Spanish physician Pedro Castagno, who wrote Ferrara's influential *'Reggimento contra la peste'* ('Regimen against the plague'), described how the oily balm should be applied to the body.

> 'Before getting up in the morning, after lighting a fire of scented woods (juniper, laurel and vine shoots), warm the clothes and above all the shirt, rub first the heart region, near the fire to ease balm absorption, then the throat. [Afterwards], wash hands and face with acqua chiara (clean water) mixed with wine or vinegar of roses, with which sometimes all the body should be cleaned, using a sponge.'

Researchers have deduced that the balm contained myrrh and Crocus sativus, both known for their antibacterial properties, as well as venom from scorpions and vipers. All this was similar to anti-plague regimens used in other parts of Italy, particularly 'Oil of Scorpions' and an ancient ointment called Theriac, also made from viper venom. Other Italian towns deployed similar public health measures but they were unable to keep a clean sheet. John Henderson (2019) suggests that Ferrara's striking success may be down to its 'level of enforcement'.

A recent study (Alfani 2019) found that this plague depressed growth in several cities and 'caused long-lasting damage to the size of Italian urban populations and to urbanization rates. These findings support the hypothesis that seventeenth-century plagues played a fundamental role in triggering the process of relative decline of the Italian economies.'

Later outbreaks of bubonic plague in Italy occurred in Florence in 1630–1633 and the areas surrounding Naples, Rome and Genoa in 1656–57.

Alfani, Guido, 2013. 'Plague in seventeenth-century Europe and the decline of Italy: an epidemiological hypothesis'. *European Review of Economic History*. 17 (4): 408–430.

Alfani, Guido, 2001. 'Plague and long-term development: the lasting effects of the 1629–30 epidemic on the Italian cities'. *The Economic History Review*. 0 (4): 1175–1201.

Cipolla, Carlo M., 1981. *Fighting the Plague in Seventeenth Century Italy*. Madison: University of Wisconsin Press.

Henderson, John, 2019. *London, Florence Under Siege: Surviving Plague in an Early Modern City*.

The 1630s are notorious for plague outbreaks. They include: Augsburg (1632–35); Dijon (1631), Nurnberg (1632), Derbyshire (1632), Venice (1633), the Netherlands (1633–37), Hull (1635), London (1636), Newcastle (1636), Nijmegen (1636–37), Northampton (1637–38), Worcester (1637), Bergen (1637) and Prague (1637).

In terms of breaking bad news, the announcement that plague was in your town probably goes down as the worst possible news you could break in the 17th century. Obviously no one wanted to hear that they had the plague, especially at a time when there was no effective treatment anyway. The news meant isolation in a vile pesthouse with your worldly goods destroyed for fear that they could carry the infection.

Announcing the first plague case anywhere had serious ramifications; not least the probability that trade with other cities would come to an abrupt end leading to significant economic dislocation. At the same time we have a tendency to shoot the messenger, sometimes literally as when 'The physician who declared the presence of plague in Busto Arsizio near Milan in 1630 was shot to death,' while at Messina in 1743 another reporting physician had a narrow escape.

Delay, of course, costs lives as when the Paduans persuaded the Venetians that the disease in the city was 'pestilential fever' and not plague. The outbreak got worse claiming the lives of 46,000 of the 180,000 residents. Similar official denial is described in Oran in Algeria in Camus' *La Peste*.

Seville (1647–1652)

The Great Plague of Seville (1647–52) was a ferocious outbreak that killed up to a quarter of Seville's population. It seems to have originated on board a boat from Algeria before attacking Valencia first with an estimated 30,000 deaths. The disease raged through Andalucía, sweeping into Catalonia and Aragon. The coast of Málaga lost upwards of 50,000 people. In Seville, quarantine measures were evaded, ignored, or went unenforced. The results were catastrophic with the city of Seville and environs losing 150,000 people out of a population of 600,000. All in all Spain lost 500,000, out of a population of just under 10,000,000, or nearly 5 per cent of its entire population.

Plague in the Kingdom of Naples (1656)

> *The entire life of the city, in its everyday economic and sociological affairs, was trampled by the violence of a disease which appeared at the time to be a divine curse announcing the end of the world.*
>
> – https://www.ilcartastorie.it/en/la-peste-del-1656/

In 1656, a plague nearly wiped out the population of Naples. It was only prevented by forcible quarantine in the many poorer districts, and the efforts of a Martinus Ludheim, a visiting physician from Bavaria. It originated in the January when a Spanish soldier who had arrived from Sardinia, was admitted to the Annunziata Hospital. The alarm was sounded by Dr. Giuseppe Bozzutto, who first diagnosed the symptoms. His promptness and efficiency was not fully appreciated by the government, which imprisoned the doctor for having spread the worst of news. The plague, however, did not recognise this as an injustice and it was only when the corpses started to pile up, when food was running low, and when people started to vote with their feet and flee the city, that the government was forced to admit that there was indeed plague in Naples. That was in May. Mortality rates overall were an astonishing 870,000 – 1.25 million within the Kingdom of Naples and about half the city's 300,000 inhabitants. It would take Naples almost two centuries to recoup its pre-plague population.

Amsterdam (1663–1664)

> '*June 22 1664: there was 'great talk' at the coffee-house of 'the plague [which] grows mightily among them [the Dutch], both at sea and land'.*
>
> *July 25 1664 'no news, only the plague is very hot still, and increases among the Dutch.'*
>
> – Samuel Pepys

Any trading centre or port in the 17th century was highly likely to experience plague. Amsterdam was no exception; its outbreak of bubonic plague from 1663 to 1666 probably originated from Algiers about the same time that plague erupted in London. According to Samuel Pepys, for a few weeks at the end of 1663, ships from Hamburg and Amsterdam were quarantined for thirty days. In 1664, 24,148 people were buried in Amsterdam when over 10 per cent of the population died in this period. People assumed the plague was caused by the digging of new canals. The city government tried to scotch rumours about the imminent threat and downplay its magnitude in a bid to prevent panic.

Tobacco smoke was seen as an effective prophylactic against the plague. What with the plague and war with England looming, the English ambassador commented in May 1664: 'there are dead this last week to the number 338 at Amsterdam and if the plague thus increases within, and a warre with His Majestie without, there will be little need of that vast new towne which they are making there'. Rich people fled the cities to avoid the disease. The *vroedschap* (city council) warned that eating salad, spinach or prunes should be avoided. They shut the theatres, only allowing performances to resume in 1666.

A combination of quarantine measures and increased mortality adversely affected economic demand impacting on: the hospitality industry with residents and visitors avoiding taverns; the housing market depressing rents; demand for energy mainly in the form of peat and even the medical market where demand for midwives was down.

There were, nevertheless a number of significant socio-economic changes wrought by the plague. To compensate for the commercial hardship local governments initiated a raft of 'welfare policies'. Every town or city had its own policy reflecting the absence of a central government in the Dutch republic but, with the arrival of plague, a 'national' policy was developed. This attempted to prevent any incoming traffic of goods and persons from plague-infested places but was compromised by a concomitant rise in smuggling. Amsterdam also gives us one of the earliest instances of official advice relating to hand hygiene when regularly washing one's hands with water and vinegar was recommended, and to stay away from the sick.

The Great Plague of London: 1665–1666

Of all the diseases wherunto the body of man is subject, the Plague or Pestilence is the most fearfull.

– the opening words of a contemporary medical textbook,
The Plagues Approved Physitian

Nathaniel Hodges, president of the Royal College of Physicians, chimed in with: people 'terrorised each other with remembrances of a former pestilence'. High mortality, rapidity of spread and swiftness to death were the hallmarks of this universal terror.

Being an island in times of pestilence presents its own unique problems in disease containment and management. There are so many potential and unguarded points of entry. As we have seen, in 1663 plague in Amsterdam and Hamburg prompted the English Privy Council to impose quarantine for those vessels coming from those two international ports. The Privy Council, the Lord Mayor of London and city aldermen were at a collective loss as to how else to contain the pestilence; they pleaded the 'unprecedented times' excuse because, oddly, they could find 'no remembrance of what course had been taken to prevent its importation from foreign parts' during previous outbreaks. Instead they did something decidedly un-English, they looked to the 'custom of other countries' with the result that, 240 years after the first *lazaretto* was set up in Venice to combat the Black Death, they established one here to isolate potential threats coming into England.

Hole Haven at Canvey Island was the location – a good distance from London with a creek that 'could take one hundred vessels'. On 23 November 1663, Samuel Pepys, slipping up on his history, remarked how it was 'a thing never done by us before'. This was only partly true because there had been ship quarantine before, in 1635, for example, when the Lord Mayor of London had recommended the prohibition of vessels landing from infected places until a proper number of days had passed.

Two naval vessels were deployed to patrol the Thames Estuary, intercepting incoming ships that were 'English or foreign'. Those from infected ports or with crews showing symptoms of plague, such as the *Convertine* in 1665, would be ordered to turn back or were sent straight to Hole Haven for thirty days quarantine. By the late 17th century 'quarantine' meant any period of isolation rather than a full forty days. Impounded ships were cleansed, all cargo was aired onshore, and crews were isolated aboard their ships. If anyone died, their body was thrown overboard.

Tilbury was a second line of defence where incoming ships were inspected again and only ships issued with a certificate of health could pass. By 1664, as the situation everywhere deteriorated, the quarantine period was increased to forty days and more foreign ports were blacklisted. Outside London, the offshore quarantine procedure was rolled out across other key ports in England and Wales.

Someone somewhere will always find a way round such measures, be it by deceit, compassion or by privilege: a Dutch captain made it inland only to be sent back to his ship; a heavily pregnant woman, who had travelled from Hamburg to Rochester was permitted to land on the proviso that she was infection free; and in the spring of 1664, a merchant travelling with fifteen horses for the royal family appealed for his daughter to bring the horses up to London, for fear they might be 'stifled' at Hole Haven.

We can attribute the origin of London's plague to trading ships bringing in bales of cotton from plague-struck Amsterdam. The first cases were two French merchants, who died in London during December 1664. The next recorded cases occur in the spring of 1665 in the parish of St Giles-in-the-Fields outside the city walls (near the modern Tottenham Court Road), which then spread through the narrow alleys to the crowded and squalid parishes of Whitechapel and Stepney on its relentless journey to within the walled city of London. A riot erupted in St. Giles when the first house was sealed up; the crowd broke down the door and freed the inhabitants. Those rioters who were caught were severely punished.

In March 1665 war was declared between the Netherlands and England so the government's focus naturally shifted away from disease mitigation and prevention towards matters of war. According to the Bills of Mortality, nearly 70,000 Londoners died of bubonic plague in 1665, although this is surely an underestimation.

Until the outbreak of war the measures appeared to work: Hole Haven was a safe distance from the crowded and insanitary urban centre that was London and quarantined ships never got close enough to allow rats and their fleas to come ashore in London's docklands.

Samuel Pepys' diary gives us a vivid account of the unusually deserted streets with almost daily references to the echoing silence broken only by the noise of the searchers, those officials paid to locate corpses or drive the dead-carts shouting 'bring out your dead', and the sound of the clattering carts carrying them away to parish churches or communal plague pits, such as Finsbury Field in Cripplegate and the open fields in Southwark. The Bedlam burial ground was in use from 1569 to at least 1738; recent excavations suggest that perhaps 30,000 Londoners are buried there; *Yersinia pestis* DNA was found in the teeth of individuals buried in pits, confirming they had died of bubonic plague. In the streets bodies were being stacked up against the walls of houses and the plague pits became mounds of decomposing corpses. In Aldgate, a huge hole was dug 50 feet long and 20 feet wide – labourers were digging at one end while the dead-carts tipped in corpses at the other. When there was no room for further extension it was dug deeper until ground water was reached at 20 feet. When finally covered with earth it accommodated 1,114 corpses.

Plague doctors prowled the streets 'diagnosing' victims, many of these oddities could claim no form of medical training whatsoever. A plague doctor had to serve a long quarantine after seeing a plague patient in his plague doctor costume. He was regarded as a 'contact' who by agreement had to live in isolation to be quarantined. As in Amsterdam, tobacco was believed to be a prophylactic; apparently no London tobacconist ever died from the plague during the epidemic.

Under order of Charles II, no stranger was to be permitted in London without a certificate of health and public funerals were outlawed, 'unwholesome Meats, stinking Fish, Flesh, musty Corn' were forbidden from the marketplace, infected homes were to be 'shut up for forty days', and warders were to be appointed to prevent the unhealthy 'from conversing with the sound'. Measures were introduced to close some ale houses in affected areas and limit the number of lodgers allowed in a household. Nevertheless, Charles II had no idea just how far the plague would shutter and shatter England's economy and social life.

As we have seen in our coverage of the Black Death, plague was essentially a disease and killer of the poor and studies reveal that there were very few upper-class victims. In 1665, the mortality rates in the poorer parishes and suburbs to the south and north-east of the city were double those in the well-heeled centre. The flight of the rich (including Charles II) to alternative accommodation in the countryside at the beginning of epidemics, would partly account for this, as would the construction of the buildings inhabited by different social groups: well-maintained houses with tiled roofs would attract far fewer rats than the tumbledown huts of the poor. This was illustrated when most of the city's aldermen and other officials stayed at their posts – yet few died as they lived in better built houses. Plague is also essentially a disease of the household: once the rats of a house were flea infected, it was likely that most, if not all, of its human inhabitants would develop the disease, be they young or old, male or female.

Daniel Defoe wrote in his *Journal of the Plague Year*: 'Nothing was to be seen but wagons and carts, with goods, women, servants, children, coaches filled with people of the better sort, and horsemen attending them, and all hurrying away.'

Arnold, Catherine, 2006. *Necropolis: London and its dead*. London

Lincoln, Margaret, 2021, *London and the 17th Century: The Making of the World's Greatest City*, London

Sumich, Christie, 2013, 'A Broom in the Hand of the Almighty': The Plague and the Unruly Poor in: Divine Doctors and Dreadful Distempers: How Practising Medicine Became a Respectable Profession, *Clio Medical*

Malta (1675–1676)

Dr Giuseppe del Cosso insisted that it was not plague but a 'malignant pricking disease'.

The 1675–76 Malta plague epidemic caused approximately 11,300 deaths; the capital Valletta and the Three Cities (the fortified cities of Birgu, Senglea and Cospicua) had a mortality rate of about 41 per cent. In the rural settlements, the mortality rate was 6.9 per cent. Infected merchandise from Libya was probably the cause since the disease first appeared in the Valletta house of a merchant who possessed goods from Tripoli.

On Christmas Eve 1675 Anna Bonnici, the 11-year-old daughter of the merchant Matteo Bonnici, developed red petechial haemorrhages and enlarged lymph nodes; she died on 28 December. She was examined by Dr Giacomo Cassia who informed the protomedicus Domenico Sciberras of the case, but they did not identify the disease as plague. Things only got worse for the Bonnicis: on 10 January 1676, Anna's 2-year-old brother Giacchino died, and a female slave in their household became sick soon afterwards but recovered. The cause of these deaths was still not identified when another member of the family, 7-year-old Teresa, died from similar symptoms on 13 January. Members of the Agius family, relatives of the Bonnicis, also became ill and died; this finally caused alarm bells to ring and the authorities closed the houses of the victims. Matteo Bonnici also caught the disease and died on 25 January.

Despite a secret meeting which concluded that the disease was probably the plague, it was too late for the islands of Malta. All suspected cases were transferred to the *lazaretto* on the Isolotto where most of them died soon afterwards. Severe penalties including capital punishment awaited those who did not report cases to the authorities, and three men were hanged as an example. Looters found to have stolen items from houses belonging to people who had died were also hanged. Residents of parts of Valletta with high infection rates were forbidden to leave their homes but they were provided with food. Barbers were ordered not to cut the hair of infected people or their relatives. When the disease spread to the countryside, the entire island was declared infected and international quarantine measures were adopted.

Some were in denial: for example, Dr Giuseppe del Cosso insisted that it was not plague but a 'malignant pricking disease'. Many blithely went about their daily lives as usual – a major factor responsible for the exceedingly high death toll. People were then forbidden to congregate in churches and hotels or in outdoor public spaces, barricades were built and isolation hospitals were enlarged. Surgeons and doctors were drafted in from Naples and Marseille; a general curfew was proclaimed on 25 May. Houses were disinfected by *profumatori*. On 24 September 1676, the end of the epidemic was celebrated with the clearing of barricades, firing of guns, ringing of bells and processions.

As ever, ministering to the sick was a dangerous occupation: among the clergy, the dead included a Knight Grand Cross, 8 other knights, 10 parish priests, 1 canon, 95 other priests and 34 monks. Ten physicians, 16 surgeons and over 1,000 other health care workers also died.

One of the lasting legacies of the epidemic was that attempts were made to improve medical teaching in Malta. This formalisation of medical training is the forerunner of the medical school of the University of Malta. Traditional Maltese mourning rites had to change as a result of the 1676 plague. Before the epidemic, mourning periods would last for one or two years, and three days after a person died no fire would be lit in the kitchen in the house of the deceased. Women were in purdah for forty days, while men would go out unshaven after eight days. These were abandoned in favour of wearing black.

Grima, Joseph F. (22 December 2019). 'The beginning of Malta's worst plague outbreak in 1675'. *Times of Malta*.
Scerri, Louis (12 March 2017). 'The plague that decimated Malta twice over'. *Times of Malta*.

Spain – Andalucia and Valencia (1676–1685)

To the Spanish it must have seemed that the plague which prostrated Seville was never going away, because just 25 years later, another plague outbreak ravaged the country. For nine years (1676–1685), wave after wave of the pestilence subdued the country, striking parts of Andalucía and Valencia particularly savagely. The poor harvest of 1682–83 conspired with the disease to create serious famine, the combined effects of which killed tens of thousands of the weakened and exhausted population. By the time it was finally all over in 1685, it is estimated to have claimed over 250,000 lives. This was the last outbreak of plague in Spain in the 17th century.

Factoring in normal births, deaths, and emigration, it is estimated that the total human death toll throughout Spain in the 17th century, was a minimum of nearly 1.25 million. As a result, the population of Spain scarcely changed between 1596 and 1696. The plagues naturally had an adverse economic effect on the country.

J. H. Elliott, J.H. 1961, 'The Decline of Spain', *Past and Present*, Vol. 20 pp. 52–75; reprinted in Elliott, Spain and its World 1500–1700 (New Haven, 1989), pp. 217–240.
J. I. Israel, J.I., 1978, 'The Decline of Spain: A Historical Myth?', *Past and Present*, Vol. 81 pp. 170–85.

The Great Plague of Vienna (1679)

'Viennese death'

Being a major trading crossroads between east and west, Vienna, home to the Habsburgs, was always susceptible to outbreaks of plague since the 14th century Black Death. Add to that the disgusting conditions in the overcrowded and densely populated city with stinking heaps of rotting garbage, human waste slopping in the streets, no drainage or sewerage systems, with numerous warehouses piled high with all manner of goods from the known world, from grain to carpets and clothing, and you have a perfect plague storm. Rats must have proliferated in these infected conditions; in fact, so unhealthy and filthy was Vienna even by the low standards of the day, that the plague often carried the title 'Viennese death' in other parts of Europe.

Doctors, as everywhere, were at a loss as to how to treat patients; they tried emetics, bloodletting and applying noxious ointments; all, of course, to no avail. Corpses were carted to the the city limits and slung into large open pits for burning. However, before that the pits were left in the open air for several days until they were full, exposing the rats to ongoing infection.

Wherever you looked there seemed to be plague. In 1666 a severe outbreak tore into Cologne lasting until 1670. France endured its last plague epidemic in 1668 while in 1675–84 a new plague originated in the Ottoman Empire centered on Turkey and areas of the Balkans before invading North Africa, Bohemia, Poland, Hungary, Austria and Saxony, progressing generally northward.

Vienna's plague was exceptionally severe, causing at least 76,000 deaths. Other cities in central Europe suffered similar levels of casualties: Prague in 1681 lost 83,000; Dresden was affected in 1680, Magdeburg and Halle in 1682. In Halle, a mortality of 4,397 out of a population of about 10,000 was recorded. Many north German city populations fell in these years. By 1683, the plague disappeared from Germany until the epidemic of 1707.

To commemorate the city's deliverance from the Great Plague and later waves of the disease, the Viennese erected monuments such as the famous Baroque Karlskirche with the associated 69-foot plague columns known as the Pestsäule. From the privileged position of having fled his city (and his people), the Habsburg emperor Leopold I vowed to erect a mercy column if only the epidemic would end.

Langdon-Davis, J., 1963, *The Plague and Fire of London*, London

Shrewsbury, J.F.D., 1970, *A History of Bubonic Plague in the British Isles*, Cambridge

Velimirovic, Boris, 1989, Plague in Vienna, *Reviews of Infectious Diseases*, 11, Issue 5, 1989, 808–826

Chapter 21

1633–1634 The Massachusetts
smallpox epidemic

'...deserted wigwams and deserted villages dotted the landscape...the loss of so many children and young people made it difficult for the Pequot populations to rebound even after the epidemics had run their course.'

– The Mashantucket Pequot Museum and Research Center laments the
annihilation of the Pequot

I f smallpox was not the disease which afflicted the native Americans in the New England 1616–19 epidemic described above then it certainly was to blame for the Massachusetts smallpox epidemic, or Colonial Epidemic, that ravaged Massachusetts in 1633.

As we have seen, Europeans brought smallpox to North America in their ships and with their crews when they first started their programme of colonisation. For example, twenty settlers on the *Mayflower* which left England in 1620 were infected, including their only doctor, Samuel Fuller, who became physician for the Plymouth Colony. Some research indicates that Fuller had no medical knowledge at the time of the voyage and mugged up on the rudiments of medicine during the journey. The *Mayflower* did, however, have three surgeons on board headed by the fittingly (or paradoxically, given the profession) named Giles Heale who had been admitted to the Guild of Barber-Surgeons in London in 1619.

By 1618, more than two thirds of the Massachusetts native Americans including the Mohawks, native people in the Lake Ontario area and the Iroquois, died from smallpox.

The *Mayflower* docked in Plymouth Bay on 20 December 1620. The settlers began building the colony's first house on 25 December but they were severely hampered when a pestilence attacked them, a pestilence which had emerged on the ship. On 11 January 1621, William Bradford (1590–1657) was helping to build houses when he was suddenly struck with great pain in his hipbone and collapsed. William Bradford of Austerfield became Governor in 1621; he recovered, but many of the other settlers were not so lucky.

During February and March 1621, sometimes two or three people died each day. In an attempt to hide their diminishing number from the native Americans who might be observing them, the settlers buried their dead in unmarked graves on Cole's Hill, often at night, and attempted to conceal the burial plots by allowing them to get overgrown.

When the first house was finished, it was requisitioned as a hospital for the sick pilgrims. Thirty-one of the company were dead by the end of February, with fatalities still rising.

Between the landing and March, only forty-seven colonists had survived the diseases they contracted on the ship. During the worst of the sickness, only six or seven of the group were able to feed and care for the rest. In this time, half the *Mayflower* crew also died.

During an expedition the settlers came across a cleared village known as Patuxet to the Wampanoag people; it had been abandoned three years earlier following a plague that killed all of its residents. The 'Indian fever' involved haemorrhaging and is assumed to have been fulminating smallpox. The outbreak had been so severe that the colonists discovered unburied skeletons in the dwellings.[1]

Relatively speaking, the European settlers remained less affected by smallpox in the 1630s. A New England colonist in 1630 said the native Americans 'fell down so generally of this disease as they were in the end not able to help one another, not to make a fire, nor to fetch a little water to drink, nor any to bury the dead...'. Yet despite the carnage wrought by smallpox, it was seen as a gift from God by some Puritans, including Increase Mather, a clergyman and one of Harvard's first presidents, who stated that the smallpox epidemic was God's solution to the native American and Puritan land disputes.

A letter dated 2 August 1630 from Samuel Fuller to Sir William Bradford describes the parlous situation in England and in North America:

> 'There is come hither a ship (with cattle, and more passengers) on Saturday last; which brings this news out of England; that the plague is sore, both in the city and country, and that the University of Cambridge is shut up by reason thereof; also, that there is like to be a great dearth in the land by reason of a dry season. The Earl of Pembroke (8 April 1580 – 10 April 1630) [Chancellor of the University of Oxford] is dead, and Bishop Laud is Chancellor of Oxford.... The sad news here is, that many are sick, and many are dead, the Lord in mercy look upon them! ..., I can do them no good, for I want drugs, and things fitting to work with... Mrs. Cottington is dead. Your loving brother in law, Samuel Fuller.'
>
> Samuel Fuller – *Mayflower Descendant*,
> Vol. 7, pg. 81–82.

Crosby (2004) points out that the first recorded outbreak of smallpox in British or French North America erupted in the early 1630s among the Algonquins of Massachusetts: 'whole towns of them were swept away, in some not so much as one soul escaping Destruction'.

---

1. Bradford Book 2, 1621

Stephanie Peters (2005) reminds us that many European settlers praised God for the disease because it gave them unopposed and unfettered access to Indian lands and thus facilitated their colonization in a way never imagined.

This is how Bradford graphically describes this outbreak:

'...they fall into a lamentable condition as they lye on their hard matts, ye poxe breaking and mattering, and runing one into another, their skin cleaving (by reason therof) to the matts they lye on; when they turne them, a whole side will flea of at once, (as it were,) and they will be all of a gore blood, most fearfull to behold ... they dye like rotten sheep. The condition of this people was so lamentable... they would burne ye woden trayes & dishes they ate their meate in, and their very bowes & arrowes; & some would crawle out on all foure to gett a litle water, and some times dye by ye way, & not be able to gett in againe...The cheefe Sachem him selfe now dyed, & allmost all his freinds & kinred. But by ye marvelous goodnes & providens of God not one of ye English was so much as sicke, or in ye least measure tainted with this disease, though they dayly did these offices for them for many weeks togeather. And this mercie which they shewed them was kindly taken.'

Duffy, John, 1951, Smallpox and the Indians in the American Colonies, *Bulletin of the History of Medicine* 25, 327

Peters, Stephanie True, 2005, *Epidemic! Smallpox in the New World*, Tarrytown NY

Snow, Dean R., 1988, European Contact and Depopulation in the Northeast: the timing of the first epidemics, *Ethnohistory* 35, 15–33

Chapter 22

The 1648 Central America
yellow fever epidemic

*'If you get yellow fever today your chances of survival are probably not much different
than they were in the 1700s or the 1800s. It's still going to be 1 out of every 5 or so who
are going to die. There is no treatment, you can prevent it but you can't treat yellow fever.'*
— Jim Writer, *Yellow Jack: How Yellow Fever Ravaged America and Walter Reed
Discovered Its Deadly Scourge.*

Yellow fever is a short-lasting viral disease with symptoms which typically
include fever, chills, loss of appetite, nausea, muscle pains particularly in the
back, and headache. These usually get better within five days but in about
15 per cent of patients, within a day of improving, the fever returns with a vengeance
and victims enter a second, toxic phase of the disease. Victims then suffer recurring
fever, accompanied by jaundice due to liver damage, as well as abdominal pain;
bleeding in the mouth, nose, the eyes, and the gastrointestinal tract triggering vomit
containing blood. Hence the Spanish name for yellow fever, *vómito negro*, 'black vomit'.
There may also be kidney failure, hiccups and delirium. The mortality rate is 20 to
50 per cent. Severe cases may have a mortality greater than 50 per cent.

Survivors enjoy lifelong immunity, and normally no permanent organ damage
results. In 1927 yellow fever virus became the first human virus to be isolated.

Yellow fever is caused by yellow fever virus and is spread by the bite of an infected
female mosquito, *Aedes aegypti*, a type of mosquito found throughout the tropics and
subtropics. But other *Aedes* mosquitoes such as the tiger mosquito (*Aedes albopictus*)
can also be a vector. The virus is an RNA virus of the genus Flavivirus. There is now
a safe and effective vaccine.

The virus probably originated in East or Central Africa whence it spread to West
Africa infecting monkeys and mosquitoes and small village population groups of
humans. As it was endemic in Africa, local populations had developed some immunity
to it: when yellow fever broke out in an African community where colonists resided,
most Europeans died, while the indigenous Africans usually developed non-lethal
symptoms resembling influenza – acquired immunity in effect. It then spread to south
and central America with the slave trade in the 17th century with mosquito larvae
flourishing in water kegs on board the slave ships: rapid transmission in the crowded
confines came when some of the slaves, infected with yellow fever, were bitten by
mosquitoes, which then bit uninfected people, spreading the disease.

It was first introduced into Recife, Brazil, between 1685 and 1690. This was preceded by the first definitive outbreaks – in Guadeloupe in 1635, on Barbados in 1647 and in Mexico's Yukatan Peninsula where it killed half the Mayan and Spanish population, and the Carribean Windward Islands in 1648. The indigenous Mayans called the illness *xekik* ('blood vomit'). The earliest mention of 'yellow fever' appears in a manuscript of 1744 by Dr. John Mitchell of Virginia. In the 18th and 19th centuries, yellow fever was regarded as one of the most dangerous infectious diseases.

Barbados had been systematically ecologically transformed with the introduction of sugar cultivation by the Dutch. Those rain forests so plentiful in the 1640s were completely levelled by the 1660s. By the early 18th century, the same sugar plantation depredation had occurred on Jamaica, Hispaniola and Cuba. Sugar plantations and the environmental and ecological disruption they caused to natural habitats have a lot to answer for: they created the perfect conditions for mosquito and viral reproduction, leading to subsequent outbreaks of yellow fever. Deforestation reduced populations of insectivorous birds and other creatures that fed on the guilty mosquitoes and their eggs.

It did not take long for the epidemic to spread north so that between 1668 and 1699 outbreaks were reported in New York, Boston and Charleston. Bermuda went on to endure four yellow fever epidemics in the 1800s which in total claimed the lives of 13,356 people, military and civilian. During the 1864 epidemic, Dr. Luke Pryor Blackburn, from Halifax, Nova Scotia, an expert on the disease, visited the island several times, to assist the local medical community. When he departed in October 1864, he left behind some trunks of soiled clothing that were to have been sent on to him in Canada.

It transpired that Blackburn's visits had been bankrolled by the Confederacy, and that a certain Union informer had been offered $60,000 to distribute Dr. Blackburn's trunks of soiled clothing to Union cities including Boston, Philadelphia, Washington and Norfolk. One trunk also went to New Bern, which was identified as having introduced yellow fever to that city, claiming the lives of 2,000 people. Blackburn was arrested and tried, but acquitted owing to lack of evidence, which still left the toxic trunks unaccounted for. In 1878, he went on to fight yellow fever in Kentucky where he had set up a practice in Louisville and was eventually elected governor.

It did not take long for West Indies postings to win a reputation as dangerous places to be sent – not just because of the conflicts there but also due to the endemicity of yellow fever throughout colonial times and during the Napoleonic Wars (1803–1815). No wonder: the majority of the British soldiers sent to Haiti in the 1790s died of disease, chiefly yellow fever, and the mortality rate in British garrisons in Jamaica was seven times that of garrisons in Canada, largely because of the ravages of yellow fever and other tropical diseases. Both English and French forces posted to the Caribbean suffered terribly with the 'yellow jack'.

In 1802–03, Napoleon Bonaparte despatched an army 40,000 strong to Saint-Domingue to suppress the slave-led Haitian Revolution; bad move: yellow fever accounted for about 35,000 to 45,000 casualties: among the victims was the expedition's commander and Bonaparte's brother-in-law, Charles Leclerc. Some scholars believe Napoleon intended to use the island as a staging point for an invasion of the United States through Louisiana, then newly regained by the French from the Spanish.

Others, more likely, believe that Napoleon was anxious to regain control of the lucrative sugar trade in Saint-Domingue (Hispaniola). Only one-third of the French troops survived to return to France, and in 1804 the new republic of Haiti declared its independence.

Napoleon gave up on the island and abandoned his plans for North America, negotiating the Louisiana Purchase to the US in 1803. This was the acquisition of Louisiana by the United States from France for 15 million dollars. Acquiring the territory doubled the size of the United States at the time, at the knock-down price of less than 3 cents per acre. But for Napoleon, without significant revenues from sugar colonies in the Caribbean, Louisiana was of little value.

Meanwhile, back in Europe, major outbreaks continued to erupt in Atlantic ports following the arrival of sailing vessels coming back from the Caribbean, usually Havana. In 1730, 2,200 deaths were reported in Cadiz, Spain, followed by outbreaks in French and British seaports. Outbreaks occurred in Barcelona, in 1803, 1821 and 1870. In the last of these, 1,235 fatalities were recorded out of an estimated 12,000 cases. Smaller localized outbreaks occurred in Saint-Nazaire in France, Swansea, and, in the most northerly case, Glasgow, as well as in other European port cities. A cargo of copper ore from Cuba was discharged at Swansea docks in mid-September 1865, during a spell of exceptionally hot weather. A small number of mosquitoes infected with the yellow fever virus, came ashore at the same time and promptly established an epidemic of yellow fever in the town. In the next 25 days, at least 27 inhabitants were infected and 15 of them died.

Espinosa, M., 2009. *Epidemic Invasions: Yellow Fever and the Limits of Cuban Independence, 1878–1930.* Chicago

Marr, John S., 2013, 'The 1802 Saint-Domingue yellow fever epidemic and the Louisiana Purchase.' *Journal of Public Health Management and Practice* 19#.1, 77–82.

Meers, P. D., 1986. 'Yellow fever in Swansea, 1865'. *The Journal of Hygiene.* 97 (1): 185–91

Sawchuk, L. A. 1998. 'Gibraltar's 1804 Yellow Fever Scourge: The Search for Scapegoats'. *Journal of the History of Medicine and Allied Sciences.* 53 (1): 3–42

Chapter 23

The 1677–1678 Boston smallpox epidemic

'In Boston burial-places never filled so fast with bells tolling for burials from sunrise, and 'corpses following each other close at their heels'.

– Cotton Mather

The state of Massachusetts, and Boston in particular, can claim a number of firsts in the control of smallpox: it was in Massachusetts that inoculation for smallpox was first experimented in the Americas. Massachusetts was the first state in which vaccination against smallpox was performed. The first medical publication in the US was a broadside on the treatment of smallpox published in Boston. The first state compulsory law for the vaccination of school children was passed in Massachusetts.

The first surviving printed map of Boston dates from 1722 and was drawn by Captain John Bonner, a navigator and a shipwright who died in 1726. Among its many interesting features it helpfully lists the smallpox epidemics occurring in Boston up to 1722: they were in 1649, 1666, 1677, 1678, 1680, 1690, 1702 and 1721. Wider New England suffered smallpox epidemics in 1677, 1689–90, and 1702. During this time, public health authorities in Massachusetts dealt with the threat primarily by means of quarantine: incoming ships were quarantined in Boston Harbor, and any smallpox patients were held under guard or in a 'pesthouse'.

Here is a roll call of smallpox and its association with Boston up to the 1677 epidemic: it only took a year after its settlement in 1630 for Boston to register smallpox related deaths. In 1633 it wiped out almost every native as far north as the Piscataqua and destroyed some 300 Narragansetts to the south; in 1636 the General Court moved out to Cambridge and later to Roxbury to escape the disease then raging in Boston; in 1638 Winthrop reports that 'two ships came in much "pestered", lost many passengers and some principal men', that, 'many fell sick after they landed and again many of these died and many inhabitants with them'; in 1659 the General Court sat at Charlestown on account of the spread of the smallpox in Boston.

In the winter of 1677–78 smallpox again reared its head, introduced as usual by English ships, with many deaths recorded. Fast days were held to stay its progress. So, by the time of the 1677 epidemic, Boston had more than enough experience of this disease, which probably emerged even before the *Mayflower* set sail in 1620. In around 1613 the Narragansetts alone were some 3,000 warriors strong and had they been at full strength they would surely have repelled with ease the invaders. The attempt to found a settlement at Plymouth would have failed, as did the similar effort at Jamestown in 1607, had not the depradations of smallpox played their deadly part. As Woodward (1932) points out: 'smallpox was the blessing in disguise that gave our emigrant ancestors an opportunity to found the state'.

It was reported that on 30 September 1677, thirty people died of smallpox. So intense was the fear and suffering caused by the 1677–78 epidemic that the Massachusetts General Court issued three proclamations, each calling for an official day of 'humiliation' and prayer and prohibiting all work on those days. The outbreak also triggered the first medical paper to be published in the American colonies. Thomas Thatcher wrote a broadside in 1677 and called it *A Brief Rule to guide the Common People of New England How to order themselves and theirs in the Small Pocks, or Measels'*, which offered advice to the public on how to deal with the disease.

Thatcher advised avoiding excessive heat or cold, desisting from meat and wine and eating watergruel made with indian-flour, not with oatmeal, supping small beer warmed with a 'tost', drinking warm milk and eating boiled apples and any other easily-digested foods. Thatcher was one of the pre-eminent preacher-physicians of the day: the combination of medicine and theology was common on both sides of the Atlantic and was well established. Medicine was not a distinct profession but was practised by the clergy, even by those in the higher echelons: for example, the Bishop of Worcester was physician to Richard II. Thatcher by his publication paved the way for a more humane treatment of smallpox in the USA; nevertheless smallpox continued to ravage. We learn of the 'boyling of the blood by which nature thrusts out the impurities from veins to flesh and from flesh to skin' and are warned of 'the danger of overhastening or overdelaying this process either by too many clothes, too hot rooms, cordials like Diascordium, Gascon's powder and such like, or by cooling by bloodletting, glysters, vomits, purges or cooling medicines, lest by the first treatment come phrenzies, dangerous sweats or flowing of the pocks together, or by the latter means there be raked away that supply of blood which should keep them out until they are ripe.'

In November 1678 Cotton Mather reported that 'Boston burial-places never filled so fast' with bells tolling for burials from sunrise, and, somewhat gruesomely, 'corpses following each other close at their heels' and 38 dying in one week, 'above 340 have died in Boston... since it first assaulted the place'. Grob (2002) tells us that the quarantine measures prevented its spread to neighbouring towns; for example Gallups Island was selected as a voluntary quarantine station.

Bostonians were aware of the contagious nature of smallpox without, of course, understanding how it was transmitted. The town records of 6 May 1677, contain specific instructions for the airing out of any clothes or bedding of a person who had smallpox.[1] There were four specific areas where linens could be laid out, during the 'dead time' of the night and not in back yards or in the street. Three citizens, the Boston Selectmen, worked with the police to ensure that these rules were followed. Sick people were also under quarantine orders to remain in their homes until they

---

1. Blake 1959, p. 20

The Reconstruction of Myrtis. Myrtis is the name given by archaeologists to an 11-year-old girl from Athens, whose remains were discovered in 1994–95 in a mass grave at Kerameikos, Greece. Forensic analysis showed that Myrtis and two other bodies had perhaps died of typhoid fever during the Plague of Athens in 430 BC. (*Tilemahos Efthimiadis*)

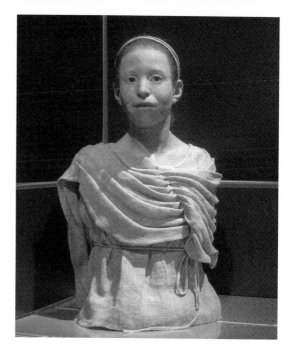

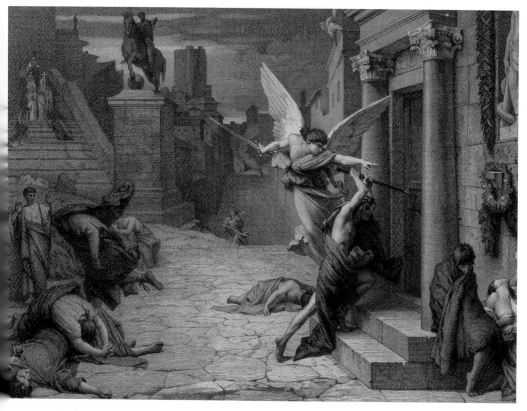

The angel of death knocking on a door during the plague of Rome. In the left background, the steps are leading up to the church of S. Maria Aracoeli. To the right, we see a shrine to Aesculapius with a statue and inscription 'AESCVLAP[IO] SERVATO[RI]'. (*Engraving by Levasseur after J. Delaunay. From the Wellcome Library*)

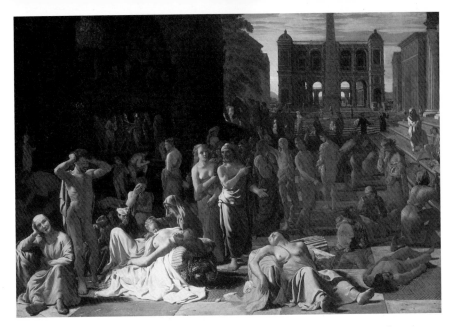

Michael Sweerts' 'Plague in an Ancient City' (ca. 1652–54). Possibly the Plague of Athens. (*Los Angeles County Museum of Art*)

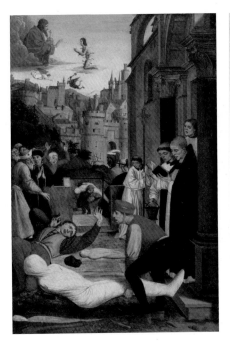
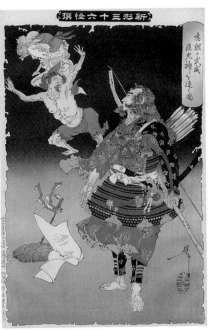

Above left: St Sebastian pleading for the life of a gravedigger afflicted with plague during the Plague of Justinian, AD 541–549. (*Josse Lieferinxe (–1508) Walters Art Museum, Baltimore*)

Above right: Tsukioka Yoshitoshi, 'Driving Away the Demons'. October 1890. From the Thirty-six Ghosts series. The print shows Minamoto no Tametomo driving away the smallpox demons.

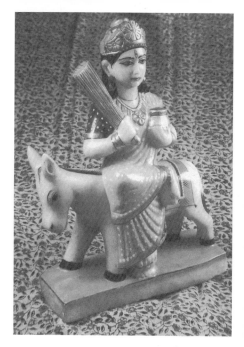 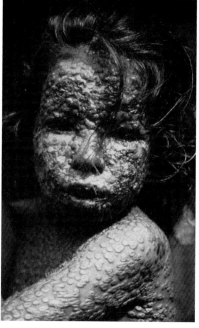

Above left: Sitala Mata. Sitala (शीतला śītalā), is a Hindu goddess; as an incarnation of Supreme Goddess Durga, she cures poxes, sores, ghouls, pustules and diseases. She gives coolness to those afflicted with fever.

Above right: A child infected with smallpox in Bangladesh, 1973.

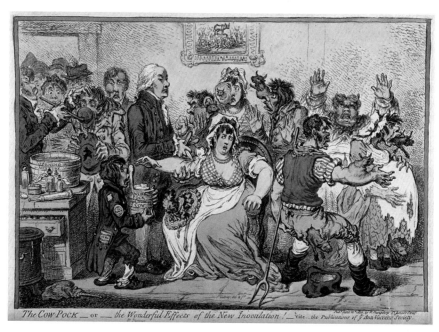

This 1802 caricature of Edward Jenner vaccinating patients against smallpox using cowpox (a procedure pioneered by Jenner in 1796) demonstrates the fears found among the population regarding new medical techniques – early anti-vaxxers. (*Wellcome Collection, V0011069*)

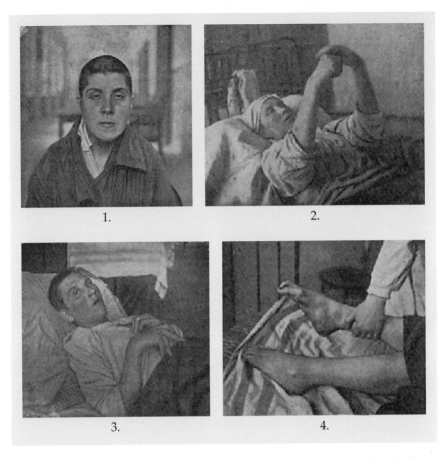

Encephalitis Lethargica. A page from Margulis MS: *Acute Encephalitis: Epidemic and Sporadic*. Moscow, Government Publishers, 1923. Photo 1: 'lethargy in both eyes'; photo 2: 'catalepsy', i.e. the patient can sleep in any position; photo 3: patient with muscle cramps in the fingers; photo 4: patient with muscle cramps in the feet.

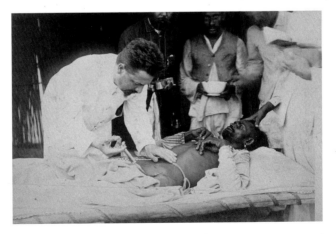

Dr. Simmonds injecting his curative serum in a plague patient during the outbreak of bubonic plague in Karachi, 1897. Karachi was placed in quarantine in 1882, during the outbreak of bubonic plague which spread from Bombay. (*Wellcome Library. Photograph probably by R. Jalbhoy*)

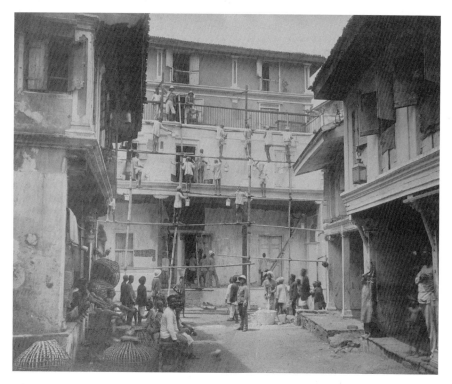

Above and below: Washing away the plague in Bombay 1896–1905. Workers clean a house in a neighbourhood affected by the 1896 bubonic plague. (*Capt. C. Moss, Wellcome Library*)

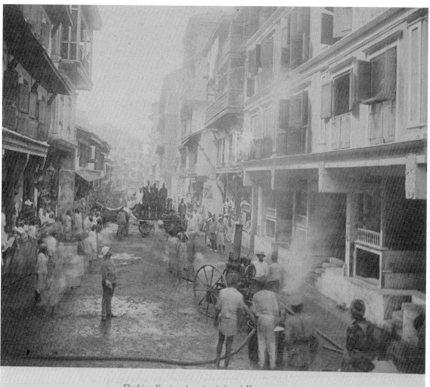

Flushing Engine cleansing infected Houses.

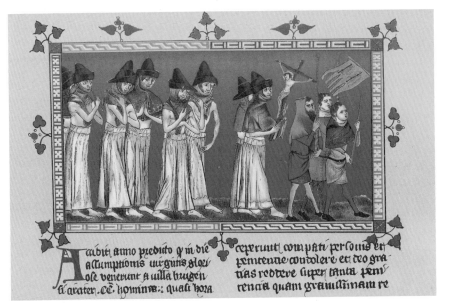

Acabit anno predicto g in die Aflumptionis uirginis glou ose uenerunt a uilla brugen si arater. CC. hominus :. quasi hora ceperunt compati personis et penitente condolere et deo gra tias redere super tanta peni renia quam grauissinam re

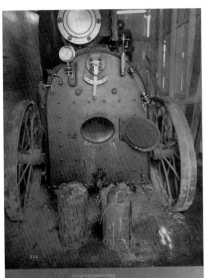

Above: Flagellants at Doornik in the Netherlands scourging themselves in atonement, believing that the Black Death is a punishment from God for their sins, 1349.

Left: The rat incinerator in Sydney.

Below: Rat catchers with a pile of dead vermin in Sydney in 1900. Rats were fetching up to 6d a head during the outbreak.

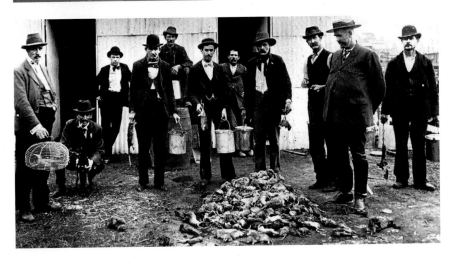

A heap of rats in Sydney; about 600 of them. Tens of thousands of rats were killed and incinerated. Captain Thomas Dudley, who worked at the Sydney wharves as a sailmaker, exhibited symptoms: he had been living near east Darling Harbour where he noticed scores of dead rats; moreover, he had been pulling dead rats from his toilet before falling ill.

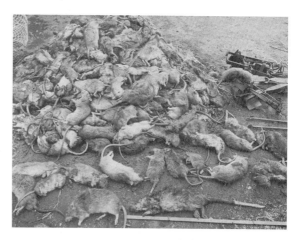

Sydney's Sutton Forest Butchery's at 761 George Street; the meat preparation area was clearly less than ideal and probably contributed to the mortality figures. Views taken during Cleansing Operations, Quarantine Area, Sydney, 1900, Vol. IV / under the supervision of Mr George McCredie. (*Pictures 14–17 courtesy of the Mitchell Library, State Library of New South Wales, [FL1087836; FL1064108; FL1064109; FL1087816]*)

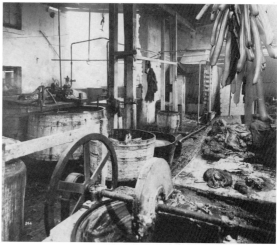

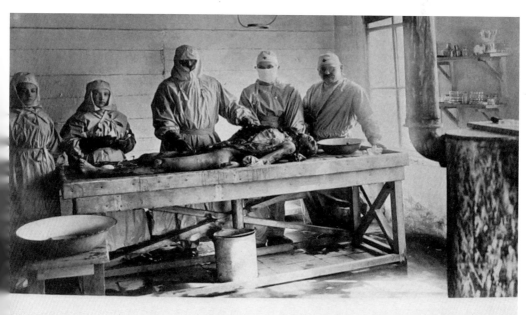

Вскрытіе труповъ чумныхъ членами русской научной экспедиціи.

A picture of a Manchurian plague victim in 1910–1911.

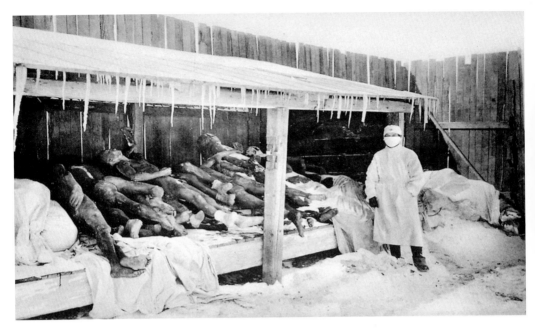

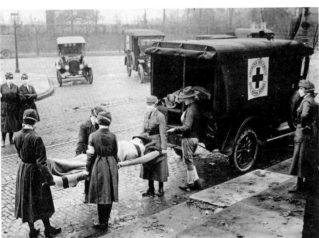

Above: Dead Manchurian plague victims held in storage awaiting scientific research.

Left: 1918 flu patients in St Louis – Red Cross Motor Corps in attendance, October 1918.

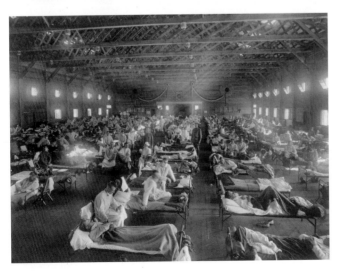

Camp Funston, Kansas emergency hospital during the 1918 flu pandemic. In March 1918, Chinese contract workers at the camp presented with influenza. Soon, the disease spread across the camp requiring hospitalization of over 1,100 soldiers within three weeks, besides thousands more receiving treatment at infirmaries around the camp.

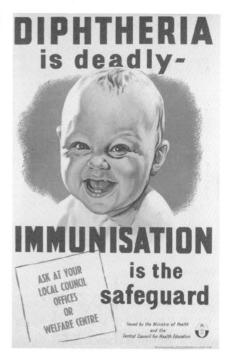

TOUT LE MONDE L'A (ter) L'INFLUENZA!

La Ronde des Médecins et des Potards.

DIPHTHERIA is deadly-

IMMUNISATION is the safeguard

ASK AT YOUR LOCAL COUNCIL OFFICES OR WELFARE CENTRE

Above left: 'Everyone has Influenza' – The Round of Doctors and Druggists. The 12 January 1890, edition of the Paris satirical magazine *Le Grelot* depicted an unfortunate influenza sufferer bowled along by a parade of doctors, druggists, skeleton musicians and dancing girls representing quinine and antipyrine. (*Wood engraving by Pépin (E. Guillaumin), 1889 via Wellcome Images*)

Above right: 'Diphtheria is Deadly' – UK poster encouraging vaccination.

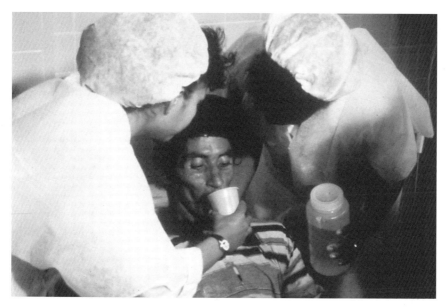

This cholera patient is drinking oral rehydration solution (ORS) in order to counteract his cholera-induced dehydration. (*Centers for Disease Control and Prevention's Public Health Image Library (PHIL), #5301*)

What You Need To Know About...
Psittacosis

Left: Precautions against psittacosis from the PBS Pet travel website.

Below: A depiction of dancing mania, on the pilgrimage of epileptics to the church at Molenbeek, drawn in 1564 by Pieter Breughel the Younger (1564–1638).

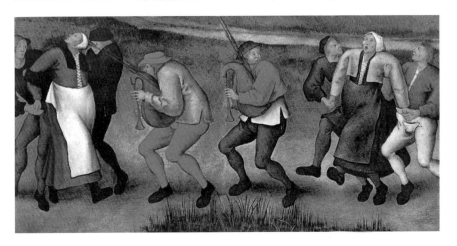

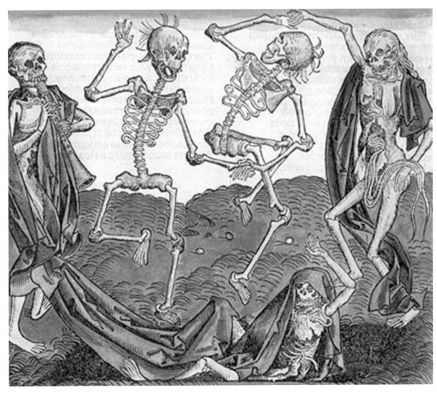

A '*danse macabre*' from 1493 by victims of the Sweating Sickness.

Right: Sign barring children under 16 from entering town, posted on a tree during the 1916 New York City polio epidemic. (*Courtesy of March of Dimes*)

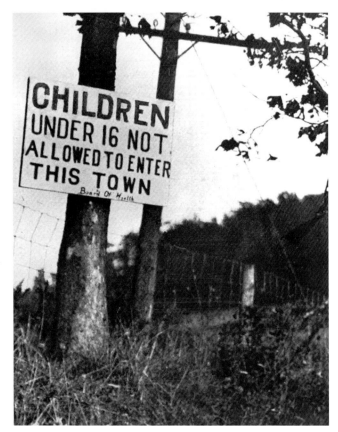

Below: March of Dimes poster of Cyndi Jones as a poster child in Saint Louis, Missouri, 1956. (*Courtesy of Cyndi Jones*)

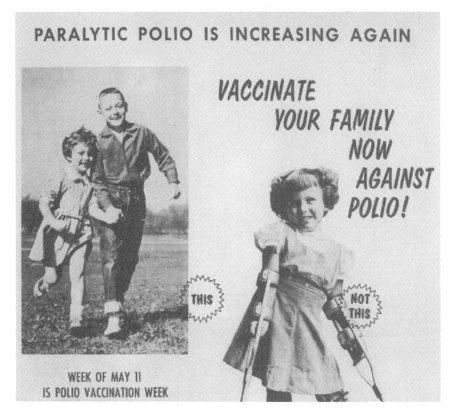

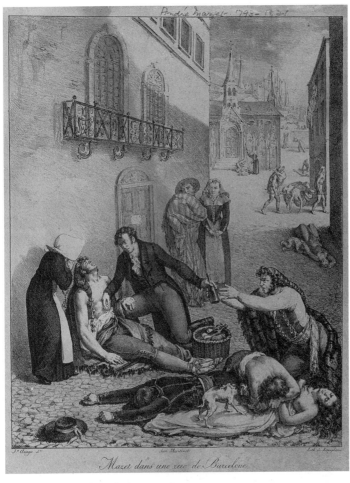

Mazet dans une rue de Barcelone.

Left: French doctor André Mazet tending people suffering from yellow fever in the streets of Barcelona. (*Lithograph by Langlumé after Martinet after J. Arago via Wellcome Images*)

Below: An Asian Flu patient (1957–1958).

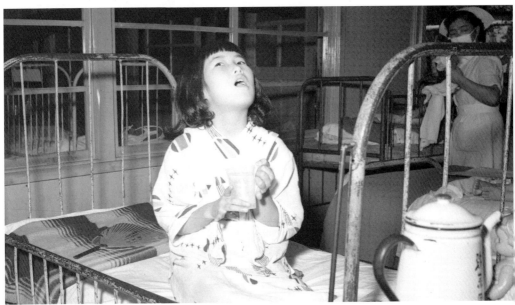

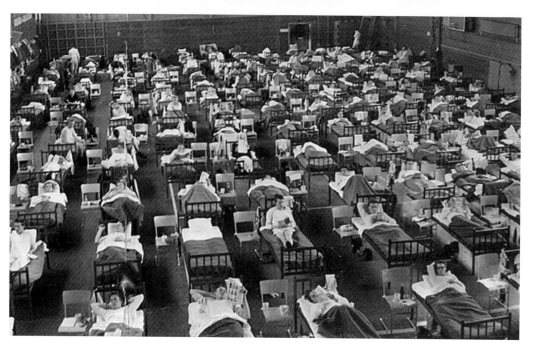

Above: Asian
Flu patients in
Sweden.

Right: Alley
outside wet
market on
Xinghu Road,
Shenzhen, China
in 2019 during
the COVID-19
pandemic.
(*Daniel Case*)

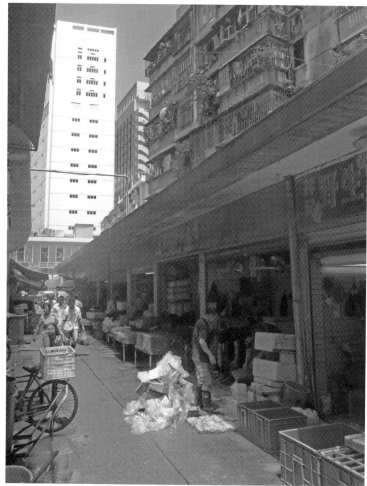

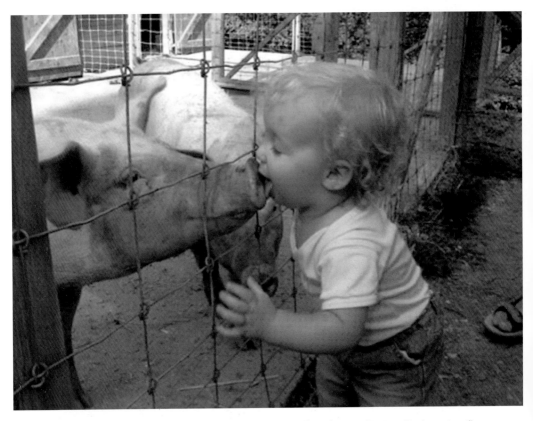

Oh dear. The only good news is that, despite what the media implied, swine flu cannot be caught from pigs, or pork.

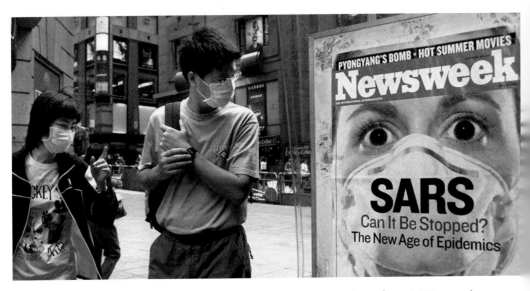

'How SARS terrified the world in 2003, infecting more than 8,000 people and killing 774'. Governments worldwide seem to have forgotten this by 2019–2020, or else they have all gone into selective memory mode. Some still can't remember the lessons from 2003 in 2021. (*Lo Sai Hung / AP*)

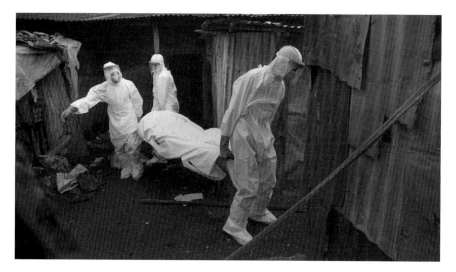

Above and below: Ebola virus victims in Liberia.

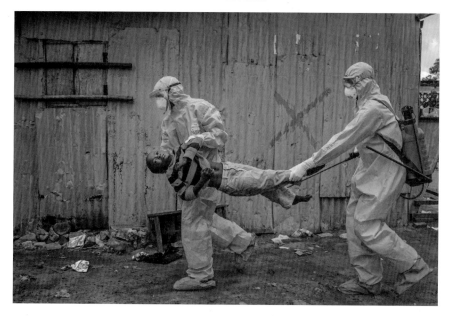

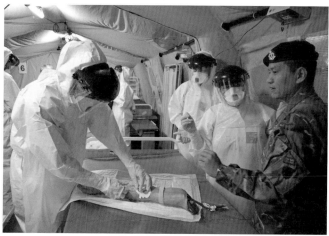

NHS medics practise taking a blood sample from a fake arm at the Army Medical Services Training Centre, at Strensall near York. (*Simon Davis/DFID*)

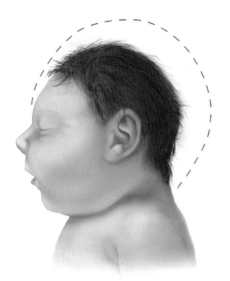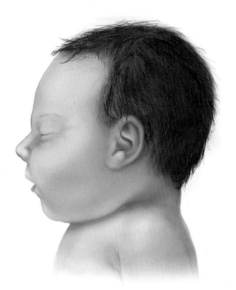

Microcephaly in Zica virus patients. The image on the left shows a significant reduction in the size of the child's head. (*Image: CDC*)

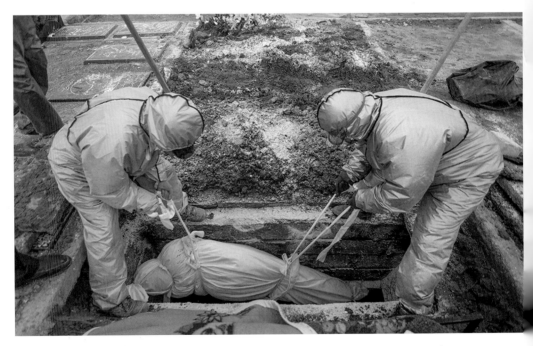

Burying the evidence? A COVID-19 victim in Iran. The number of deaths from coronavirus in Iran is nearly triple what Iran's government claims. Leaked data suggest that 42,000 people had died with COVID-19 symptoms by 20 July 2020, compared to 14,405 officially reported for that date.

were considered well enough to go out. A watch of twelve men was ordered to monitor that the quarantine orders were being followed.

In 1690 the disease, which had prevailed in Boston before the departure of Sir William Phips' doomed expedition up the St Lawrence to attack Quebec, spread through the fleet and many died both during the advance and the retreat, while even more perished on shore after its return. In 1697 smallpox was back, carrying off in that and in 1698 some 1,000 of the 7–8,000 inhabitants of Boston.

In 1701 the first smallpox prevention act authorized the requisitioning of houses for the isolation of patients. Three hundred died in 1702; the tolling of bells at funerals was to be limited, and it was suggested that the price of coffins be moderated, as well as the digging of graves and wages of porters to carry the corpses. The constable was still required 'to attend the funerals of those dying of the smallpox' and to walk before the corpse to give notice to 'any y't may be in danger of ye infection'. The next outbreak was in 1721 when, famously, inoculation was introduced.

Behbehani, Abbas, December 1983. 'The Smallpox Story: Life and Death of an Old Disease' (PDF). *American Society for Microbiology*. 47 (4): 464.

Kass, Amalie, M., 2012. Boston's Historic Smallpox Epidemic. *Massachusetts Historical Review*, 14, 1–51.

Kelly, Thomas, 2015. Tracing Smallpox Through the Burying Grounds, *Historic Burying Grounds Initiative Newsletter* 4, 2015, 1, 5–11

Woodward, Samuel Bayard, 1932, 'The Story of Smallpox in Massachusetts.' *New England Journal of Medicine* 206, no. 23, 1181–91.

Chapter 24

The US yellow fever epidemics

'[I am] firmly convinced that the disease at present in our city is not by any means epidemic.'
– The president of the New York City Board of Assistant Aldermen,
Dr S.W. Dalton, after studying the yellow fever cases closely.

1699 Charleston and Philadelphia yellow fever epidemic

Before the end of the 19th century medical opinion persisted in the belief that yellow fever was spread by human to human. It was not until 1881 when a Cuban epidemiologist, Carlos Finlay (1833–1915), acting on a theory that mosquitoes carried the virus, was the first to postulate that a mosquito was the disease vector: a mosquito that bites a victim of the disease could subsequently bite and thereby infect a healthy person. He presented this theory at the 1881 International Sanitary Conference at Havana's Academy of Sciences, 'The Mosquito Hypothetically Considered as the Transmitting Agent of Yellow Fever'. A year later Finlay identified a mosquito of the genus *Aedes* as the organism transmitting yellow fever. His theory was followed by the recommendation to control the mosquito population as a way to control the spread of the disease.

Finlay (son of a Scots physician) is the author of forty papers on the disease. His theory that an intermediary host was responsible for the spread of the disease was treated with ridicule for years. Nevertheless he remained a humane and compassionate man, often taking on patients who could not afford medical care. As a result of his work, Finlay was nominated seven times for the Nobel Prize in Physiology or Medicine. Although he was never awarded the prize, he received the National Order of the Legion of Honour of France in 1908.

Viruses, of course, have no respect for international boundaries so it is little surprise that at least twenty-five major yellow fever outbreaks occurred in North America: the 1693 Boston yellow fever epidemic – the first irrefutable outbreak of yellow fever – took root in Boston when a British fleet from Barbados docked in the harbour, although there had been some evidence of earlier outbreaks. For the next 200 years, the disease regularly re-visited Boston and other cities in North America. These included 1699 in Charleston; 1702 New York City and 1793 in Philadelphia where it struck during the summer and recorded the highest fatalities in the United States.

In September 1668, Samuel Megapolensis, the pastor of the Dutch church in the new city that was New York, wrote to a friend about how the Lord had 'visited us with dysentery, which is even now increasing in virulence. Many have died of it, and many are lying sick.' What Megapolensis was actually describing was probably the city's first outbreak of yellow fever, which would devastate the city on and off for over 100 years. He went on, his words freighted with the supernatural and with superstition which would not have been out of place in ancient Greece or Rome:

> 'It appears as if God were punishing this land for its sins. Some years (ago) there appeared a meteor in the air. Last year we saw a terrible comet in the west, a little above the horizon, with the tail upward, and hanging over this place. It showed itself for about eight days, and then disappeared. So we fear God's judgements, but supplicate his favor.'

With regards to the blight that was yellow fever, New York was virgin territory, an easy prey with inhabitants living without immunity and dying as a consequence. There were rich pickings to be had here. This was in contrast with that other plague of the north east, smallpox, which, although it tore mercilessly through American Indian communities, was mitigated since many colonists had acquired immunity to the disease before they left Europe. In 1702, Lord Cornbury, New York's colonial governor, wrote that 'in ten weeks time, sickness has swept away upwards of 500 people of all ages and [both] sexes'. With a population of around 5,000 that means that 10 per cent of the city died in less than three months.

As we know, the cause, origin and transmission of yellow fever were still very much a medical mystery: in the 17th and 18th centuries the disease was attributed to bad vapours (the 'miasma' theory of disease), poor sanitation and increased immigration – so that it came to be known as the strangers' disease. It was believed to be spread through infected clothing. Urban areas burned tar, enveloping cities in belching, choking smoke in an effort to cleanse the air. Quarantine, lockdowns and isolation, combined with the asphyxiating smoke, reduced outbreak sites to virtual ghost towns. To combat the miasma in the 1730s, New York began to regulate livestock inside city limits, and slaughterhouses and leather tan yards were moved out. This had no effect whatsoever, so, galvanised by an outbreak in 1793, New York City created its first Department of Health, which 'enacted a series of increasingly stringent quarantine laws, created a three-man Health Office Commission to administer them, and authorized the Common Council to pass sanitary ordinances, abate nuisances, and appoint a sanitary inspector'. Here are some of the measures forced on the authorities by the epidemic in 1702:

> *Burying the Dead:* A Proclamation instituting a penalty of five pounds to anyone who does not bury their dead after 12 hours.

> *Ban on Burning Oysters:* A Proclamation instituting a penalty of five pounds for burning oysters and shells within the city of New York.

> *Prayer & Fasting on Wednesdays:* A Proclamation instituting every Wednesday henceforth as a day of prayer and fasting in light of the epidemic calamity.

In 1798 one quarantine location, a farm outside the city limits called 'Belle Vue', was purchased in 1798 by the city's hospital and soon, as Bellevue Hospital, became a facility for isolating victims. In 1799, responding to calls to clean up the city's dirty wells, Aaron Burr established a water supply firm called the Manhattan Company, better known for its financing arm (the Bank of the Manhattan Company, forerunner of today's J.P. Morgan Chase); Burr's business did lay some wooden pipes in lower Manhattan, and for the first time, a few New Yorkers had running water. However, there was one crucial thing wrong with Burr's project: it was itself unsanitary so in 1803, the Common Council voted to drain and fill the pond, which had become polluted by the nearby slaughterhouses.

The final major yellow fever epidemics to strike the northeastern cities came to an end in 1805, a year in which serious outbreaks occurred in both New York and Philadelphia. Although the disease re-emerged sporadically in the succeeding years, it did not recur as an epidemic until 1819, when it struck at Boston, Philadelphia and Baltimore. It hung over Philadelphia and Baltimore for three summers before making one final visit to New York in 1822. Yellow fever effectively stopped afflicting the states north of Virginia. Infected sailors and passengers were constantly being landed, but the quarantine and isolation measures appear to have been effective in checking the disease.

In the south, though, things were different – in the coastal area from Virginia south to Florida and west along the Gulf nearly 700 people in Savannah, Georgia, died from yellow fever in 1820, including two local physicians who lost their lives caring for the sick. Several other epidemics followed, including 1854 and 1876.

New Orleans

'Only our mosquitoes keep up the hum of industry.'
– The New Orleans Picayune.

New Orleans – a major port for the slave trade and a city with a climate hospitable to the *Aedes aegypti* mosquito – endured a long history of yellow fever epidemics. Between 1839 and 1860, some 26,000 people in New Orleans contracted yellow fever. The first yellow fever epidemic was in 1796 which killed 300 people. The disease came back in 1799 with similar effect; three relatively mild outbreaks hit in the following decade, followed by a more severe one in 1811 which claimed 500 people. For the next six years New Orleans was yellow fever free, but the disease returned with a vengeance in the summer and autumn of 1817, burying more than 800 victims. A minor outbreak the following year was succeeded by a major epidemic in 1819 which had a death toll of 2,200.

Nevertheless, New Orleans was prospering: by 1820 the population exceeded 27,000, up from 5,000 in 1785, and 1840 saw the city with 100,000 inhabitants. Much of this explosion was due to the annual influx of European immigrants and newcomers from other states; but wherever the people came from they were all fodder for yellow fever. Until the outbreak of the American Civil War, barely a year passed without a recurrence of the disease with virulence steadily increasing: between 1835 and 1860, the annual number of deaths from yellow fever exceeded 1,000 on twelve occasions.

In the 1853 epidemic the authorities – civic and medical – were beyond irresponsible; on July 23 the president of the Board of Assistant Aldermen, S.W. Dalton, a leading physician, informed one local newspaper editor that after studying the yellow fever cases closely he was 'firmly convinced that the disease at present in our city is not by any means epidemic'. The fever was merely sporadic, he thought, and in any case it was restricted largely to immigrants and other new arrivals. This statement was made in the face of the official weekly burial return, which attributed 17 of the city's 617 deaths to yellow fever. In August, as the disease reached its peak, the mayor desperately clutched at straws: up until then he had focused on trying to clean and drain the city: massive quantities of quicklime had been spread in the gutters, privies and sewers and also liberally sprinkled in the graveyards and on the corpses; the rooms and buildings in which the sick had died were cleansed and fumigated and pools of stagnant water were drained.

The high point of the epidemic of 1853 was reached on 21 August when more than 300 burials were reported in one day. The 1853 outbreak had claimed 7,849 lives in New Orleans.

Meanwhile, steamboats continued blithely to carry passengers and the disease upriver from New Orleans to other cities along the Mississippi River. The epidemic was dramatized and featured in the plot of the 1938 film *Jezebel*, starring Bette Davis. From the beginning of the 19th century river boats had consistently and effectively spread yellow fever from New Orleans to the many river towns in Louisiana and Mississippi. Natchez, Missouri, more than 200 miles upriver was first assailed in 1817 and suffered repeatedly in the following years. Vicksburg, further north, suffered its first outbreak in 1841.

From 1859 to 1867 New Orleans enjoyed some respite with only a few sporadic cases but 1867 saw a major epidemic with over 40,000 cases and 3,100 deaths; 1870 saw a flare up of epidemic proportions, killing upwards of 600 citizens. In the 1870s the disease revisited every summer, but only twice became epidemic, in 1873 and 1878, the latter was the third worst in the history of the city. From July to December some 27,000 people were infected and over 4,000 died.

The contagion was exacerbated by thousands of infected refugees fleeing Cuba at the end of a war of independence from Spain. Many came to New Orleans. In an attempt to prevent the disease from entering the city, a quarantine station on the Mississippi River south of the city was set up to inspect incoming ships. The *Emily B. Souder* arrived there in late May: one sick sailor, diagnosed with malaria, was removed from the ship. The ship was duly fumigated and cleared to dock in New Orleans. The night the ship docked, another crew member fell sick and died and another four days later. When the *Souder* left to return to Havana, another vessel, the *Charles B. Woods* docked. Within six weeks every member of the families of the *Woods'* captain and engineer had contracted yellow fever. They recovered, but a 4-year-old girl living in the same neighbourhood died in July.

The bad news that yellow fever had again struck New Orleans drove one-fifth of the city's population out of the city, leaving the usual ghost town. 'Only our mosquitoes keep up the hum of industry,' reported the *New Orleans Picayune*. Physicians desperately attempted treatments with bloodlettings, carbolic acid, purging, teas, cold baths and quinine – all useless. The state board of health declared an epidemic on 10 August after 431 reported cases and 118 deaths. The mayor convened the College of Physicians, which on 27 August advised people to avoid infected cases if possible and keep the streets clean, among other measures. The hapless mayor implored all 'that can move, to quit the city'. About 20,000 people fled.

By the 1870s an unfortunate combination of railroad extensions and faster Mississippi boats and the inexorable spread of *Aides aoegypti*, meant that yellow fever would inevitably reach as far north as St. Louis. The 1878 epidemic struck first at Baton Rouge and Vicksburg, then drove on to Memphis, and to Cairo, Illinois, eventually reaching St. Louis. At the same time the Tennessee River carried the pestilence to Chattanooga, and up the Ohio River as far as Louisville.

In 1878, the outbreak in New Orleans spread into the lower Mississippi Valley infecting at least 120,000 and killing between 13,000 and 20,000. On 27 July a towboat dropped two crew members with yellow fever in Vicksburg. Another infected crew member died on the boat that night. Vicksburg reported more than 3,000 cases and more than 1,000 deaths in a population of about 12,000. In August, 100 cases of yellow fever were reported in Grenada, Mississippi, about 100 miles south of Memphis.

But the self-interested press and the dilatory health authorities had failed to alert New Orleans citizens of the outbreak until the middle of July, after more than 1,000 people had already succumbed. New Orleans businesses feared lest word of an epidemic would cause a quarantine to be placed on the city, and that their trade would suffer accordingly. John Duffy (1968) describes this astonishing situation as follows:

> 'In New Orleans, as in other 19th century cities, the newspaper editors, municipal officers, and leading physicians often compounded the tragedy by their refusal to face up to reality. Despite appalling casualty lists from cholera, yellow fever, and the perennial summer fluxes and fevers, they stoutly maintained that their city was a veritable health spa. The only ones falling prey to sickness, they asserted, were strangers and the intemperate and immoral poor. Medical journals and newspapers proclaimed that newcomers could protect themselves from yellow fever if they would only leave during the summer season and not return until the cool temperatures of fall had banished the disease. The editor of the New Orleans City Directory early in 1853 expressed the prevailing opinion of civic and professional leaders when he declared that the New Orleans physicians now considered yellow fever to be an obsolete idea. Ironically, as already mentioned, almost 9,000 of the city's residents died of fever in the five-month period from June to October of that same year.'

Duffy goes on to highlight the venal commercial interests of the media which had 'a vital economic stake in playing down the significance of epidemics', fearful that even the slightest rumour would spark a mass exodus of the beleaguered city and with it the newpapers' readership and advertising revenues: 'Almost by reflex action, newspaper editors in the 18th and 19th centuries either denied the existence of the first few cases of a communicable disorder or else casually dismissed the danger.' To make matters worse, doctors and scientists still did not have a clue how this and other communicable diseases were spread: yellow fever, like other diseases spread by insect vectors, was as much a baffling mystery in 1853 as it had been since Europeans first encountered it in the 16th and 17th centuries. The following is typical of the ignorance and confusion, from *Treatment of Yellow Fever* by Surg. R.D. Murray:

> 'I have seen yellow fever in twenty-one summers (including 1870) and in every month except February. The elimination of yellow fever from our nomenclature will follow when there is a proper conception of the influence of clothing, bedding, and unclean bedrooms as transmitters. The disease is air borne for some distance…it may be diluted, and is transmitted by clothing, bedding and related articles. Hair from the dead has transmitted it; corn sacks; blankets and old newspapers have carried it; mountains of filth will not produce it; they may give it a new nidus or garden from which it goes out 'seeking whom it may devour'. The cleanest town in the South may have a severe prevalence if the people insist on disobeying the advice of the health officials.
>
> In 1875 as a result of several post-mortems and an attack of the disease, I came to the conclusion that yellow fever was an inflammation of the duodenum, primarily, and wanted to call it epidemic duodenitis'.

The following features some cautionary lessons which would be of value today for getting the balance right between public health and economics as laid out in *Inspection Service* by P.A. Surg. G.B. Young:

> 'In conducting a system of trained inspection for the purpose of preventing the spread of disease and of facilitating intercourse and trade as far as is consistent with safety, it is most important to always keep in mind that the limitation of the spread of the disease should be paramount to every other consideration, the facilitating of traffic being of only secondary importance…Next to preventing the actual spread of the disease the most important thing to do is to strive to minimize the distress that the fear of its coming brings to all within the threatened territory…only those should be permitted to travel who can give a good sanitary history; and that while en route they shall be preserved from contact with any infected or suspected person, place, or thing.'

Yellow Fever: Its Epidemiology, Prevention, and Control, Lecture, 1914 was a landmark event in the understanding of yellow fever and its transmission:

> 'In 1914, Dr. Henry Rose Carter gave a series of lectures on yellow fever at the United States Public Health Service School… Carter discussed theories of yellow fever with Walter Reed. In his first lecture on March 26, Carter makes immediately clear and unequivocally the method of infection that his colleague had proven: yellow fever is transmitted by mosquitoes.'

Memphis, Tennesee and the shotgun barricades

Yellow fever should be dealt with as an enemy which imperils life and cripples commerce and industry. To no other great nation of the earth is yellow fever so calamitous as to the United States of America.
    – John Woodworth, the Marine Hospital Service Surgeon General

Memphis, which had a population of about 35,000 suffered 15,000 yellow fever cases in 1878 leaving about 10 per cent, 3,500 dead. This despite half of the residents fleeing the city for rural areas or north and east away from the river. While some places accommodated them, others established 'shotgun barricades', with armed men ensuring that no one could enter their towns. The disease would travel with fleeing refugees as far away as Kentucky, Indiana, Illinois and Ohio. In response to the rampant epidemic, the mayor of Memphis on 28 July imposed a quarantine, which blocked railroad lines. Local businessmen threatened a lawsuit unless the city released a train of goods from New Orleans which city leaders allowed to enter. In August, a steamboat crew member who had avoided the quarantine died in a Memphis hospital. On 13 August a local resident who operated a food stand near the riverfront also died from yellow fever.

Such was the toll that those who remained in a depopulated Memphis relied on volunteers from religious organizations to care for the sick. The madame of a local brothel, Annie Cook, converted her bordello into a hospital, where she nursed the ill. She died from the disease that September. By the end of the year, more than 5,000 were confirmed dead in Memphis.

The $15 million in losses the epidemic caused bankrupted Memphis. The federal government convened a commission to investigate the outbreak and established the National Board of Health in 1879. In a report to Congress John Woodworth, the Marine Hospital Service surgeon general, emphasized the gravity of the situation: 'Yellow fever should be dealt with as an enemy which imperils life and cripples commerce and industry. To no other great nation of the earth is yellow fever so calamitous as to the United States of America.'

That same year President Rutherford B. Hayes signed the Quarantine Act giving the Marine Hospital Service responsibility for stopping disease from entering the country through shipping. On 18 December the Committee of the Senate and House of Representatives on Epidemic Disease established the Board of Experts authorized by Congress to investigate the Yellow Fever Epidemic. Six weeks later, the board recommended a quarantine system to prevent yellow fever from entering the country. In 1879, responding to calls for a federal public health agency, Congress established the National Board of Health.

Throughout the 1880s and early 1890s the United States was relatively free from yellow fever. Apart from an outbreak in Florida in 1888, the disease did not attain epidemic proportions. The Florida epidemic, which was centred around Jacksonville on the Atlantic coast, managed to spread 70 miles inland to Gainesville and 40 miles north to Fernandina before cool weather stopped it in its tracks; however, cases still were in the thousands and deaths in the hundreds.

In 1897 it was widely believed that yellow fever was a thing of the past, but no, the disease flared again in New Orleans when 2,000 cases resulted in about 300 deaths. After another brief respite, the disease resurged with epidemic force in 1905. The only consolation was that by now the nefarious and insidious role played by *Aedes aegypti* was understood and decisive action by city, state and federal authorities led to an effective program for eradication of mosquitoes. Workmen covered cisterns with screens and treated standing water with kerosene. Residents burned an estimated 300 tons of sulphur to fumigate their premises. That year further spread was prevented and there were no future outbreaks. Whereas former epidemics in New Orleans had reached their peak in August and September, the 1905 epidemic was largely ended before the end of August. Nevertheless, in its dying throes *Aedes aegypti* took with it 452 of the 3,402 residents who contracted the disease (13.29 per cent).

In 1878 the entire Mississippi River Valley south from St. Louis was afflicted, and tens of thousands fled the stricken cities of New Orleans, Vicksburg, and Memphis. An estimated 120,000 cases of yellow fever resulted in some 20,000 deaths. Memphis suffered several epidemics during the 1870s, culminating in the 1878 epidemic (called the 'Saffron Scourge' of 1878), with more than 5,000 fatalities in the city. Some contemporary accounts said that commercial interests had again prevented the rapid reporting of the outbreak of the epidemic, increasing the total number of deaths.

The 1878 epidemic was the worst that occurred in Mississippi. 'Yellow Jack' or 'Bronze John', devastated Mississippi socially and economically. Entire families were killed, while others fled their homes for the presumed safety of other parts of the state. Quarantine regulations brought trade to a stop: some local economies never recovered. By the end of the year, 3,227 people had died from the disease.

Clearly the virus always had profound social as well as health and economic impacts, unravelling the social fabric of the communities it struck – creating refugee populations, undermining trusted institutions, and severing familial bonds. During the American War of Independence (1775–1783) disruption of trade between the United States and the rest of the world limited the spread of yellow fever from endemic regions to the nation's seaports. However, after the war, the formation of the federal government encouraged an expansion in international trade and expedited the migration of large non-immune populations to the prospering coastal cities. These factors together contributed greatly to the spread of yellow fever. Outbreaks occurred in nearly all the major coastal cities of the nation.

About 1,000 miles away from New Orleans, Charleston, South Carolina on the Atlantic coast – only a third the size of New Orleans – was experiencing a very similar pattern of outbreaks as New Orleans. Epidemics hit in the 1790s and in the early years of the 19th century: in 1804, 1807 and 1809, then nothing until 1817 and 1819 followed by a relentless series of epidemics nearly every summer and autumn until the peak in the 1850s. In 1854, out of a population of less than 50,000, 675 deaths were recorded, a shocking number which rose further in 1858 to 717 (1.43 per cent).

Further north after 1792 the most northerly ports of Norfolk and Portsmouth in Virginia were worst affected with a series of epidemics starting in the 1790s after which there was a hiatus until 1855 when yellow fever ravaged the two cities which had a combined population of 25,000. Half of these panicked and fled, but almost all of the 10,000 who remained contracted the disease resulting in a death toll close to 2,000. In June 1855 after two seamen died of yellow fever during the voyage, the steamship *Ben Franklin* arrived outside Norfolk, Virginia. The port doctor, unaware of the deaths, allowed the ship to dock for repairs. The black population had some immunity, but although it did not escape the infection, it did have a lower case-fatality rate than the white population. In Norfolk one third of this population died, while in Portsmouth more than 40 per cent succumbed. The Howard Association, a benevolent organization, was formed to help coordinate assistance in the form of funds, supplies, medical professionals and volunteers, who poured in from many other areas, particularly the Atlantic and Gulf Coast areas of the United States.

In North Carolina several outbreaks struck Wilmington and New Bern between 1796 and 1862. In Georgia, Savannah suffered a series of yellow fever epidemics from 1800 to 1858. Florida's Atlantic coast was sparsely settled and had no major ports, so it escaped much of the pestilence, but St. Augustine and Jacksonville suffered occasional epidemics in the years before the Civil War. However, Key West, at the tip of the Florida peninsula, and Pensacola, on the Gulf coast, were frequently afflicted by the disease.

Clearly from 1820 to 1867 almost every town on the Gulf coast lived in dread of yellow fever as the disease relentlessly and remorselessly made its deadly way down the coast, laying low cities like Mobile, Gulfport, New Orleans, Galveston and other Texas ports westward to Brownsville, as well as towns on the Mississippi River and its tributaries. In 1839 the fledgeling state of Texas, just two years old, suffered when yellow fever struck Galveston, with a population of just over 2,000. This single outbreak slaughtered one tenth of the population.

As with the American War of Independence, the American Civil War (1861–65) saw a reduction in outbreaks caused by the suppression of trade, thanks largely to the effectiveness of the Northern blockade of Southern ports. Consequently, yellow fever killed only 436 of the 233,786 Union soldiers who died of disease during the conflict.

By the end of the 19th century, during the 1898 Spanish-American War, fewer than 1,000 soldiers died in battle, but more than 5,000 died of disease in Cuba, and most of those deaths were due to yellow fever according to the US Army Yellow Fever Commission. The Commission was set up by the US military in response to these deaths. Walter Reed offered advice to a friend who expected to be posted there. Surmising that the germ for yellow fever was inhaled, Reed wrote that a 'plug of cotton in the nostrils would be advisable'.

Led by Major Walter Reed, working in Cuba, the commission confirmed in 1900 what Dr. Finlay suspected: yellow fever was transmitted by mosquito bites. To prove it, thirty men, including Spanish immigrants, soldiers and two civilians, volunteered to be deliberately infected with such mosquito bites. Four doctors served on the board: Walter Reed, James Carroll, Aristides Agramonte and Jesse Lazear. The board began testing Finlay's theory, allowing mosquitoes to feed on volunteers. For the first nine subjects, the results were negative. On August 27 the sceptical James Carroll volunteered to be exposed to a mosquito that had fed on an active case of yellow fever twelve days before. Carroll contracted the disease, became seriously ill but recovered. On 25 September Lazear, bitten by a mosquito used in his experiments, died.

On 20 November Camp Lazear, named in tribute to the sacrifice made by Jesse Lazear, was established outside Havana. The Yellow Fever Board paid volunteers consisting of army personnel and Spanish immigrants to expose themselves to mosquito bites in order to show incontrovertibly that the insect transmits the disease. Each volunteer was paid $100 for participating and received an additional $100 if infected. Fourteen volunteers contracted the disease; all recovered. The commission started mosquito control programs in Cuba using improved sanitation, fumigation with insecticides and reduction in standing water areas where mosquitoes bred. The number of yellow fever cases dropped dramatically.

Finlay's landmark discovery helped William C. Gorgas reduce the incidence and prevalence of mosquito-borne diseases in Panama during the American campaign, and from 1903 onwards, to construct the Panama Canal, progress on which was being threatened by the disease. Up until then, about 10 per cent of the workforce had died each year from malaria and yellow fever. By 1906, roughly 85 per cent of canal workers were hospitalized with the two diseases. The French hospitals contained numerous pools of stagnant water, such as basins underneath potted plants, in which mosquitoes could breed. Workers were so terrified of yellow fever that they fled the construction site in droves at the first hint of the disease. Tens of thousands of workers died.

According to Susan Brink (2016)

> 'Dr. William Gorgas, who had worked on mosquito eradication in Cuba, convinced President Roosevelt to grant funding on an eradication effort in Panama. In the summer of 1905, Gorgas, along with 4,000 workers in what he called his 'mosquito brigade', spent a year working to stop mosquitoes from laying their eggs. They fumigated private homes with insecticides and sprayed areas of standing water with oil to interrupt mosquito breeding. The efforts cut the number of yellow fever cases in half by September, and in October there were only seven new cases. Finally, on 11 November 1906, the last victim of yellow fever on the Panama Canal died. The yellow fever epidemic was over.'

After the Second World War, DDT was a powerful weapon in mosquito control measures, and mosquito eradication became the primary method of controlling yellow fever.

War and the slave trade both had a role to play in the depradations caused by yellow fever in the US – not least the American War of Independence and the American Civil War. Often, vessels from Europe crammed with slaves would call in at Caribbean ports to water and reprovision before continuing to the Gulf coast ports like New Orleans; these ports, as we have seen, were often reservoirs of infection. As Duffy points out, 'A fairly close correlation exists between the European and colonial wars and the existence of yellow fever in North America. The Seven Years' War (1756–1763) between England and France, and others was fought on a wide front, which included the West Indies and all of North America'. The next period of yellow fever in America began in 1793 and lasted to 1805 which coincides with the start of the French Revolution, while 1805 was the year in which Nelson defeated the French fleet and gave England virtual control of the seas for the remainder of the Napoleonic Wars. He also shows how it was more than a coincidence that the first yellow fever epidemics in British North America came during the years from 1693 to 1710, a period which included the War of the League of Augsburg and the War of the Spanish Succession.

By 1815 the United States had of course won its independence from Great Britain (in 1783). This obliged the US to seek new trade deals, some of which crucially involved commerce with the West Indies which not only effected the importation of goods but also of infectious and tropical diseases. As we have seen, the Civil War suppressed the commercial activities of southern ports and may have been a contributory factor in ending or reducing the devastating outbreaks of yellow fever of the preceding ten years. The Spanish-American War led to the American occupation of Cuba, a hot-bed of yellow fever, and in all probability responsible for the final series of outbreaks in the United States.

The persistence and ubiquity of yellow fever in the US also played a significant role in American medical history, public health and in preventative medicine. The first epidemics of yellow fever in the late 17th and early 18th century, which hit at a time when smallpox was also rampaging, led to the formulation of some early quarantine laws. Massachusetts, for example, passed a law in 1699 intended to prevent ships carrying infected persons or persons coming from ports where contagious diseases were prevalent from landing in the colony. When an indignant British government disallowed this measure, the colonial legislature resolved the matter by authorizing justices of the peace to prohibit individuals from disembarking.

At the dawn of the 19th century there was an upsurge in public health measures; for example In direct response to the first major epidemic in 1793, a board of health was set up in Philadelphia; health boards and health commissions were established in New York and Baltimore; in Charleston quarantine powers were invested in the city council and in New Orleans the Spanish governor and attorney general instituted rigorous quarantine measures and recommended draining stagnant pools and cleaning the city streets. The devastating Louisiana epidemic of 1853 was the reason for the creation in 1855 of the Louisiana State Board of Health, the first of its kind in the United States. The correlation between yellow fever and the emergence of health boards was particularly evident in the Southern states where, for example, the Florida State Board of Health was a direct reaction to the 1888 outbreak.

It is hard to quantify the net impact of the continual attacks of yellow fever. New Orleans, which suffered more than most in the 19th century still became the main entrepôt of the South. Other Gulf coast cities and towns emerged, thrived and rapidly increased in population and wealth. Nevertheless, many European immigrants did avoid southern ports, and there is little doubt that the epidemics of yellow fever were a drag on the development of the southern coastal cities. Effective public health programs can be attributed to the rising standards of living, advances in medical and scientific knowledge, 'an increasing sensitivity to human misery', and the development of more effective government. Yellow fever and Asiatic cholera, the two most significant plagues in 19th century America, honed social awareness of problems in public health. Reforms obviously played their part but yellow fever was often the catalyst which expedited the change.

Bloom, Khaled J., 1993, The Mississippi Valley's Great Yellow Fever Epidemic of 1878, *Louisiana State University Press*.

Fenner, E.D., 1854, *History of the Epidemic of Yellow Fever at New Orleans, Louisiana, in 1853.* New York.

Keating, J.M., 1879, *A History of the Yellow Fever: The Yellow Fever Epidemic of 1878 in Memphis*, Memphis

Stephens Nuwer, Deanne, 1999. 'The 1878 Yellow Fever Epidemic along the Mississippi Gulf Coast'. *Gulf South Historical Review*. 14 (2): 51–73.

Chapter 25

The 1702–1703 St. Lawrence Valley smallpox epidemic

'The French intruders took most of the blame and were snubbed in every way; they were "dreaded as the greatest sorcerers on earth". Death threats were made to the missionaries and one was clubbed, another threatened with a cleaver to the head; the mission house was burnt almost to the ground.'

One of the earliest references to smallpox in Canada comes in 1635 and relates to an outbreak among the Montagnais Indians who lived on the banks of the St Lawrence at Three Rivers, as related in the Jesuit *Le Jeune's Relation* of that year. Le Jeune tells how he witnessed that many of the Indians were sick and many died; indeed 'it [smallpox] was so universal amongst the savages of our acquaintance that I do not know of one who has escaped its attacks…many crops are lying beneath the snow'. Later, when a mission was established with the Hurons at Ihonaturia near Georgian Bay, smallpox broke out and decimated the tribe; the Hurons put it down to the 'medicine' of the black robes. The following year 'the pestilence which for two years past had from time to time visited the Huron towns, now returned with tenfold violence and with it soon appeared a new and fatal scourge – the small-pox. Terror was universal'.[1] The season of Huron festivity turned into the season of mourning; suicides increased, 'Silent dejection' prevailed and 'Everywhere was heard the wail of the sick and dying children…at the sides of the house[s] crouched squalid men and women, in all the stages of the distemper.'

The French intruders took most of the blame and were snubbed in every way; they were 'dreaded as the greatest sorcerers on earth'. Death threats were made to the missionaries and one was clubbed, another threatened with a cleaver to the head; the mission house was burnt almost to the ground. Especially tragic was the high mortality amongst children in the three villages worst affected: St. Michel, St. Ignace and St. Joseph: 260 had been baptised here – more than 70 children under 7 years died – the Jesuit baptisers got the blame. The smallpox went on intermittently until 1640.

In 1661 the Attikamegues, or Nation of the White Fish, were almost wiped out by the Iroquios and those the Iroquois did not kill the ravages of the smallpox took.

---

1. Heagerty 1926

Indeed 1661 and 1662 provided a 'rich harvest' for the disease: of the more than 200 who received holy baptism that winter over 120 'died soon after to take their flight to heaven'. In 1663 the Iroquois were savagely afflicted by 'sad havoc' resulting in deserted villages and half-tilled fields. 'More than 300 dying children were baptised by some captive Frenchmen.' Smallpox persisted until 1665 and by 1680 war, smallpox and alcohol 'swept away more than 1,000 souls' reducing the once proud tribe to a shadow of its former self.

The carnage continued with horrific descriptions of 'monsters rather than human beings, their bodies were so hideous, emaciated and full of corruption'; there were cabins 'full of the dying…living skeletons and bodies all disfigured'.

Smallpox also took its atrocious toll in 1702 and 1703 along the St. Lawrence Valley. By the end of 1702 between 6 and 6.5 per cent of the European settlers had died of the disease; if we add the 25 per cent of newborns who succumbed, the death toll reaches about 1,300. Women of childbearing age were particularly badly hit with 10 per cent mortality; this would inevitably impede population growth in the short term. The high rate of deaths generally may be accounted for by the fact that in the 17th century smallpox was not prevalent amongst the non native population so the 1702 epidemic fed on a demographic that offered little or no immunity.

The epidemic started in October 1702 when an Iroquois chief from Orange (now Albany NY) died in the Hôtel-Dieu Hospital. Sister Jean-Françoise Juchereau de St Ignace, superior of the Religious Hospitallers of the Hôtel-Dieu at Quebec and author of *Les Annales de l'Hôtel-Dieu de Québec, 1636–1716* gives us some detail. Her work during a series of epidemics, of influenza, measles and fevers which ravaged New France in 1688 was highly commended and emulated during the epidemics of 1703 and 1711. Her kindness and charity were demonstrated in the hospitality extended to Sarah Garrish, an English girl ransomed from the Abenakis who had killed her family and enslaved her, and to a renegade Benedictine. Juchereau describes a pestilence which spread 'with incredible fury', sparing no house and wiping out entire households, compromising any significant care that could be extended to victims. Priests were overwhelmed by the number of burials and demands of the dying so that traditional burial protocol was abandoned for many months. Juchereau estimated that 2,000 died in the city of Québec but that, given the city's population at the time, must be an overestimate. Approximately half that number may be nearer the true figure.

Registered burials for 1703 reveal that 1,148 deaths were recorded – 3.6 times the average for the period, and 4.7 times the number for 1701, making it easily the worst epidemic to strike the colony since its founding. In January 1702 in Québec 267 deaths were registered, twenty-five times the number the previous year. By the time it relented in May the number of fatalities was 767 compared with 61 a year before. In Montreal where the epidemic lasted a little longer the death toll was 353 compared with 51 the previous year.

Desjardins. B., 1996, Demographic Aspects of the 1702–1703 Smallpox Epidemic in the St. Lawrence Valley, *Canadian Studies in Population* 23, 49–67

Heagerty, J.,1926. The Story of Small-Pox Among the Indians of Canada. *The Public Health Journal*, 17(2), 51–61

Marble, Alan Surgeons,1993, *Smallpox, and the Poor: a History of Medicine and Social Conditions in Nova Scotia, 1749–1799*, McGill-Queen's University Press

Chapter 26

The 1707–1709 Iceland smallpox epidemic

O ver the centuries isolated Iceland has endured hard winters, especially during the Little Ice Age, and these, with rough northern seas have effectively cut Icelanders off from the European mainland, allowing them to develop their distinctive culture. It also shielded generations of Icelanders from crowd diseases, albeit at the expense of immunity.

The first recorded smallpox epidemic in Iceland was in 1241, arriving via what is now roughly Denmark. In 1707 the absence of immunity created a calamitous disaster for the remote Icelanders when a ship from mainland Europe brought with it that most unwelcome of imports, smallpox. The island had suffered with several smallpox epidemics before, but the last outbreak ended in 1670, so almost no-one under 40 in 1770 had acquired any immunity to protect them. Iceland had more or less reverted to virgin country for the virus.

As is typical with smallpox epidemics, the disease made its way inexorably through the island so that by 1709, when the last cases of sickness were recorded, the virus, *variola*, had killed 12,000 people, nearly a quarter of Iceland's population. The only benefit to accrue from this carnage was the immunity conferred to the survivors.

Cliff, A., & Haggett, P., 1984. Island Epidemics. *Scientific American*, 250(5), 138–147.

Chapter 27

Plague in the 18th century

The 1710–1712 Great Northern War plague outbreak: Denmark, Sweden, Lithuania

> *'The plague is met by order; its function is to sort out every possible confusion: that of the disease, which is transmitted when bodies are mixed together; that of the evil, which is increased when fear and death overcome prohibitions. It lays down for each individual his place, his body, his disease and his death, his well-being, by means of an omnipresent and omniscient power that subdivides itself in a regular, uninterrupted way even to the ultimate determination of the individual, of what characterizes him, of what belongs to him, of what happens to him.'*
>
> – Paul-Michel Foucault (1926–1984)
> *Discipline and Punish: The Birth of the Prison*

The Great Northern War (1700–21) was a war in which a coalition led by the Tsar of Russia, Peter I, overcame the supremacy of the Swedish Empire in Northern, Central and Eastern Europe. Along with the usual collateral of war it brought with it plague which peaked between 1710 and 1712 having arrived from Anatolia and Constantinople. It then spread to Pińczów in southern Poland, where it was first recorded in a Swedish military hospital in 1702, moving on to affect the Baltic Sea region by 1711, reaching Hamburg by 1712. Once again we find war and plague inextricably bound together with the pestilence dictating military policy and influencing outcomes, with military action exerting a similar impact on the trajectory of the plague.

The course of the war and the course of the plague mutually affected each other: soldiers and civilian refugees were often agents of the plague while the death toll in the military as well as the depopulation and devastation of towns and rural areas could and did severely impact the ability to resist enemy forces or to supply troops. On the eastern coast from Prussia to Estonia the average death toll for wide areas was up to two thirds or three quarters of the population, with many farms and villages left completely desolated. However, it is difficult to distinguish between deaths directly due to plague and deaths due to plague's companion, famine and starvation, and between other diseases, dysentery, smallpox and spotted fever, that came along with the plague.

Containment was the only real way of combating the plague, and so *cordons sanitaire* were established around infected towns like Stralsund and Königsberg; one was also established around the whole Kingdom of Prussia from 1707 and those crossing into the

Prussian exclave were quarantined. Bridges were demolished, lesser roads blocked, and orders were given to hang people avoiding the guarded crossings and burn or fumigate all incoming goods. Unfortunately for effective disease containment there were too many exemptions, not least for people with cross-border estates or occupations, who were allowed to pass over freely. 'Plague houses' to quarantine infected people were established, an example being the Charité of Berlin.

In 1707 the plague reached Cracow, where 20,000 people died within three years; in Warsaw, 30,000 people perished between 1707 and 1710. Poznań lost around 9,000 people, about two thirds of its 14,000 inhabitants, to the plague between 1707 and 1709. The port of Danzig (Gdansk) gives us another example of a city in denial and pursuing a less than transparent policy to preserve its international trade. While not involved in the war, the city had suffered a reduction in trade, rising taxes and food shortages. The city council downplayed the plague to the outside world, especially to Danzig's trading partners, thus keeping the city open and allowing international and local trade to continue with few restrictions.

Controls on burials were eased due to a coffin shortage and the deaths of many grave diggers; a 'health commission' was set up to, among other things, provide the plague victims with food. The health commission's reports were later kept secret: Danzig eventually lost about half of its inhabitants. Stettin too adopted a policy of opacity to protect its trade; restrictions were also imposed on travellers, especially soldiers' families returning from Swedish-occupied Poland after defeat at the Battle of Poltava (8 July 1709), and a ban on fruits in the town's markets, since fruits were believed to transmit the disease. These returning soldiers' wives who had contact with the plague-stricken areas around Poznań were most likely the transmitters of the plague to Pomerania.

In November 1709, when the Prussian king Frederick I returned to Berlin after a meeting with Russian tsar Peter the Great, the king had a strange encounter with his mentally ill wife Sophia Louise, who in a white dress and with bloody hands pointed at him, Lady Macbeth-like, pronouncing that the plague would devour the king of Babylon. Mindful that there was a legend of a White Lady foretelling the deaths of the House of Hohenzollern, Frederick took his wife's outburst seriously and ordered that precautions be taken in Berlin amongst which was the construction of that pest house outside the city walls, the Berlin Charité.

From Livonia and Estonia, refugees took the plague to central Sweden and Finland, introducing it to Stockholm via a ship from Pernau. Here the health commission (Collegium Medicum) at first denied that the affliction was indeed the plague, despite buboes being clearly visible on the bodies of victims from the ship and in the town. The plague raged in Stockholm until 1711, affecting primarily women (45.3 per cent of the dead) and children (38.7 per cent of the dead) in the poorer quarters outside the Old Town. Of Stockholm's approximately 55,000 inhabitants, about 22,000 succumbed. In Altona, the plague killed 1,000 people, among them 300 Jews. Malmö suffered losses of 30 to 40 per cent. The Russian army led by Peter the Great entered the town; the tsar 'frolicked in Hamburg while his troops plundered the suburbs'.

When the plague broke out in Hamburg in 1712, it was carried there from the Danish troops by a prostitute from Hamburg's Gerkenshof Lane, where out of 53 people

35 fell ill and 18 died. The lane was blocked off and isolated. In March 1714 when the plague finally abated in Hamburg, 10,000 people had succumbed.

Frandsen, Karl-Erik, 2009. *The Last Plague in the Baltic Region. 1709–1713.* Copenhagen

The Great Plague of Marseille: 1720–1723

'...the accumulation of small negligence led to one of the worst epidemics in the city (about 30% of casualties among the inhabitants). This is an excellent model to illustrate the issues we are facing with emerging and re-emerging infectious diseases today and to define how to improve biosurveillance and response tomorrow.'
                    – Christian Devaux (2013) *Small oversights that led to the Great Plague of*
                                        Marseille: Lessons from the past

The Great Plague of Marseille has the distinction of being the last major outbreak of bubonic plague in western Europe. The disease certainly did not go out with a whimper: it killed 100,000 people: 50,000 in the city during the next two years and another 50,000 to the north in surrounding provinces and towns. Estimates indicate an overall death rate of between 25–50 per cent for the population in the wider area, with Marseille at 40 per cent, Toulon at above 50 per cent, and the area of Aix and Arles at 25 per cent.

The port city also has the much rarer distinction of actually learning from the past: at the end of the plague of 1580 Marseille prudently took measures to control the spread of disease in any future outbreaks. The city council established a sanitation board, whose members included doctors of the city; it is first mentioned in a 1622 text of the Parliament of Aix and included the establishment of a public health infrastructure which saw the opening of the first public hospital in Marseille with a full complement of doctors and nurses. Because of the plethora of fake news, quackery and misinformation that is often pedalled during a plague, the Sanitation Board took on responsibility for the accreditation of local doctors to provide citizens with a list of doctors who were believed to be genuine.

The Board established an effective three-tiered control and quarantine system. Members inspected all incoming ships and gave them one of three 'bills of health' which then determined the level of access to the city by the ship and its cargo. A delegation of members of the board was empowered to greet every ship. They reviewed the captain's log, which recorded every city where the ship had landed, and checked it against the sanitation board's master list of cities throughout the Mediterranean that had rumours of recent plague incidents. The delegation also inspected all the cargo, crew and passengers, looking for signs of possible disease. If the team detected disease, the ship was not allowed to dock. Even a clean bill of health was no guarantee of entry; all ships were required to undergo a minimum of eighteen days' quarantine at one of the off-island lazarettos/lazarets that were built around the city. If crew members or passengers were suspected of plague, they were sent to one of the more isolated quarantine sites where they would be held for fifty to sixty days to ensure they were clean.

In 1720, *Yersinia pestis* arrived at Marseille from the Levant on board the *Grand-Saint-Antoine* which had sailed from Sidon in Lebanon, having previously called at Smyrna, Tripoli and plague-ridden Cyprus. A Turkish passenger was the first to be infected and soon died, followed by several crew members and the ship's surgeon. The ship had been refused entry to Livorno. When it arrived at Marseille, it was promptly placed under quarantine in the lazaret by the port authorities. However, pressure was applied by influential city merchants who wanted to get their hands on the silk and cotton cargo for the great medieval fair at Beaucaire; they pressured authorities to lift the quarantine.

A few days later, the disease flared up in the city with the usual train of events: hospitals were overwhelmed and townsfolk panicked, driving the sick from their homes and out of the city. Mass graves were dug but were quickly filled. Despite all the good work over the last 140 years the fatalaties swamped all public health efforts, until thousands of corpses lay in putrifying piles around the city.

Marseille soon assumed the appearance of a city at war and under siege: the death penalty awaited anyone who attempted communication between Marseille and the rest of Provence. This was physically enforced by a plague wall, *mur de la peste*, which was built to cut off or defend the port; it was made of dry stone, 2m high and 70cm thick, with guard posts set back from the wall. Remains of the wall can still be seen.

International infectious disease specialist Nicolas Roze was appointed General Commissioner: he established quarantine by setting up checkpoints and built gallows to deter looters; he also had five large mass graves dug out, converted La Corderie into a field hospital and organised distribution of humanitarian aid to the population. In September Roze personally headed a 150-strong group of volunteers and prisoners to remove 1,200 corpses in the poor neighbourhood of the Esplanade de la Tourette. Some of the corpses were three weeks old and contemporary sources describe them as 'hardly human in shape and set in movement by maggots'. The rotting, stinking corpses were thrown into open pits that were then filled with lime and covered with soil. Of 1,200 volunteers and prisoners deployed to fight the plague generally, only three survived according to Roze who himself caught the disease, but survived.

When the plague subsided the city made another attempt at forestalling any future outbreak: the plague defences were reinforced; the waterside Lazaret d'Arenc was built where a double line of 15-foot walls ringed the whitewashed compound, punctured on the waterside to permit the offloading of cargo. Merchantmen were required to pass inspection at an island further out in the harbour where crews and cargoes were examined.

Devaux, Christian, 2013. 'Small oversights that led to the Great Plague of Marseille (1720–1723): Lessons from the past'. *Infection, Genetics and Evolution*, 169–185.

The Moscow plague riots of 1771

The Russian plague epidemic of 1770–72 claimed between 52,000 and 100,000 lives in Moscow alone – between one sixth and one third of its population. It started in the Moldovan theatre of the 1768–1774 Russian-Turkish war and in January 1770 swept up into Ukraine and central Russia, peaking in Moscow in September 1771 and sparking the Plague Riot. The epidemic redrew the map of Moscow when new cemeteries were established beyond the 18th-century city limits.

Russian troops in Focşani, Moldova were the first to see signs of plague; the disease, indigenous to the area, was contracted through prisoners of war and booty. Unsurprisingly the bad news was exaggerated by enemies of Russia, but Catherine II wrote a reassuring letter to Voltaire, arguing that 'in spring those killed by plague will resurrect for the fighting'. Skullduggery ensued: General Christopher von Shtoffeln coerced army doctors to conceal the outbreak, which was not made public for some time when Gustav Orreus, a Russian-Finnish surgeon identified it as plague and enforced quarantine in the troops. Shtoffeln, however, refused to evacuate the infested towns and himself fell victim to the plague in May 1770. Of 1,500 cases recorded in his troops in between May and August 1770, only 300 survived.

August 1770 came and Catherine still refused to admit the plague in public. Moscow had been deposed by St Petersburg as state capital and its suburbs became a magnet for vast numbers of serfs and army deserters. The increasing population generated escalating amounts of waste but there was no real solution for getting rid of it. There was human waste, horse waste and waste from tanneries, slaughterhouses and other polluting industries, all of which was steadily piling up. Catherine made strenuous efforts to clean up the city, but found herself in a losing battle against the plague. Creating quarantine stations on Russia's southern border proved ineffective.

In December 1770, Doctor A.F. Shafonskiy, the chief physician at the Moscow General Hospital, identified a case of the bubonic plague and promptly reported it to German physician A. Rinder, who was in charge of the public health of the city. Unfortunately, Rinder ignored the report. Shafonskiy submitted a further report in February but the officials chose to side with the German instead. In March, there were definitive signs of the disease, and so Moscow's government began implementing the established procedures, including setting up field hospitals. In June 1771, Rinder died after contracting the disease from a patient and by September the city was in its worst shape yet: the plague had peaked with 20,401 people dying in that month alone, and roughly three quarters of Moscow's population fled the city. The poor were terrified by the summary destruction of their contaminated homes without compensation or control, and so hid dead bodies, burying the deceased at night or simply slinging them out on the streets. This was one of the reasons that, in the aftermath, Catherine ordered the removal of all cemeteries to the suburbs.

Governor Saltykov could not control the situation and deserted Moscow for his country estate; the chief of police followed. Jacon Lerche, the newly appointed sanitary inspector of Moscow, declared a state of emergency, shutting down shops, inns, taverns, factories and even churches; the city was placed under quarantine.

Huge groups of people were literally thrown onto the streets and denied their regular trade and recreation.

On 15 September 1771, Moscow residents revolted against the authorities. The mob interpreted emergency measures by the state as a conspiracy to spread the disease. An attempt by Archbishop Ambrose to prevent the citizens from gathering at the Icon of the Virgin Mary of Bogolyubovo (Икона Боголюбской Богоматери) in Kitai-gorod as a quarantine measure ignited the Plague Riot. On 15 September huge crowds of Muscovites streamed towards Red Square; sweeping aside a military unit, they burst into the Kremlin and destroyed the Chudov Monastery (archbishop's residence) and its wine cellars. Archbishop Ambrose managed to escape to the Donskoy Monastery. Archbishop Amvrosy, however, who removed a revered icon from the public to stem transmission of the disease by worshippers, was accused of conspiracy, hunted down and killed as 'enemy of the people'. Active rioting continued for three days; the remaining unrest was finally subdued by Grigory Orlov at the end of September.

Things deteriorated further when on 16 September rioters captured the Donskoy Monastery, killed Archbishop Amvrosy, and destroyed two quarantine zones at Danilov Monastery and one beyond the Serpukhov Gates. In the afternoon, most of the rebels who approached the Kremlin were confronted by military units. As soon as the Muscovites tried to attack the Kremlin's Spasskiye Gates, the army opened fire with buckshot, dispersing the crowd and capturing some of the rebels. On the morning of 17 September, around 1,000 rebels reconvened at the Spasskiye gates, demanding the release of captured rebels and elimination of quarantines. The army managed to disperse the crowd yet again and finally suppressed the riot.

Some 300 people were brought to trial. A government commission headed by Grigory Orlov took some measures against the plague and provided citizens with work and food, which finally pacified the people of Moscow. The commission improved services in quarantines, put an end to the burning of property, reopened public baths, permitted trade, increased food deliveries and organized public works. At the same time four rioters were executed while 165 adults and 12 teenagers were subjected to other punishment. Around 200,000 people died in Moscow and its outskirts during the plague.

There was another unlikely victim – by order of Catherine II, one of the executors cut the tang from the church bell that was used to toll the riot alarm. For more than thirty years, the emasculated bell hung silent on the bell tower. Eventually, in 1803, it was removed and sent to the Arsenal and, in 1821, to the Kremlin Armoury.

Beneficially, the plague and the riot provoked local research in disease prevention, which was boosted by discovering indigenous plague in newly conquered territories of the Caucasus. The research relating to the epidemic was revealed to western European academia through *An account of plague which raged in Moscow 1771*, published in 1798 in Latin by Belgian physician Charles de Mertens; an English translation was published in 1799.

The depradations caused by the plague forced the government to reduce taxes and military conscription quotas in affected provinces; both measures debilitated the military capabilities and forced Catherine to seek a truce with the Ottoman Empire.

Here are some excerpts from de Mertens' account which give a flavour of the disaster as it unfolded; note the insistence on fair pay for medical staff and on PPE.

The havoc was still greater during the time of the riots, which began on the 15th September, in the evening when an outrageous mob broke open the pest-houses and quarantine hospitals, renewing all the religious ceremonies which it is customary for them to perform at the bedside of the sick, and digging up the dead bodies and burying them afresh in the city...the people began to embrace the dead, despising all manner of precaution, which they declared to be of no avail, as the public calamity (I repeat their own words)was sent by God, to punish them for having neglected their ancient forms of worship [and] whose wrath was only to be appeased by their refusing all human assistance...physicians, surgeons and nurses must be appointed to take care of the impested, and have handsome salaries allowed them...those who are employed in burying the dead should be protected from the contagion by having cloaks and gloves of oil cloth which should be frequently washed with vinegar...they should be provided with hooks and other instruments for lifting [the bodies] up.

Alexander, John T., 2003. *Bubonic plague in early modern Russia: public health and urban disaster.* Oxford

Melikishvili, Alexander, 2006. 'Genesis of the anti-plague system: the Tsarist period.' *Critical Reviews in Microbiology.* 36: 19–31.

Mertens, Charles de, 1799. 'An account of plague which raged in Moscow 1771.' *Oriental Research Papers.* 8 (2): 37–127

Chapter 28

The 1713–15 North America measles epidemic

'...*the largest child killer in history.*'
– C.J. Clements, 2004

The story of measles goes back as far as 5,000 years in the civilizations of the Tigris and Euphrates river valleys. It is an acute illness caused by a virus in the paramyxovirus family and is one of the most contagious diseases known to man. Measles has been called the 'largest child killer in history'.[1] If exposed, almost all non-immune children contract measles with up to 99 per cent of susceptibles contracting the virus after first contact with an infected person. It spreads with ease from person to person through the coughs and sneezes of those infected.

Symptoms usually develop 10–12 days after exposure to an infected person and last 7–10 days. Initial symptoms typically include fever, often greater than 40°C, cough, runny nose and inflamed eyes. Small white spots, Koplik's spots, may form inside the mouth soon after the onset of symptoms. A red, flat rash which usually starts on the face and then spreads to the rest of the body typically begins three to five days after the start of symptoms. Common complications include diarrhoea (in 8 per cent of cases), middle ear infection (7 per cent), and pneumonia (6 per cent) – all due in part to measles-induced immunosuppression. Less commonly, seizures, blindness, or inflammation of the brain may occur. It can and does affect people of any age; most people do not get the disease more than once. Mortality is about 0.2 per cent, but may be up to 10 per cent in people with malnutrition. Most of those who die from the infection are under 5 years old. Other names for measles include morbilli, rubeola, red measles and English measles. Both rubella, also known as German measles, and roseola are different diseases caused by unrelated viruses.

The measles vaccine is effective and is exceptionally safe. Vaccination resulted in an 80 per cent decrease in deaths from measles between 2000 and 2017, with about 85 per cent of children worldwide having received their first dose by 2017. Measles affects about 20 million people a year mainly in the developing areas of Africa and Asia. In 1980, 2.6 million people died of it and in 1990, 545,000 died. By 2000, vaccine coverage reached about 72 per cent of the children in the world through national immunization programs; by 2014, global vaccination programs had reduced the number of deaths to 73,000. Despite these trends, rates of disease and deaths increased

---

1. Clements, 2004

from 2017 to 2019 due to lower immunization levels and the ill-advised, selfish and imprudent attitudes of anti-vaxxers.

The first systematic description of measles, and its distinction from smallpox and chickenpox, was by the Persian physician Muhammad ibn Zakariya al-Razi (860–932) in his *Book of Smallpox and Measles*. This chimes with the observation that measles requires a susceptible population of at least >250,000 to sustain an epidemic, a situation that occurred following the growth and development of medieval European cities. In 1676 English doctor Thomas Sydenham MD, published his *Observationes medicae circa morborum acutorum historiam et curationem (Medical observations on the history and cure of acute diseases)* in which he distinguished smallpox from the measles. He also recorded details about and distinguished the disease from scarlet fever.

The death rates effected by measles are terrifying: in 1529, an outbreak in Cuba killed two-thirds of those natives who had previously survived smallpox. In 1531 measles claimed half the population of Honduras; it also tore through Mexico, Central America and the Inca civilization. Measles' risk to Pacific Islanders was particularly acute in the 19th century as traders and travellers crisscrossed the globe. In 1824, Hawaii's King Kamehameha II and Queen Kamamalu traveled to London to meet King George IV, but swiftly contracted measles. Both died within a month. The virus, along with several other diseases, struck Hawaii in 1848, killing up to a third of the native population.

Between roughly 1855 and 2005 measles has been estimated to have killed about 200 million people worldwide. It despatched 20 per cent of Hawaii's population in the 1850s and in 1875 over 40,000 Fijians died from it, approximately one-third of the population, courtesy of the visiting crew of HMS *Dido*. In the 19th century, the disease killed 50 per cent of the Andamanese population. In 1846 Danish physician Peter Ludwig Panum visited the Faroe Islands to study a measles outbreak that had infected more than 75 per cent of the islands' 7,782 residents – killing at least 102. Panum observed that 'not one' of the elderly residents who had been infected in 1781 'was attacked a second time'. Awareness of such immunity would later become key to defeating the virus.

Samuel de Champlain founded the colony of New France in Canada in 1608; originally intended as a hunting and fishing outpost, it was many years before it became a permanent settlement. Early Québec could boast a low population density (24,564 in 1714.) and was relatively isolated from the outside world – both useful characteristics which limited the spread of communicable diseases which thrive on large host populations to survive. Old Québec, with its comparatively healthy and fertile population, unlike France and Colonial America, was, for a time untroubled by plagues and epidemics. But things began to change in the early 18th century: the colonists were no longer so isolated from outside contact with the rest of North America. Colonial America was growing and due to a long period of immigration, had a much larger population than New France. Serial warfare with Britain and native tribes also led to more frequent encounters with the outside world. Additionally, the fur trade saw trade routes open up with local aboriginal tribes. Epidemics began to break out with greater frequency and severity throughout the colony resulting in many fatalities because the lack of exposure in earlier days meant that the Canadians had no acquired immunity to infectious diseases introduced into the colony.

Measles had afflicted the north east of America since the mid 17th century. In 1657 in Boston, John Hull wrote in his diary that 'the disease of measles went through the town; fortunately there were very few deaths'. In 1693 Virginia Governor Edmund Andros issued a proclamation for a 'day of Humiliation and Prayer' due to measles there. Later, in 1757, Scottish physician Francis Home, transmitted measles from infected patients to healthy individuals via blood, demonstrating that the disease was caused by an infectious agent.

> …Francis Home… attempted to produce mild measles by mimicking the variolation process. This process involved taking blood from an infected patient and inoculating it through the skin of an uninfected person. In this way he was able to transfer measles to ten of twelve patients. This experiment clearly demonstrated the presence of measles virus in human blood…
> – Michael B. A. Oldstone, *Viruses, Plagues, & History*

Records from Colonial America reveal that a serious measles epidemic took place between 1713 and 1715: residents of Boston suffered badly during the outbreak, which began in the late summer of 1713 and had gone by the end of January 1714. By February, the virus had spread to New York, New Jersey, Connecticut and Pennsylvania. It probably arrived in New France around April through native traders travelling to and fro from Colonial America.

Cotton Mather would later introduce smallpox variolation to the colonies. However, in 1713 he was more preoccupied with measles: he wrote in his diary of an impending measles epidemic: 'The Measles coming into the Town, it is likely to be a Time of Sickness, and much Trouble in the Families of the Neighbourhood.' Tragically, measles infected most of his family members: it killed his wife, his newborn twins, another daughter, six other children and the family's maid within six weeks. Mather had often preached on the topic of death, and held that 'the dying of a child is like the tearing off of a limb.'

> His diary entry for 23 December tells how…
> 'I have given to the Printer, a Letter about the Right Management of the Sick under the Distemper of the Measles which is now spreading and raging in the Countrey. I propose to scatter it into all parts… to save many lives….'

The letter Mather referred to was 'published for the benefit of the poor' in December 1713. It told those disadvantaged citizens without access to a doctor all about the typical signs and symptoms of measles, and simple treatments for it. They were essentially generic remedies for unbalanced 'humours', recommending Syrup of Saffron and Treacle Water, Syrup(s) of Maiden-hair or Hyssop, Tea of Sage or Rosemary, Sugar-Candied, or Buttered Pills, Hot Beer and Rum, Hot Cyder, Hot Honey, Water with Roasted Apples in it, Shavings of Castile Soap in a Glass of

Wine or Beer, or Tea made of Rhubarb, and sweetened with a Syrup of Marshmallow (*Althaea officinalis*). These were all ingredients within the budgets of the poor and which might at least provide some comfort, if not survival.

Although written for the the poor, it has been called by *Pediatrics*, the official journal of the American Academy of Pediatrics[2] 'a classic of American pediatrics and compares favourably with any description of measles written on the continent'. Cotton was 'the first writer in America to write a general treatise on medicine' (Beall 1952), despite being a theologian and preacher by profession with little medical training.

During the Second World War in England, some people believed that German measles was being sent over by the Germans. One diarist with the Mass-Observation Archive from Rotherham recorded how one of her pupils had been told that 'the experts' told him this.

Aaby, P., 1984. 'Overcrowding and intensive exposure as determinants of measles mortality'. *American Journal of Epidemiology* 120: 49

Black, F.L., 1982. 'The role of herd immunity in control of measles'. *The Yale Journal of Biology and Medicine* 55: 351–360.

Clements, C.J., 2004. *The Epidemiology of Measles: Thirty Years of Vaccination*, London

Morens, D.M., Measles in Fiji, 1875: thoughts on the history of emerging infectious diseases. *Pacific Health Dialog.* 1998; 5:119–28.

2. February 1978, 61 277

Chapter 29

The 1721 Boston smallpox outbreak and the inoculation war

'...the opposition to our present laws and their improvement would seem but the blowing of a summer zephyr to those who endured the hurricane of abuse hurled against the advocates of inoculation in 1721 and of vaccination in 1800. For 180 years smallpox was responsible for more deaths than any other one cause. Almost always sporadically present, coming in epidemic form every few years, few indeed escaped its ravages.'

So said Samuel Bayard Woodward MD in his 1932 address to the Massachusetts Medical Society entitled *The Story of Smallpox in Massachusetts;* his paper neatly crystallised the storm of controversy which accompanied the introduction of inoculation in the midst of the 1721 Boston smallpox outbreak. Indeed such was the furore that it almost eclipsed the terrible death toll of some 844 Bostonians over ten months in 1721 and 1722.

We have a slave to thank for providing the catalyst for inoculation and in so doing saving the lives of ten of thousands. In 1706, Onesimus, one of Cotton Mather's slaves, explained to Mather how he had been inoculated as a child in Africa. Mather was transfixed. By 1714 his enthusiasm for inoculation was rekindled when he read in the *Philosophical Transactions of the Royal Society* an endorsement in Dr Emmanuel Timoni's description of a similar procedure witnessed while serving as Great Britain's ambassador in Constantinople. Mather then wrote in a letter to Dr John Woodward of Gresham College in London, that he planned to urge Boston's doctors to adopt inoculation should smallpox reach the colony again. This was actually followed by a second encouraging letter by Pylarinus, a Venetian physician, on the same subject published in the *Philosophical Transactions of the Royal Society* in 1715.

These authoritative reports were ignored in England, but in the US things were very different: Lady Mary Wortley Montagu, wife of the English Ambassador to Turkey, described the practice in a letter to a friend in 1716, had her son inoculated soon afterwards, and in 1718 returned to England determined to do what she could to bring what she calls 'this useful convention' into use as a first line treatment. She told anyone she could that smallpox, so fatal in England, was entirely harmless in Turkey, that women organised parties in order to have the disease together, that patients were rarely bedridden for more than two or three days, patients never had more than twenty or thirty pocks on their faces and no scars, and that there was no example of anyone who had died of it. However, it was not until April 1721, three years after her return to England that, under the protection of the Princess of Wales, later Queen Charlotte, she arranged the first inoculation in England, and that was of her own child, Mary Alice.

Smallpox did reach the colony again. The vector was HMS *Seahorse* which arrived from Barbados on 22 April after a stop at Tortuga, part of Haiti, with a crew who had survived smallpox: HMS *Seahorse* was unwittingly incubating smallpox on board. One of *Seahorse*'s sailors fell ill in Boston Harbour a day after arrival and exposed other sailors to the virus. Boston's water bailiff inspected *Seahorse* and discovered another two or three cases of smallpox in various stages before ordering the ship to leave the harbour. Despite the infected sailor being hurriedly quarantined in the lodging house where he fell ill, nine other sailors at Boston Harbour exposed to him came down with smallpox in early May. The sailors were quarantined in Spectacle Island's rudimentary hospital, but staff and customs officials were unable to contain the virus – by mid-June, the disease was spreading rapidly.

Boston's previous smallpox outbreak was in 1703, so a new generation of non-immune children and young adults were vulnerable. As it continued to spread, 900 or so residents fled to outlying rural settlements, no doubt increasing the scope of the disease. The public became increasingly concerned that they were the subjects of divine punishment. The combination of exodus, quarantine and the fears of outside traders meant that commerce was disrupted for weeks. The newly inaugurated *New England Courant* was ordered in early October by the town council to publish a house-by-house count on those affected so far by smallpox: 2,757 cases, 1,499 recoveries and 203 deaths were counted.

Guards were posted at the House of Representatives to prevent Bostonians from entering without authorisation. The death toll reached 101 in September, and the Selectmen, powerless to stop it, 'severely limited the length of time funeral bells could toll'. £1,000 was awarded from the treasury to help people who could no longer support their families. The outbreak peaked in October when 411 people died; 8 per cent of Boston's population would succumb during the epidemic and hundreds of other Bostonians would recover but with severe scarring or disabilities.

The first hundred years of blight by smallpox had passed. Twelve times an epidemic with sporadic cases a constant, the only escape was to flee: smallpox during this century had done more to hinder the growth of the Massachusetts colony than Indian raids, foreign wars or any other general disaster.

On 6 June 1721, Mather circulated that abstract of reports on inoculation by Timonius and Jacobus Pylarinus to the other fourteen local physicians, urging them to wage a medical war against smallpox by inoculating their own patients or volunteers. But he received no response. Next, Mather pleaded his case to Harvard physician Zabdiel Boylston, who courageously tried the inoculation procedure on his youngest son and two slaves – one adult and one a boy. All recovered in about a week. Boylston inoculated seven more people by mid-July. The epidemic peaked in October 1721 with 411 deaths; by 26 February 1722, Boston was again free from smallpox. The total number of cases since April 1721 amounted to 5,889, with 844 deaths – more than three-quarters of all the deaths in Boston during 1721. Meanwhile,

Boylston had inoculated 287 Boston people, with only 6 resulting deaths. On the 25 November 1721, he inoculated 15 individuals at Harvard: 13 Harvard students, Professor Edward Wiglesworth and tutor William Welsted. They, too, survived. Cotton Mather wrote in a letter detailing Boylston's work in Boston: 'The experiment has now been made on several hundreds of persons, upon both male and female, upon both old and young, upon both strong and weak, upon both white and black.'

Boylston's programme is actually one of the earliest clinical trials on record, and the use of both experimental and control groups to demonstrate the effectiveness of inoculation significantly aided the adoption of the practice.

The pious outrage levelled at Lady Montagu's trial innoculation was beyond belief. The clergy thundered from the pulpit on the impiety of taking things out of the hands of the Almighty, of trying to alter the course of nature in the manner of the atheist, the scoffer, the heathen and the unbeliever, and, concluding that Satan was the first inoculator, quoted Job 2:7, 'So went Satan forth from the presence of the Lord and smote Job with sore boils from the sole of his foot unto his crown.' The people jeered the good lady in the streets as an unnatural mother while she herself feared for the safety of her daughter, not from the disease, but from the 'Four great physicians... deputed to watch the progress of the experiment with an evident unwillingness to have it succeed, manifesting such a spirit of rancour and malignity.'

The reaction is all the more staggering, even by the standards of the time, given the pervasive quackery, the folk medicine and the superstition, when we remember that inoculation had been practised in India since time immemorial, and in China for hundreds of years where routine practice was to blow dried and ground variola scabs into the nostrils of the patient – the right side being used for males, the left for females. Just as strange is that inoculation was unknown in England and indeed in Europe generally forty years after it had been practised in Turkey where inoculation involved inducing a less serious form of the smallpox disease by exposing an incision to the variola pus.

Eleven years before Lady Montagu's experiment the best the west could offer was a Thomas Hawkins who 'was paid 8d. for whipping two people who had ye smallpox'. Was this as a cure or a punishment?

Boylston was forbidden to continue his inoculation campaign beyond November due to opposition from Boston's Selectmen, as well as occasional violence from the public. But a tutor at Harvard inspired by his research, Thomas Robie, continued vaccinating patients at Spectacle Island. One of his patients was another tutor, Nicholas Sevier, who returned to Harvard sixteen days after he was inoculated to report on the success of his procedure. Harvard's academic community became more accepting of inoculation after the successful experiments of Boylston and Sevier.

It took a Scotsman – and an anti-inoculation physician, William Douglass – to introduce The Royal Society's editions containing the Timonius and Pylarinus letters to Boston in 1718. For many years he was the sole medical graduate in the Colony. 'Always positive and sometimes accurate', he lent the journals to a friend he calls 'a vain, credulous preacher'. This preacher was the irrepressible Cotton Mather; Mather made use of the papers immediately. To many Boston physicians, inoculation must have appeared as unscientific and quackish as other contemporary treatments

Table 4: The primary difference between the methods of inoculation and vaccination, which both generate an immunity against smallpox, was in the viral source. Inoculation used actual smallpox material, while vaccination used immunologically-related cowpox, and now Vaccinia virus.

Modes of exposure to smallpox		
Natural infection	Inoculation	Vaccination
Prolonged contact with an infected person, especially during the first stages of the smallpox rash when virus levels are very high. Also, contact with infected bodily fluids or contaminated objects. http//www.bt.cdc.gov/agent/smallpox/overview/disease-facts.asp	Deliberate exposure to the smallpox virus using material from a smallpox scab – for example rubbed into a small cut on the skin. Generally results in a milder form of disease, but still carries a risk of death. http//en.wikipedia.org.wiki/inoculation	Induction of a much milder, acute infection through direct exposure, using a virus related to smallpox. Originally vaccines used the pus of cowpox. Modern smallpox vaccines contain vaccinia virus.

such as bleeding and purging, which were still common practice during the early 18th century.

Meanwhile, while Mary Alice lay ill in London, HMS *Seahorse* duly unloaded her deadly cargo in Boston harbour: a year later, 5,759 of the 12,000 inhabitants of Boston had been infected and 844 died; neighbouring Roxbury, Cambridge and Charlestown were particularly affected, 100 dying in Charlestown alone.

The fact that Mather was neither liked nor respected did not help his cause – Samuel Woodward (1932) gives the background:

'He inextricably mixed piety and medicine in many of his publications, thought disease the result of sin, sickness *Flagellum Dei pro peccato Mundi*, advised the scattering of wens by the laying on of a dead hand and eulogized the healing virtues of a solution of sowbugs [woodlice]. He believed in witch marks and the application of the water ordeal which, as Oliver Wendell Holmes puts it, means 'Throw your grandmother into the water, if she has a mole on her arm. If she swims she is a witch and must be hanged; if she sinks the Lord have mercy on her soul.'

Woodward describes the uproar amongst the medical fraternity and the people:

'The storm broke; the other physicians would have no part in the matter; the mob, believing that inoculation was simply giving smallpox to those who might otherwise escape, were roused to fury. A legion of incendiary pamphlets appeared. Men declared that it was impious to interfere between the Creator and his creatures, that multiplying smallpox by artificial means was a wilful tampering with death... The clergy almost unanimously supported Boylston. The physicians almost as unanimously derided his efforts. There were times when Boylston was truly in great peril...men patrolled the town with halters threatening to hang him to the nearest tree, that he once remained secreted in a 'private place' in his own house for fourteen days, while parties entered by day and by night in search of him and that even after the madness of the multitude had to some degree subsided he was forced to visit his patients by night and in disguise.'

Despite all the vilification, the demonization, the accusations that 'infusing such malignant filth into the mass of the blood is to corrupt and putrify it', of papers 'prostituted in hellish servitude', of the card tied to the improvised explosive device thrown through a window into his house which read, 'Cotton Mather, you dog. Damn you! I'll inoculate you with this with a pox to you' – despite all of this Mather and Boylston and their inoculation programme eventually won through. In 1723 on the invitation of Dr. Hans Sloan, President of the Royal Society, Boylston went to England, and spoke before both the College of Physicians and the Royal Society to which he was in 1726 elected a member. In eight months he had inoculated one third as many persons as were subjected to the procedure in all England in the seven years 1721–1728. The figures speak for themselves: the mortality rate after inoculation in the 1721 epidemic was 2.4 per cent, after natural smallpox 14.8 per cent.

Sadly, this was not the end of smallpox in Massachusetts, but inoculation was to prove a great life-saver: in 1751, introduced as usual by an infected ship, smallpox struck 124 individuals of whom 22 died. It spread slowly until May of the next year, but in December was out of control. Fences were built across streets near infected houses, flags of warning hung out, the tolling of bells at funerals suppressed, burials carried out at night, town meetings held in the open; 2,124 persons were inoculated, of whom 30 died – 1 in 70. Of the 5,545 who acquired it in the natural way, 539 died – 1 in 11.

In 1764 in five weeks, 4,977 persons were inoculated, 46 died – one in 109; 669 elected for the natural way, of whom 124 died – one in 5. Inoculation hospitals were opened at Point Shirley and Castle William. In 1769 and again in 1773 new outbreaks forced the opening of more hospitals. In 1775, during the British occupation, Washington's army was so blighted that wholesale inoculation was resorted to – 4,988 men were treated, and 18 died.

During 1778, 2,121 inoculations were performed with 29 deaths, 9 per cent; 122 other cases were recorded with 42 deaths, 34 per cent. In 1792, smallpox was brought in by a vessel from Ireland, practically the whole town was inoculated within a few days. The absolute need for this procedure was now almost universally accepted. Life-saving apart, the inoculation debate had a profound impact on Western society's medical treatment of the disease. The outbreak also permanently changed social and religious public discourse about disease.

The use of inoculation laid the foundation for the modern techniques of infectious disease prevention; the contentious public debate that accompanied the introduction of this poorly understood medical procedure has alarming similarities to modern day misunderstandings over vaccination. It was a pivotal milestone in the history of vaccination and smallpox eradication, paving the way for Edward Jenner to develop effective smallpox vaccination by the end of the century.

The Boston epidemic is significant for other reasons: this was the first time in US medicine where the press was used to inform, or alarm, the general public about a health crisis. The *New England Courant*, under its owner James Franklin and fledgeling editor, a 16-year-old Benjamin Franklin (1706–1790), using the *nom de plume* Silence Dogood, continued to publish satirical articles about Mather and inoculation in the months following the epidemic. Boylston retorted with *An Historical Account of the Small Pox Inoculated in New England*. The controversy had a profound influence on Franklin, changing the way he thought about politics, the press and freedom of the press.[1] Coss tells us:

> ' …it was the first real experiment that Benjamin Franklin, the great experimenter, had ever witnessed firsthand; and…it made Boylston a hero. Boylston, like Franklin, was a man of humble origins. He didn't have a Harvard College education, like most of the other doctors in town. He didn't come from a prominent family or a wealthy family. I think Ben Franklin walked away from this experience realizing the potential of his own life.'

In Philadelphia, Franklin became a fervent supporter of inoculation – arguably the number one proponent of inoculation in all of the Colonies – and Philadelphia became the cutting edge centre of inoculation. In 1777, George Washington made the critical decision to have all his soldiers inoculated. Many historians believe that this was perhaps Washington's greatest contribution as a general in the Revolution. In the end, variolation became a widespread and accepted technique in the West, decades before Jenner's discovery of vaccination with cowpox.

Best, M., 2004. 'Cotton Mather, you dog, damn you! I'll inoculate you with this; with a pox to you': smallpox inoculation, Boston, 1721. *Quality & Safety in Health Care.* 13 (1): 82–83.

Coss, Stephen (2016-03-08). The Fever of 1721. New York

Farmer, Laurence, 1958. 'The Smallpox Inoculation Controversy and the Boston Press 1721–2'. *Bulletin of the New York Academy of Medicine.* 34 (9): 599–601, 608.

Minardi, Margo, 2004. 'The Boston Inoculation Controversy of 1721–1722: An Incident in the History of Race'. *The William and Mary Quarterly* 61 (1): 57–82.

Willett, Jo, 2021, *The Pioneering Life of Mary Wortley Montagu*, Barnsley

---

1. Coss 2016

Chapter 30

1735–1741 'Throat distemper' (diphtheria) epidemic: New England, New York, New Jersey

The January 1975 issue of *Pediatrics* – official journal of the American Academy of Pediatrics – begins its article, *On the Treatment of Diphtheria in 1735* with:

> 'The most frightful epidemic of any childhood disease in American history began in 1735. The disease was diphtheria ... the most characteristic feature of this epidemic was the occurrence of multiple deaths in families. There were at least six instances of eight deaths at a time due to diphtheria in a single family.'

And in so doing the paper encapsulates perfectly the one most terrible and terrifying characteristic of this 'plague of the throat'.

So, in 1735, when a young child in Kingston, New Hampshire came down with what to all intents and purposes initially looked like a regular cold, no one could have imagined that most of New England would fall sick. Folk tradition in Kingston attributes the outbreak in April 1735 to when Joseph Clough skinned a pig, which had died of a throat ailment. Clough himself became ill and later died of a similar sickness. The Great Throat Distemper of 1735 to 1740 (now termed diphtheria) was one of the most ferocious epidemics ever to terrify New England. 'Distemper' told everybody, doctors included, that the humors were out of sync; germs and infectivity did not come into it, only bloodletting and purgation (which made it all much worse).

Every New England state was attacked, none more so than New Hampshire. Exeter suffered 127 deaths, with 105 of them children under the age of 10. Kingston, with a small overall population, lost 113 people, 96 of whom were children. The town that suffered most was Hampton Falls, a very small community compared to the others. It endured 210 deaths, 160 of which were children.

Diphtheria is an infectious disease, caused by a contagious bacterium, *Coryne-bacterium diphtheria* passed on by close contact with an infected person, which primarily affects the mucous membranes of the respiratory tract, as well as the skin and other sensitive areas of the body, including ears, eyes and genital areas. We get our first descriptions in Aphorisms 24 and 31 in the Hippocratic treatise *Dentition*. In the first we read that 'in the ulceration of the tonsils the presence of something resembling a spider's web is not good'. The second describes the voice change when the ulceration spreads over the uvula, that is the paralysis of the upper palate after an ulcerous sore throat. Aretaeus of Cappadocia (fl. AD 130–140) described the diphtheric sore throat and explained that it was called Egyptian or Syrian ulcers since it was rampant in these countries. The physician Rufus of Ephesus (fl. late 1st and early 2nd centuries AD) and Aëtius of Amida (fl. mid-5th century to mid-6th century) added to our knowledge.

More recently it was first reported in the early 1600s and became more virulent with the urbanisation of the west; in 1826 it received its official name, diphtérite, after the Greek for a hide or leather, describing the thick coating of the throat patients present with. The name came from French physician Pierre Bretonneau (1778–1862); he also distinguished diphtheria from scarlet fever.

'As the disease worsens, a pseudomembrane often develops over the tonsils and nasopharynx. In other words, the bacterium collects and coagulates into a film, which covers the lining of the throat, causing swelling of the neck and difficulty breathing. As the pseudomembrane gets larger, swelling worsens and lymph nodes become enlarged, giving the neck a 'bull-neck' appearance. In untreated cases, this pseudomembrane will become large enough to obstruct the larynx and the trachea, slowly cutting off the airway, causing suffocation and death.'
– *The Strangling Angel of Children – The Birth of Endotracheal Intubation* by Elizabeth Roberts, MA, CPC May 12, 2011

The pseudomembrane is formed from waste products and proteins caused by the toxin secreted by the bacteria. The pseudomembrane sticks to tissues and may obstruct breathing. The toxin itself may travel to the heart, muscle, kidneys and liver, where it may temporarily or permanently damage these organs. Complications may include myocarditis (damage to the heart muscle), neuritis (inflammation of nerves, which may contribute to nerve damage, paralysis, respiratory failure and pneumonia), airway obstruction and ear infection.

In 1858, Parisian paediatrician Eugene Bouchut (1818–1891) developed the method of endotracheal intubation, which involved introducing a small straight metal tube into the larynx, securing it by means of a silk thread and leaving it there for a few days until the pseudomembrane and airway obstruction has resolved sufficiently. Bouchut presented this technique along with the results he had achieved in the first seven cases at the Académie des Sciences conference on 18 September 1858. The Académie initially rejected Bouchut's ideas, despite the method having the benefits of being less invasive than the previous first line intervention, tracheotomy, and often resulted in a higher survival rate.

The New England epidemic moved northeastward, affecting many small towns in New Hampshire to Maine. From July 1735 to July 1736 the death records of fifteen New Hampshire towns revealed that 984 people died from the disease, mostly children. On the Isles of Shoals, 8 miles out to sea, the isolated fishing community lost 36 children.

Burial records show that in Ipswich, all eight children in the household of Mark and Hephzibah Howe died during November 1735; town records record that they died of 'cancre quinsy', an 18th century term for laryngeal obstruction. A neighbouring family also reported losing all eight children. One family afflicted was that of the Reverend Samuel Danforth. Danforth wrote: 'The Lord sent a general visitation of Children by coughs & colds, of which my three children Sarah, Mary & Elisabeth Danforth died, all of them with[in] the space of a fortnight.' Often, as many as four children were buried in a single grave. Church records reveal parents pressurised ministers into performing early baptisms 'By Reason of Dangerous Sickness'. Rowley, Massachusetts lost one-eighth of its population; nearby Byfield would lose one seventh. What quarantine there was, was rather ad hoc: in Exeter, New Hampshire, for example, the townspeople seized the house where a young man had died of the disease and quarantined his brother until he too died. Self-isolation was not an option and the communal graves cruelly mirrored the fact that often children in Puritan New England would routinely sleep four to a bed, infected or not. They went to school together; they sat together in pews at church; they carried the small bodies of their deceased friends and siblings to the graveyard as a reminder of their own mortality. They were discouraged from grieving because to grieve or mourn the dead was to turn away from God. The comforting ministrations of clergy and doctors only helped to spread the disease from one family to another. There was, in short, no escape.

Physicians were at a complete loss; as with other contagions their confusion is reflected in the number of names or misdiagnoses the distemper was given: cynanche, angina, canker, bladders, rattles or throat distemper. More commonly the illness was 'the strangling angel of children'. To compound the chaos scarlet fever was also rampant during 1735, and children were dying of both.

In 1735, with a vaccine for diphtheria more than a hundred years away, treatment of the disease was primitive and painful. When the throat distemper tore through Boston, a notice in the *Boston Gazette* offered some truly frightening home-based treatment advice which typified the best the frantic world could offer:

> 'First be sure that a vein be opened under the tongue, and if that can't be done, open a vein in the arm, which must be first done, as all other means will be ineffectual. Then take borax or honey to bathe or annoint the mouth and throat, and lay on the Throat a plaister Vngiuntum Dialthae. To drink a decoction of Devil's bitt or Robbin's Plantain, with some Sal Prunelle dissolved therein, as often as the patient will drink. If the body be costive use a clyster agreeable to the nature of the Distemper. ... But be sure and let blood, and that under the tongue. We have many times made Blisters under the arms, but that has proved sometimes dangerous.'

Superstition, and its frequent stablemate, fake news were rampant: the New England Historical Society takes up the story:

> 'In Newbury, Massachusetts people speculated that the disease was related to an explosion in the population of caterpillars in the summer of 1735. The noxious caterpillars covered the roads and houses. They could even float across streams. They crackled when carriage wheels crushed them and caused the wheels to grow slippery. A prayer and sermon seemed to extinguish the caterpillars, but doubts persisted that they also caused the throat distemper.

In Haverhill, Mass., a pamphlet explained that children's wailing and coughing showed God or supernatural beings spoke through them. In 1738 the throat distemper epidemic entered its third year and a 17-page poem about it appeared in pamphlet form. AWAKENING CALLS TO EARLY PIETY suggested the disease resulted from impious behavior.'

In the end across New England some 5,000 people died of diphtheria between 1735 and 1740. More than 75 per cent were children. Overall, it killed 22 of every 1,000 people. In New Hampshire, where it struck first and worst, 75 out of every 1,000 people died.

Caulfield, Ernest, 1939, A History of the Terrible Epidemic, Vulgarly Called the Throat Distemper, as It Occurred in His Majesty's New England Colonies Between 1735 and 1740, *Yale J Biol Med.* 11(3): 219–272.

Fitch, Jabez, 1736, An account of the numbers that have died of the distemper in the throat, within the province of New-Hampshire: with some reflections thereto; July 26. 1736. *U.S. National Library of Medicine.*

Chapter 31

1775–1782 North American smallpox epidemic and the prison ships

'At the end of the war [of Independence] in 1783, the remains of those who died on the British prison ships were left to rot along the Brooklyn shore. Nathaniel Scudder Prime reported on "skulls and feet, arms and legs sticking out of the crumbling bank in the wildest disorder" while Edwin G. Burrows described the skulls on the coast 'as thick as pumpkins in an autumn cornfield'.

If, as Captain George Vancouver did in 1792, you were to cruise down the northwest coastline of America hugging the shore you would have been concerned, as indeed Captain Vancouver and his officers were. Where have all the natives gone? he must have pondered. The land was fertile, with abundant salmon and fresh water, but there were so few people, only deserted villages like the first he encountered south of his soon to be namesake Vancouver Island on the shores of Discovery Bay. This was 'over-run with weeds; amongst which were found several human skulls, and other bones, promiscuously scattered about'. A dystopian scene the like of which seasoned explorer George Vancouver had never before witnessed.

Futher exploration in the Strait of Juan de Fuca between Vancouver Island and the Washington state mainland, from 29 April 1792, revealed more depopulation and devastation; one crew member Thomas Manby noted, 'we saw a great many deserted villages some of them ... capable of holding many hundred Inhabitants'. Manby concluded that 'By some event, this country has been considerably depopulated, but from what cause is hard to determine.' Vancouver concurred. All the evidence, he believed, indicated 'that at no very remote period this country had been far more populous than at present'.

To the sailors this was the fallout from a disaster to end all disasters. The cataclysm, it turned out, was depradation on a comprehensive scale wreaked by, *terribile dictu*, smallpox.

The first ominous signs came during the early days of the American War of Independence in 1775–76: catalysed by the siege of Boston, the siege of Quebec and the failed mobilisation of Dunmore's Ethiopian regiment, these episodes, particularly the first two, compelled General George Washington, commander-in-chief, and his medical staff to make important policy decisions regarding smallpox control in the Continental Army.

In 1775, Lord Dunmore, Royal Governor of Virginia, issued a proclamation offering to emancipate all slaves of revolutionaries who were willing to join him under arms against the rebels; 500 or so Virginia slaves promptly abandoned their masters and joined Dunmore's ranks. The governor formed them into Lord Dunmore's Ethiopian Regiment.

After their failure at Quebec, Washington and the British took the war to New York City: Washington's retreat after the battle of Pell's Point had marooned his remaining forces and the British captured Fort Washington on 16 November taking 3,000 prisoners – it was Washington's most disastrous defeat. The American prisoners were subsequently sent to the infamous prison ships where more American soldiers and sailors died of disease and neglect than died in every battle of the war combined. In total more than 11,500 American prisoners of war died aboard sixteen British prison ships during the war which were nothing less than floating British concentration camps. The British disposed of the bodies by swift interment or just dumping them overboard.

At the end of the war in 1783, the remains of those who died were left to rot along the Brooklyn shore. Nathaniel Scudder Prime reported on 'skulls and feet, arms and legs sticking out of the crumbling bank in the wildest disorder' while Edwin G. Burrows floridly described the skulls on the coast 'as thick as pumpkins in an autumn cornfield'. The most infamous British prison ship was the HMS *Jersey* or Old Jersey, referred to by its inmates simply as 'Hell'. More than 1,000 men were kept aboard the *Jersey* at any one time on a vessel designed for 400, and about a dozen died every night from diseases such as smallpox, dysentery, typhoid and yellow fever, as well as from starvation and torture.

This was typical in wars of many periods: diseases such as smallpox claimed more lives than battle. Between 1775 and 1782, a smallpox epidemic broke out throughout North America, killing an estimated 130,000 among all its populations in those revolutionary war years.[1] As noted, Joseph Ellis suggests that Washington's decision to have his troops inoculated against the disease was one of his most important and shrewdest decisions.[2] Between 25,000 and 70,000 American patriots died during active military service. Of these, approximately 6,800 were killed in battle, while at least 17,000 died from disease. The majority of the latter died while prisoners of war of the British, mostly in those prison ships in New York Harbour.

Around 171,000 sailors served in the Royal Navy during British conflicts from 1775–1784; approximately a quarter of whom had been press-ganged into service. Around 1,240 were killed in battle, while an estimated 18,500 died from disease between 1776 and 1780. The greatest killer at sea, of course was scurvy, although smallpox enjoyed rich pickings.

Fenn, Elizabeth A., 2003, The Great Smallpox Epidemic. *History Today* 53, Issue 8 August.
The Destructive Operation of Foul Air, Tainted Provisions, Bad Water, and Personal Filthiness, upon Human Constitutions; Exemplified in the Unparalleled Cruelty of the British to the American Captives at New-York during the Revolutionary War, on Board their Prison and Hospital Ships, *Medical Repository*, volume 11, 1808

---

1. Clodfelter 2017
2. 2004 p.87

Chapter 32

The Andamanese measles
tragedy (1789–93)

T he Andamanese are the various indigenous peoples of the Andaman Islands, part of India's Andaman and Nicobar Islands union territory in the Bay of Bengal. Until the late 18th century, the Andamanese culture, language and genetics were shielded from external influences by their rather unfriendly reaction to visitors, which included murdering any shipwrecked foreigners, and by the remoteness of the islands. Survival International, which campaigns for tribal groups says that 'that tribe, once 5,000-strong, now numbers only 41 people'.

British colonialism of the worst kind effectively did for the Andamanese's protective isolation, and for the Andamanese. Devoid of immunity against common infectious diseases from the Eurasian mainland, the southeastern regions of South Andaman Island were depopulated by disease within four years of the initial British arrival in 1789. Epidemics of pneumonia, measles and influenza exacted heavy tolls, as did alcoholism. By 1875, the Andamanese were already 'perilously close to extinction', yet the persistent attempts by the British to reach, subdue and enslave them continued unrelentingly. Worse still there is evidence that some sections of the British Indian administration were working deliberately to annihilate the tribes. After the mid-19th century, the British established penal colonies on the islands and an increasing number of mainland Indian and Karen settlers arrived, encroaching on former territories of the Andamanese. This only accelerated the decline of the tribes.

Sita Venkateswar (2004), maintains that it is probable that some disease was introduced among the coastal groups by Lieutenant Colebrooke and Blair's first settlement in 1789, resulting in a marked reduction of the Andamanese population. The four years that the British occupied their initial site on the south-east of South Andaman were sufficient to have decimated the coastal populations of the groups referred to as Jarawa by the Aka-bea-da.

Venkateswar, Sita, 2004, Development and Ethnocide: Colonial Practices in the Andaman Islands, IWGIA

Chapter 33

Philadelphia yellow fever epidemic, 1793

'At the first sign of symptoms, 'more especially if those symptoms be accompanied by a redness, or faint yellowness in the eyes, and dull or shooting pains about the region of the liver, take one of the powders in a little sugar and water, every six hours, until they produce four or five large evacuations from the bowels...'

– Part of the discredited purge and bleed regime
recommended by Dr Benjamin Rush

This was one of the most severe epidemics in United States history. During the 1793 yellow fever epidemic 5,000 or more people were listed in the Philadelphia, population 50,000, official register of deaths between 1 August and 9 November. Most died of yellow fever. By October, 20,000 people had fled the city. The mortality rate peaked in October, before frost finally killed off the mosquitoes and brought an end to the epidemic in November. Doctors knew neither the origin of the fever nor that it was transmitted by mosquitoes.

The mayor organized a fever hospital at Bush Hill and other crisis measures. The assistance of the Free African Society was requested by the city and readily agreed to by the members, based on the mistaken assumption that native Africans would have the same partial immunity to the new disease as many had to malaria. Black nurses tended the sick, both black and white, and the Society hired men to remove corpses, which most people would not touch. A total of 240 black people died, in proportion to their population at the same rate as whites. Despite what many thought, most of the city's black people were not immune to the fever although many slaves could have gained immunity before being transported from Africa. People who survived one attack gained immunity.

The disease was probably imported to Philadelphia by refugees and mosquitoes on ships from Saint-Domingue. It rapidly spread in the port city, in the crowded blocks along the Delaware River. About 5,000 people died, 10 per cent of the population of 50,000. The city was the temporary capital of the nation and three outbreaks of yellow fever during this period shut down the new federal government and paralyzed commerce. As noted, many, including President George Washington, fled the city.

The eminent physician Benjamin Rush was aware of of Dr. John Lining's observation during the 1742 yellow fever epidemic in Charleston that African slaves appeared to be affected at rates lower than whites; he thought they had a natural immunity. Writing an open letter to the press under the pseudonym 'Anthony Benezet', a Quaker who had provided schooling for blacks, Rush suggested that the city's black people had immunity and urged them 'to offer your services to attend the sick to help those known in distress'. Rush, though, was no yellow fever specialist: he treated patients with bleeding, calomel (mercurous chloride, a white powder formerly used as a purgative) and other crude medicinal techniques that usually were ineffective and actually brought many patients closer to death.

Rush decided that a powder of ten grains of calomel and ten grains of the cathartic drug jalap (the poisonous root of a Mexican plant, *Ipomoea purga*, related to the morning glory, which was dried and powdered before ingesting) would create the elimination he was seeking. On 10 September he published a guide to treating the fever: *'Dr. Rush's Directions for Curing and Treating the Yellow Fever'*, outlining a regimen of self-medication. At the first sign of symptoms, 'more especially if those symptoms be accompanied by a redness, or faint yellowness in the eyes, and dull or shooting pains about the region of the liver, take one of the powders in a little sugar and water, every six hours, until they produce four or five large evacuations from the bowels...' He urged that the patient stay in bed and 'drink plentifully' of barley or chicken water. Then after the 'bowels are thoroughly cleaned', it was proper to take 8 to 10 ounces of blood from the arm if, after purging, the pulse was full or tense. To keep the body open he advised more calomel or small doses of cream of tartar or other salts. If the pulse was weak and low, he recommended camomile or snakeroot as a stimulant, and blisters or blankets soaked in hot vinegar wrapped around the lower limbs. To restore the patient he prescribed 'gruel, sago, panada, tapioca, tea, coffee, weak chocolate, wine whey, chicken broth, and white meats, according to the weak or active state of the system; the fruits of the season may be eaten with advantage at all times'. The sick room should be kept cool and vinegar should be sprinkled around the floor.

Rush's ideas on yellow fever treatments were at odds with those of many experienced French doctors, who came in from the West Indies where they dealt with yellow fever outbreaks on an annual basis. Rush's claim that his remedies cured 99 out of 100 patients only brought ridicule from historians and modern doctors. The newspaper editor William Cobbett attacked Rush's therapies and called him a Sangrado, after a character in *Gil Blas*, who bled patients to death. In 1799 Rush won a $5,000 libel judgment against Cobbett.

Rush's therapy was dismissed as 'purge and bleed', and as long as the patient remained debilitated, Rush urged further purging and bleeding. Some of his patients became comatose. The calomel in his pills soon brought on a state of constant salivation, which Rush urged patients to attain to assure a cure. A characteristic sign of death was black vomit, which salivation seemed to ward off. Other doctors began seeing patients who suffered severe abdominal distress brought on by purging. Post-mortems revealed stomachs destroyed by such purges.

Neighbouring towns banned refugees from Philadelphia, and port cities such as Baltimore and New York imposed quarantines against refugees and goods from Philadelphia; New York established a 'Committee appointed to prevent the spreading and introduction of infectious diseases in this city', which set up citizen patrols to monitor entry to the city. Stage coaches from Philadelphia were not allowed into many cities. Some cities did send food aid and money; for example, New York City sent $5,000 to the Mayor's Committee.

Sadly, two leaders of the Free Africa Society, Richard Allen, a Methodist preacher, and Absalom Jones found it necessary to report on the events, *A Narrative of the Proceedings of the Black People during the late awful calamity* ... in a bid to set the record straight and defend themselves against the spurious inflammatory pamphlet published by Mathew Carey and cited above, after he had fled the city for much of September 1793. He accused black people of starting the epidemic, charging high prices for nursing, taking advantage of whites, and even of stealing from them during the epidemic. His pamphlet was entitled *A Short Account of the Malignant Fever* (1793). Allen and Jones responded that it was the whites who charged high rates for nursing during the crisis. They noted that white nurses also profited and stole from their patients. 'We know that six pounds was demanded by and paid to a white woman, for putting a corpse into a coffin; and forty dollars was demanded and paid to four white men, for bringing it down the stairs.' Many black nurses served without remuneration:

'A poor black man, named Sampson, went constantly from house to house where distress was, and no assistance, without fee or reward. He was smitten with the disorder, and died. After his death his family were neglected by those he had served. Sarah Bass, a poor black widow, gave all the assistance she could, in several families, for which she did not receive any thing; and when any thing was offered her, she left it to the option of those she served.'

Here they describe their own courageous and invaluable work:

'The first we visited was a man in Emsley's alley, who was dying, and his wife lay dead at the time in the house, there were none to assist but two poor helpless children. We administered what relief we could, and applied to the overseers of the poor to have the woman buried. We visited upwards of twenty families that day – they were scenes of woe indeed! The Lord was plentiful to strengthen us, and removed all fear from us.'

Carey may have been less prejudiced and more objective when he also recorded, amongst the population in general, rumours of greed, especially by landlords who threw convalescing tenants into the street to repossess.

How did the epidemic start? In spring 1793, French colonial refugees, some with slaves, arrived from Cap Français, Saint-Domingue. The 2,000 immigrants were fleeing the slave revolution in the north of the island and thronged in the port of Philadelphia; it seems likely that the refugees and ships were carrying the yellow fever virus and mosquitoes. In 2013 Billy G. Smith, professor of history at Montana State University, contended that the principal vector of the 1793 plague in Philadelphia (and other Atlantic ports) was the British merchant ship *Hankey*, which had fled the West African colony of Bolama (an island off West Africa, present day Guinea-Bissau) the previous November, depositing infected mosquitos and yellow fever at every port of call in the Caribbean and eastern Atlantic seaboard. The *Hankey*, a small British vessel that circled the Atlantic in 1792 and 1793, transformed the history of the Atlantic world, impacting upon people from West Africa to Philadelphia, Haiti to London.

The story began with a group of well meaning British colonists who planned to establish a colony free of slavery in West Africa. With the colony failing, the ship set sail for the Caribbean and then North America, carrying, as it turned out, those infected mosquitoes; in the United States, tens of thousands died in Philadelphia, New York, Boston, and Charleston. The voyage and its deadly cargo can be linked to some of the most significant events of the era – the success of the Haitian slave revolution, Napoleon's decision to sell the Louisiana Territory and a change in the geopolitical situation of the new United States.

The Philadelphia cases began to rise: after two weeks Benjamin Rush soon realised that yellow fever was back and pronounced that the city faced an epidemic of 'highly contagious, as well as mortal... bilious remitting yellow fever' adding to the alarm by declaring that, unlike with most fevers, the principal victims were not the very young or very old but would be teenagers and heads of families in the dockside areas. Believing that the refugees from Saint-Domingue were carrying the disease, the city imposed a quarantine of two to three weeks on immigrants and their goods, a quarantine that the authorities were unable to enforce. Cases of fever proliferated at first around the Arch Street wharf; Rush attributed them to 'some damaged coffee which putrefied on the wharf near Arch Street'.

The College of Physicians published a letter in the city's newspapers, written by a committee headed by Rush, suggesting eleven measures to prevent the 'progress' of the fever: avoid fatigue, the hot sun, night air, too much liquor, and anything else that might lower resistance. Vinegar and camphor in infected rooms 'cannot be used too frequently upon handkerchiefs, or in smelling bottles, by persons whose duty calls to visit or attend the sick'. They outlined measures for city officials: stopping the tolling of church bells and making burials private; disinfecting streets and wharves; exploding gunpowder in the street to increase the amount of oxygen. Everyone should avoid unnecessary contact with the sick.

Dr. Kuhn advised drinking wine, 'at first weaker wines, such as claret and Rhenish; if these cannot be had, Lisbon or Madeira diluted with rich lemonade. The quantity is to be determined by the effects it produces and by the state of debility which prevails, guarding against its occasioning or encreasing the heat, restlessness or delirium.' He placed 'the greatest dependence for the cure to the disease, on throwing cool water twice a day over the naked body. The patient is to be placed in a large empty tub, and two buckets full of water, of the temperature 75 or 80 degrees Fahrenheit's thermometer, according to the state of the atmosphere, are to be thrown on him.'

Many of those who could left the city. Since the normal practice was for hospitals not to admit infectious disease patients, Philadelphia Hospital included, the Guardians of the Poor commandeered Bush Hill, where yellow fever patients were accommodated in the outbuildings. Nurses were hired. Panic began to spread throughout the city; more people fled. Between 1 August and 7 September, 456 people died; 42 deaths were reported on 8 September. Some 20,000 people left the city through September. President Washington and his cabinet continued to meet until, astonishingly, he left the city on 10 September for his scheduled holiday. The state legislature cut short its September session after a corpse was found on the steps of State House. On 14 September Mayor Clarkson was joined by twenty-six men, who formed a committee to reorganize the fever hospital, arrange visits to the sick, feed those unable to care for themselves, and arrange for wagons to carry the sick to Bush Hill hospital and the dead to Potter's Field. The committee acted quickly: after a report of 15-month-old twins being orphaned, two days later the committee had identified a house for sheltering the growing number of orphans.

When the Mayor's Committee inspected Bush Hill fever hospital, they found the nurses unqualified and arrangements chaotic. 'The sick, the dying, and the dead were indiscriminately mingled together. The ordure and other evacuations of the sick, were allowed to remain in the most offensive state imaginable... It was, in fact, a great human slaughter-house.' On 15 September, Peter Helm, a barrel maker, and Stephen Girard, a merchant and shipowner born in France, volunteered to personally manage the hospital and represent the Mayor's Committee. Broken bedsteads were repaired and more brought from the prison so patients would not have to lie on the floor. A barn was adapted as a place for convalescing patients. On 17 September, the managers hired nine female nurses and ten male attendants, as well as a female matron. They assigned the fourteen rooms to separate male and female patients. With the discovery of a spring on the estate, clean water was pumped into the hospital. Helm and Girard informed the committee that they could accommodate more than the 60 patients then under their care, and soon the hospital had 140 patients. Jean Deveze, a French doctor with experience treating yellow fever in Saint-Domingue admired Girard's selfless devotion to the patients. In a memoir published in 1794, Deveze wrote of Girard:

'I even saw one of the diseased ... [discharge] the contents of his stomach upon [him]. What did Girard do? ... He wiped the patient's cloaths, comforted [him] ... arranged the bed, [and] inspired with courage, by renewing in him the hope that he should recover. — From him he went to another, that vomited offensive matter that would have disheartened any other than this wonderful man.'

Nevertheless, it soon became clear that mortality at the hospital remained high; about 50 per cent of those admitted died and the daily death toll remained above 30 until 26 October. The worst seven-day period was between 7 and 13 October when 711 deaths were reported.

This is how Mathew Carey (1793) described the scene in the city, the paranoia and the fear:

'Those who ventured abroad, had handkerchiefs or sponges impregnated with vinegar of camphor at their noses, or smelling-bottles full of the thieves' vinegar. Others carried pieces of tarred rope in their hands or pockets, or camphor bags tied round their necks.... People hastily shifted their course at the sight of a hearse coming towards them. Many never walked on the footpath, but went into the middle of the streets, to avoid being infected in passing by houses wherein people had died. Acquaintances and friends avoided each other in the streets, and only signified their regard by a cold nod. The old custom of shaking hands fell in such general disuse, that many shrunk back with affright at even the offer of a hand. A person with crape [mourning crepe], or any appearance of mourning, was shunned like a viper.

The consternation of the people of Philadelphia, at this period, was carried beyond all bounds. Dismay and affright were visible in almost every person's countenance. Acquaintances and friends avoided each other in the street, he noted. In some households, family members were banished into the street when they complained of a headache, a common precursor to yellow fever. 'Parents desert their children as soon as they are infected, and in every room you enter you see no person but a solitary black man or woman near the sick.'

Doctors, preachers, and laymen all looked forward to the advent of autumn to end the epidemic. Since the deadly mosquito was never implicated in their destruction, they hoped a seasonal 'equinoctial gale', or hurricane, common at that time of year, would simply blow away the fever. The Mayor's Committee took a census of the dead, they found, no surprise, that the majority of victims were poor people, who died in homes up the alleys, behind the main streets. When the contagion finally did start to abate in October, the Mayor's Committee advised people outside the city to wait another week or ten days before returning. It published directions for cleaning houses which had been closed up, recommending that they be aired for several days with all windows and doors open. 'Burning of nitre will correct the corrupt air which they may contain. Quick lime should be thrown into the privies and the chambers whitewashed.'

On 31 October a white flag was hoisted over Bush Hill with the legend, 'No More Sick Persons Here'.

Philadelphia suffered further yellow fever epidemics in 1797, 1798, and 1799. Other major ports also had epidemics, beginning with Baltimore in 1794, New York in 1791, 1795 and 1798, and Wilmington in 1798.

Deveze, Jean, 1794. 'An Inquiry into and Observations upon the Causes and Effects of the Epidemic Disease Which Raged in Philadelphia'.

Miller, Jacquelyn, 2005, 'The Wages of Blackness: African American Workers and the Meanings of Race during Philadelphia's 1793 Yellow Fever Epidemic.' *The Pennsylvania Magazine of History and Biography* 129, no. 2 (April 2005): 163–94.

Powell, John Harvey 1993 *Bring Out Your Dead: The Great Plague of Yellow Fever in Philadelphia in 1793*. Philadelphia

Stough, Mulford 1939. 'The Yellow Fever in Philadelphia 1793. *Pennsylvania History* 66–13 6–13

Chapter 34

The 1802–1803 Saint-Domingue yellow fever epidemic

'Throughout the Haitian countryside, guerrilla warfare continued and the French staged mass executions by firing squads, hanging, and drowning Haitians in bags. Rochambeau invented a new means of mass execution, which he called 'fumigational-sulphurous baths': killing hundreds of Haitians in the holds of ships by burning sulphur to produce sulphur dioxide to gas them.'

E pidemics, as we have so often seen, have been pivotal in altering the course of world history; this yellow fever epidemic clearly altered New World geopolitics at the dawn of the 19th century. By the end of the previous century, yellow fever was widespread throughout the Caribbean and particularly ferocious in Saint-Domingue. From 1793 to 1798, case fatality rates among British troops in the West Indies, including Saint-Domingue, were as high as 70 per cent. An even worse death toll awaited the French army when it arrived in 1802 ostensibly sent by Napoleon to suppress a rebellion and to re-establish slavery. Historians have disagreed on why Napoleon initially posted nearly 30,000 soldiers and sailors to the island. Evidence suggests the troops were actually an expeditionary force with plans to invade North America through New Orleans and to establish a major holding in the Mississippi valley. However, the Napoleonic forces were hampered by a crucial lack of basic knowledge relating to disease prevention and control measures, allowing the disease to leave only a small and shattered fraction of troops alive, thus thwarting Napoleon's ambition to colonize and hold French-held lands; this expansion later became better known as the Louisiana Purchase.

Toussaint L'Ouverture

Toussaint L'Ouverture (1743–1803), Haitian general and standout leader of the Haitian Revolution was largely responsible for the establishment of the Haitian Republic. His charismatic leadership enabled former slaves to succeed in their struggle against French oppression, transforming their slave revolt into a revolutionary movement. The revolt began on 22 August 1791 and ended in 1804 with the former colony's independence. It involved black people, mulattoes, French, Spanish and British participants. The revolution was the world's only slave uprising that led to the founding of a state which was both free from slavery, and ruled by non-whites and former captives. It was therefore a defining moment in the history of the world. However, yellow fever was at least as important as L'Ouverture in defeating the French army in Haiti and must share some significant credit for this pivotal event.

L'Ouverture did not escape the notice of Napoleon; Napoleon needed to reassert French control of Haiti and had ambitious plans for the New World in general. As noted, his aim was to create an empire of the Mississippi Valley in North America to disrupt British interests in the region.

The obscene rigours of sugar production slavery and the unhealthy Caribbean climate fostered infectious diseases such as malaria and yellow fever, causing high mortality. In 1787 alone, the French imported about 20,000 slaves from Africa into Saint-Domingue, while the British shipped about 38,000 slaves to all of their Caribbean colonies: fertile breeding and feeding grounds for both diseases in which the death rate from yellow fever was such that at least 50 per cent of the slaves from Africa died within a year of arriving. The pragmatic, inhumane response from the white planters was to work their slaves to the point of death while providing them with the barest minimum of food and shelter. To them it made good economic sense to get the most work out of their slaves at the lowest cost possible, since they were probably going to die of yellow fever anyway.[1] The death rate was so high that polyandry became a common form of marriage among the slaves; rape by planters, their unmarried sons, or overseers was common.

Late in 1801 Napoleon sent his brother-in-law, General Victor-Emmanuel LeClerc and 20,000 troops to seize Haiti and eradicate the pretender, L'Ouverture. The beginning of the end for the French came in February 1802 when LeClerc landed at Le Cap. With March came the rainy season and as stagnant water collected, the mosquitoes began to breed, leading to yet another outbreak of yellow fever. Le Clerc was right to be worried: many of his troops were falling ill with a high fever. He expressed his concern to Napoleon, writing, 'I have 600 men on my sick list.' A week later, he noted, 'I have already 1,200 in hospital.'[2] Things would only get worse. By the end of April 5,000 French soldiers had died of yellow fever and another 5,000 were hospitalized with the disease; Leclerc dolefully wrote in his diary: 'The rainy season has arrived. My troops are exhausted with fatigue and sickness.'[3] LeClerc had lost one-third of his original force to yellow fever; in desperation he wrote to his brother in law:

> 'A man cannot work hard here without risking his life and it is quite impossible for me to remain here for more than six months...my health is so wretched that I would consider myself lucky if I could last for that time!...the mortality continues and makes fearful ravages.'[4]

By June, the French were dying at a rate of 30 to 50 per day. Neither the disease nor the rebel menace attenuated and LeClerc's forces were falling apart.

---

1. Dubois, 2005
2. Parkinson 1978
3. Perry, 2005
4. Parkinson 1978

The humid weather, the enemy, the proliferation of mosquitoes in the marshy lowlands around the port cities and the crucial fact that Napoleon forbade LeClerc from decamping to the highlands after his initial successes in controlling the port towns, all made the situation impossible: every general knew that mortality from yellow fever and malaria in the Caribbean could be substantially reduced by moving troops to mountain camps.[5] For strategic reasons, however, the troops needed to remain in the low lying port towns.

L'Ouverture saw this as an opportunity to negotiate with the French. In May, LeClerc proposed that L'Ouverture retain his title and staff and retire to a place of his choosing. L'Ouverture accepted, but the settlement was short-lived. The French general Brunet, after inviting L'Ouverture to a dinner meeting, double-crossed his guest who was seized by the French and shipped to France. He died months later in prison at Fort-de-Joux in the Jura Mountains.

Throughout the Haitian countryside, guerrilla warfare continued and the French staged mass executions by firing squads, hanging and drowning Haitians in bags. Rochambeau invented a new means of mass execution, which he called 'fumigational-sulphurous baths': killing hundreds of Haitians in the holds of ships by burning sulphur to produce sulphur dioxide to gas them. The rebels, now led by Jean-Jacques Dessalines, resumed hostilities against the French, doubtlessly buoyed up by the scourge of yellow fever on the Europeans: yellow fever was killing four-fifths of LeClerc's soldiers. Moreover, France had restored the hated slave trade, which gave the entire black population a cast iron resolve to unite and drive out the French.

Many of the 'French' soldiers were not French, they were Polish, as 5,000 Poles were serving in two demi-brigades in the French Army. Many Poles believed that if they fought for France, Bonaparte would reward them by restoring Polish independence, which had been ended with the Third Partition of Poland in 1795. Of the 5,000 Poles, about 4,000 died of yellow fever. A French planter wrote of their plight: 'Ten days after the landing of these two beautiful regiments, more than half their number were carried off by yellow fever; they fell down as they walked, the blood rushing out through their nostrils, mouths, eyes...what a horrible and heart-rending sight!'

As Leclerc lay dying of yellow fever he reacted by ordering all of the black slaves living in Le Cap to be murdered by drowning in the harbour. In November, Leclerc died along with most of his army. He was replaced by Rochambeau, who also was powerless to prevent yellow fever from taking its toll. The disease consumed 20,000 additional reinforcements and Rochambeau capitulated in November 1803. The last land battle of the Haitian Revolution, the Battle of Vertières, was on 18 November 1803 near Cap-Haïtien, fought between Dessalines' army and the remaining French colonial army; the slave rebels and freed revolutionary soldiers won the day. The Haitians had paid a high price for their freedom, losing about 200,000 dead between 1791 and 1803, and unlike most of the European dead, who were killed by yellow fever, the majority of the Haitian casualties were the victims of violence.

---

5. Buckley 1985

As we have seen, the resistance and yellow fever made it impossible for Napoleon to regain control over Haiti, so he gave up his dream of rebuilding a French New World empire and decided to sell Louisiana to the US. The Haitian Revolution brought about two unintended consequences: the creation of a continental America and the virtual end of Napoleonic rule in the Americas.

Chippaux, J.P., 2018. Yellow fever in Africa and the Americas: a historical and epidemiological perspective. *J Venom Anim Toxins Incl Trop Dis*. 2018;24:20.

Geggus, D., 1979. Yellow fever in the 1790s: the British army in occupied Saint Domingue. *Med Hist*. 1979; 23(1):38–58.

Girard, Philippe., 2011. *The Slaves who Defeated Napoléon: Toussaint L'Ouverture and the Haitian War of Independence, 1801–1804*. University of Alabama Press.

Marr, J.S., 2013. The 1802 Saint-Domingue yellow fever epidemic and the Louisiana Purchase. *J Public Health Manag Pract*.;19(1):77–82.

Chapter 35

Plague in the 19th century

1812–19 The Ottoman plague epidemic

'One of Europe's last major epidemics of the bubonic plague devastated the city of Odessa. A look back at a time of unprecedented paranoia, mass quarantine, corrupt plague-profiteers and 19th century debauchery reveals we haven't learned very much from crises past.'

– Lily Lynch, *Odessa, 1812: Plague and Tyranny at the Edge of the Empire*

Odessa's fearsome reputation for contagion was notorious in the region. Well before reaching the port sailors still way out on the Black Sea could spot the plague flags. A yellow flag meant purification; a red flag meant plague was waiting for them. These seafarers, many arriving from the buzzing slave markets of Constantinople, were well versed in rumours about the dreadful conditions crews of other ships had encountered in the quarantine of the port city. And Odessa was supposed to be a liberal, if decadent city.

French civil engineer and Knight of the Order of St. Vladimir of Russia, the well-named Xavier Hommaire de Hell described his trip from Constantinople to Odessa and his first sight of the city with its dreaded quarantine.

'It was, indeed, a European town we beheld, full of affluence, movement, and gaiety,'.
'But alas! Our curiosity and our longings, thus strongly excited, were not for a long while to be satisfied. The dreaded quarantine looked down on us, as if to notify that its rights were paramount.'

All crews were obliged to undergo a period of confinement. Armed guards shot dead anyone who attempted to escape before they were cleared. In 1839, *The Lancet* called Odessa's Lazaretto 'one of the severist [sic] in the world'. The *New York Times* said the city's quarantine was 'a hateful political tyranny'.

How did the plague start? Who really knows, but predictably there are the usual scapegoats: foreigners and women of the night: there is the plague infected crew of an Austro-Hungarian ship who bribed a guard to escape quarantine, then got drunk in the city's brandy shops; then there was the Turk who evaded quarantine and spread the infection among the 'female dancers at the opera'. Finally, a more romantic explanation is a contaminated ring, wrapped in cotton wool which was smuggled out of quarantine to 'an actress' in town.

On 22 November 1812, all 32,000 residents of Odessa were forcibly imprisoned in their homes for an unrelenting 66 days. The city's popular governor-general, Duke de Richelieu, posted 500 Cossacks to 'restrain' the entire population and ensure its complete isolation. 'All exterior displays of friendship were forbidden,' one survivor wrote. The plague was soon killing up to 40 people each day. No one was permitted to open their windows or doors, except when authorities delivered water-soaked meat and fumigated bread twice a day. Tar-smeared galley-slaves were deployed to push carts carrying the plague-afflicted through the streets raising a red flag when transporting the dying, and a black flag when conveying the dead. As Lily Lynch (2015) writes: 'Those stricken with symptoms of the plague were labelled "suspected" and taken to special quarantine quarters, where they were forced to dig graves, possibly for themselves.'

When it was all over, the plague had claimed the lives of 2,656 people out of a population of 32,000 – about one in twelve inhabitants. Among the dead were four of Odessa's five doctors, who had all fallen ill after caring for the sick. Any houses the dead left behind were burned to the ground.

New arrivals were made to undress, with some men gazing upon the bodies of other men in a decidedly un-English way. Lynch gives us a fascinating extract from the 1833 travel diary of British Admiral Aldolphus Slade (1804–1877) 'an intimate recollection of his preliminary health inspection':

> 'The individual commences his quarantine *in puris naturalibus*. He strips naked in the presence of the director and the surgeon of the Lazaretto, and having passed their inspection, puts on clothes, supplied either by a friend in pratique, or hired from the spenditore, and wears them till his own garments are smoked. I expressed as an Englishman a natural reluctance to submit to such exposure… My medical companion was then introduced, and as no scruples were supposed in him, similar forebearance was not observed. Either being used to the occurrence, or not caring about it, he exhibited the beauties of his person very leisurely… Next came the German watchmaker and the Jew. The son of Levi was shy, but his scruples were unheeded, and he was bid to extend his arms. Lastly, our soldier guardian walked in. He did not care about the affair. He threw off his clothes with military promptitude, and stood erect — a figure for a sculptor to have gazed on with pleasure.'

But stiff upper lip embarrassment should have been the least of the admiral's problems if the 1819 account of the sleeping quarters by the Rev. Dr. Pinkerton of the British and Foreign Bible Society is anything to go by:

> 'The cell which I occupy is 16 feet by 13: I found it very damp and cold when I first entered it, and containing nothing but two old wooden bedsteads, and a small dirty

table, and swarming with rats, mice, fleas, and other vermin. However, I procured some firewood with part of which I filled up the holes in the floor...it was several days before I succeeded in keeping out the rats and mice.'

Dr. Meissner, a German physician, tells us 'The whole scene forcibly reminded me of the lines of Dante on the eternal living death, beginning':

'Here sighs, with lamentations and loud moans, Resounded through the air pierced by no star, That e'en I wept at entering. Various tongues, Horrible languages, outcries of woe, Accents of anger, voices deep and hoarse...'

And ending:

'I then: Master! What doth aggrieve them thus, That they lament so loud? He straight replied: That will I tell thee briefly. These of death No hope may entertain.'

Where there is dirt there is usually money: Odessa and its quarantine were no exception: Lynch draws our attention to Elizabeth Abosch, Russian language instructor at the University of Maryland: 'Just as money could be made off of war, money could be made for the crafty merchants of Odessa from a terrifying epidemic,' and their captive market. Admiral Slade obviously saw a very different Odessa to the unfortunate Rev. Dr. Pinkerton: 'The *Lazaretto* is on a superb scale, containing cafes, restaurateurs, and billiards, to assist the captains and mates in spending their cash,' he wrote. A picture confirmed by Pushkin in *Eugene Onegin*, which he worked on while living in exile in Odessa:

'What novel goods and merchandises Have now arrived in quarantine? Have the expected wine casks come? What of the plague, where conflagration? And haven't there been famines, wars, or other such-like novelties?'

Meanwhile in Constantinople plague broke out in July 1812; by September around 2,000 people were dying every day. By the end of the epidemic, the Sublime Porte, the central government of the Ottoman Empire, estimated that there were 320,955 deaths, which included 220,000 Turks, 40,800 Armenians, 32,000 Jews, 28,000 Greeks, 50 Aleppines, 80 islanders and 25 Franks. The plague was nothing if not thorough, spreading throughout most of the empire including Alexandria, the Ottoman vassal state of Wallachia (Caragea's plague named after the country's ruler); Bosnia, reaching Dalmatia in 1815. In 1814–15 it reappeared in Egypt, Bosnia and Albania.

Lynch, Lily, Odessa, 1812: Plague and Tyranny at the Edge of the Empire, *Balkanist Magazine*, December 5, 2015
White, S., 2010. Rethinking disease in Ottoman History. *International Journal of Middle East Studies*, 42(4), 549–567

1813–14 Malta plague epidemic

'A statue of Saint Sebastian, patron saint of the plague-stricken, was erected on the outskirts of Qormi (facing Marsa and the harbour) after the outbreak.'

Plague returned to Malta with the 1813–1814 epidemic; it was to be the last major outbreak of plague on the islands of Malta and Gozo. It hit Malta in March 1813 and Gozo in May 1814; the epidemic was declared over in September 1814. It resulted in approximately 4,500 deaths, which was about 5 per cent of the islands' populations.

Malta's free port status meant that it was well connected with other Mediterranean ports. The disease came to Malta from Alexandria on board the brigantine *San Nicola*; two of the crew died *en route*, and although the vessel and crew were quarantined in Marsamxett Harbour for two weeks, the disease spread to the local population when guards on *San Nicola* stole infected linen from its cargo. This was stored in a wine shop in Sliema before being sold to Salvatore Borg, a shoemaker, spiv and smuggler who lived in Valletta.

The British colonial government took strict measures but these were too late: the area around the Grand Harbour was isolated and settlements with high mortality rates were cordoned off. Violations of these regulations brought harsh penalties including death by firing squad: several people were executed for concealing their infection including another Borg, Anthony.

The crew of the *San Nicola* were taken to the *lazaretto* on nearby Manoel Island on 29 March. On 1 April, the ship's captain Antonio Maria Mescara became ill, as did a servant who had looked after the two infected crew members. Mescara and the servant died on 7 April, post mortems confirmed that they died of the plague. The *San Nicola* was sent back to Alexandria under the escort of HMS *Badger*.

Sadly on 19 April Borg's 8-year-old daughter Anna Maria died but no one attributed this to the plague so she was given a normal funeral. Soon after, her mother developed a fever, causing consternation among doctors who reported the case to the authorities. The woman died on 3 May; Salvatore Borg died too. Plague was confirmed as cause of death.

Panic erupted and many people deserted Valetta for the countryside or left the islands on ships. Most of the British and some Maltese self-isolated within their homes. The disease initially spread slowly, so that people began to doubt its existence, but the outbreak picked up pace: Borg's father died and by 17 May, the disease had spread throughout the whole city. The guards who stole the linen, as well as those who stored and purchased the stolen goods, were among the first people to contract the plague and die.

On 19 June, various *barrière* were set up in and around Valletta, Floriana and the Three Cities. These were railings which were spaced such that they allowed people on opposite sides to be able to talk without coming in contact with each another. They also permitted the supply of food from the countryside to the cities. Valletta was subdivided into eight districts and movement of people was restricted under pain of death. Shops selling food were only allowed to open for four hours a day. Prisoners were forced to carry the dead from their homes to burial sites in specially-made carts known as *beccamorti*. Many died in the process, so the authorities brought prisoners from Sicily to continue the work, but these unfortunates also died.

Caragea's (Caradja's) plague, Romania 1812

> *'Public morgue officials wheeled their carts from house to house collecting corpses for disposal, indiscriminately piling up the sick together with the dead. Many "were eaten by dogs and other beasts". Some were buried alive but if they resisted they were clubbed to death. Sometimes those strong enough retaliated and killed the undertakers.'*

In 1812 Phanariote Prince John Caradja was appointed governor of Bucharest in Ottoman Wallachia. On the way from Constantinople to take up his post one of his retainers died of plague, a case which may have been responsible for introducing the disease to Bucharest. Caradja prepared for the worst; he established two quarantine hospitals in January 1813, and waited...

On 11 June the first case was officially notified and Caradja sprang into action implementing emergency measures and putting Bucharest into lock-down: the city gates were guarded to prevent people coming in and roaming around; all foreigners and non-residents were expelled and the beggars were sent to monasteries outside Bucharest. Money had to be washed in vinegar and the number of gravediggers was increased to 60; all markets, schools, bars and cafes were closed and alcohol could only be sold for home consumption; fatalities had a simple burial with no attendants. Those who hid sick people or the peddlers ('both Jewish and Christians') were expelled from the city and their belongings were torched. In August, due to the spread of the plague, the request to allow Bucharest people to flee the city was approved; most judicial proceedings were stopped, and inmates in the debtors' prison were freed. Well intentioned as they were, the measures were largely fruitless; the quarantine hospitals were soon filled to overflowing and effectively became charnel houses.

Many of the rules were flouted anyway: the distribution of public health information printed fliers was ignored. By August, the city became almost deserted, with even the doctors fleeing, as did Caradja, who relocated from Bucharest to Cotroceni. The French consul said that two-thirds of the Bucharesters fled.

Public morgue officials wheeled their carts from house to house collecting corpses for disposal, indiscriminately piling up the sick together with the dead. Many 'were eaten by dogs and other beasts'. Some were buried alive but if they resisted they were clubbed to death. Sometimes those strong enough retaliated and killed the undertakers.

An estimated 60,000 people died of the plague in the two years, 20–30,000 of them in Bucharest where the population at the time was about 120,000.

The 1894 Great Plague of Hong Kong

*'In 1894, in Hong Kong, Swiss-born French bacteriologist Alexandre Yersin isolated the bacterium responsible for plague (*Yersinia pestis, *named for Yersin) and determined the common mode of transmission.'*

The third plague pandemic started in Yunnan province in the 1850s and, over several decades, progressed along trade routes until it reached Canton (now Guangzhou) in 1894; inevitably, given the daily water traffic between Canton and Hong Kong, plague was certain to spread to the colony: in May 1894 patient zero was a national hospital clerk. From May to October 1894, the plague killed more than 6,000 people and one third of the population fled Hong Kong. In the thirty years starting in 1926, the plague recurred in Hong Kong almost every year and slew more than 20,000 people.

There were several reasons for the rapid outbreak and ferocious spread of the plague here. After the British arrived in the 1840s they established Tai Ping Shan as a settlement for Chinese workers. As the population grew, the district's tenements were sub-divided into tiny, windowless dwellings with large multi-generational families crammed into them. Houses there, up in the mountains, had no drainage channels, toilets, or running water. James Lowson, a Scottish doctor and acting superintendent of the Civil Hospital, described in unsparing prose the horror he found:

'On a miserable sodden matting soaked with abominations there were four forms stretched out. One was dead, the tongue black and protruding. The next had the muscular twitchings and semi-comatose condition heralding dissolution … Another sufferer, a female child about ten years old, lay in the accumulated filth of apparently two or three days … The fourth was wildly delirious.'

Secondly, during the Ching Ming Festival in 1894, many Chinese living in Hong Kong returned to the countryside to sweep the graves, which coincided with the outbreak of the epidemic in Canton. Thirdly, in the first four months of 1894, rainfall decreased and soil dried up, giving impetus to the spread of the plague.

Sarah Lazarus (2014) reports how:

'The colonial authorities imposed a strict regime on the local population involving the rapid disposal of corpses, the isolation of infected patients and the disinfection of houses. Later, they forcibly evicted the remaining residents and razed Tai Ping Shan to the ground. Their actions fostered mutual distrust, heightening pre-existing political and racial tensions and amplifying the panic on both sides.'

Main preventive measures included setting up plague hospitals and deploying dedicated medical staff to treat and isolate plague patients; conducting house-to-house search operations, discovering and transferring plague patients, cleaning and disinfecting infected houses and areas, setting up designated cemeteries and assigning a person responsible for transporting and burying the plague dead.

In 1894, in Hong Kong, Swiss-born French bacteriologist Alexandre Yersin isolated the responsible bacterium (*Yersinia pestis*, named for Yersin) and determined the common mode of transmission. His discoveries led in time to modern treatment methods, including insecticides, the use of antibiotics and eventually plague vaccines. In 1898, French researcher Paul-Louis Simond demonstrated the role of fleas as a vector.

From Hong Kong the plague penetrated India, Australia, the west coast of the United States, South America, Africa and Europe.

Lazarus, Sarah, When death came calling: how the plague swept through Hong Kong. *Post Magazine*, 21 June 2014.

Pryor, E.G., 1975. 'The Great Plague of Hong Kong' *Journal of the Hong Kong Branch of the Royal Asiatic Society*. 15: 61–70.

Chapter 36

The 1817–1824 cholera pandemic

'The Indian origins of cholera and its almost global dissemination from Bengal made the disease a convenient symbol for much that the west feared or despised about a society so different from its own. One of the strongest expressions of this antipathy arose from the epidemiological connection between cholera and Hindu pilgrimage.'

David Arnold, *Past & Present*, 1986

The word cholera means a bilious disease and is derived from the Greek term 'chole' or bile which is a nonspecific word that has been used in past centuries for various gastro-intestinal diseases. Cholera caused more deaths, more rapidly, than any other epidemic disease in the 19th century. It is caused by the bacteria *Vibrio cholera* as discovered in 1883 by anatomist Filippo Pacini and bacteriologist Robert Koch. The disease first emerged in the 1800s from what was then Calcutta; since then, seven cholera pandemics have swept through the world. Sixteen strains of *Vibrio cholera* have been discovered, with the deadliest being the 01 and 0139 strains. The bacterium secretes chloride to block the small intestine's ability to absorb sodium, which produces thin, grayish brown, mucoid diarrhoea in the victims who lose between 2–10 litres of fluids a day. Epidemics tended to occur after wars, civil unrest, or natural disasters, when water and food supplies become contaminated with *Vibrio cholerae*, and are fostered by crowded living conditions and poor sanitation.

Asia had seen cholera many times before this pandemic which is remarkable for the extensive geographical range it infected – from China in the east to the Mediterranean in the west, taking in the Indian subcontinent, the Middle East and eastern Africa. It started at the Kumbh Mela, a major Hindu pilgrimage and festival on the upper Ganges River, near what was Calcutta in September 1817 at Jessore; infected rice is believed to have been the initial culprit, by 1818 the disease had broken out in Bombay, on the west coast. Hundreds of thousands of people died all across Asia but what brought it to European attention and concern were the 10,000 or so British soldiers serving in India who succumbed. The list of places afflicted is endless and includes, in March 1820, Siam (Thailand), Bangkok and Manila; in spring of 1821 it reached Java, Oman, and Anhai in China; in 1822 it was in Japan, in the Persian Gulf, in Baghdad, in Syria, and in the Transcaucasus; and in 1823 cholera reached Astrakhan, Zanzibar and Mauritius.

The British Army (marching overland to Nepal and Afghanistan) and the Royal Navy and merchant shipping must take some of the blame for such extensive transmission with their seemingly unchecked movements by land and sea throughout the region. Hindu pilgrims too made a contribution, carrying cholera within the subcontinent, as on many previous occasions.

The pandemic brought out the worst (again) in British colonialism and supremacist dogma when the disease gave rise to an explosion of anti-Asian sentiment and xenophobia. Indian people and their culture were the targets: in the west the disease was subsequently associated with Asia, and South Asia, in particular, was seen as in some way to blame for cholera. There was derision towards Indian cultural practices and hygiene, especially Hindu pilgrimages following the initial outbreak. Medical professionals of the time were also noted for relying on moral judgments and generalisations of Indian people on pilgrimages. The sanitary commissioner of Bengal, Dr. David Smith, said, 'the human mind can scarcely sink lower than it has done in connection with the appalling degeneration of idol-worship at Pooree'. During the outbreak, British authorities launched inquiries into the conditions of South Asian people on pilgrimages and eventually classified pilgrims as a 'dangerous class' who were then placed under surveillance.

Cholera as a Biological Weapon

During the Second World War, the Japanese biological weapons programme, Unit 731, located in Pingfan Manchuria (24 kilometres south of Harbin) experimented with *Vibrio cholera* as a weapons agent. It was reported that the Japanese dropped cholera and typhus cultures into more than 1,000 Chinese wells and reportedly caused 10,000 cases in 1941. However, in an unusual case of friendly fire an estimated 1,700 of the deaths were among Japanese soldiers, indicative of the difficulty of protecting one's own troops from biological agents and controlling infections in acts of bioterrorism.

South Africa's biological weapons programme, Project Coast (1981–1994) developed cholera as a potential biological agent. During South Africa's civil war, cholera, anthrax and other bacteria were released into water in rebel-held areas. Iraq's biological weapons programme reportedly began at the Al-Hazen Institute in 1974 where cholera was one of the biological agents under study. North Korea has reportedly also studied cholera as a possible biological weapons agent.

Arnold, David, 1986, Cholera and Colonialism in British India, Past & Present, 113, 118–151
Arnold, David, 1993. *Colonizing the Body: State Medicine and Epidemic Disease in Nineteenth-Century India*. University of California Press. 161–163.
de Bretton-Gordon, Hamish, 2020, *Chemical Warrior: Syria, Salisbury and Saving Lives at War*, London
Eggleston, William G., 1892, Oriental Pilgrimages and Cholera, *The North American Review* 155, No. 428 126–128

Chapter 37

The Second Cholera Pandemic 1826–1837

'Vomiting or purging, or both these evacuations of a liquid like rice-Water or whey, or barley-water, come on; the features become sharp and contracted, the eye sinks, the look is expressive of terror and wildness.'
– *The London Gazette* regaling its readers with symptoms of cholera (1831)

Much of the known world was struck by the the Second Cholera Pandemic between 1826 and 1837. It spread from India to Afghanistan by 1827, and Hungary (100,000 deaths), Germany, France and the British Isles by 1831 (55,000 died). Russian soldiers brought the disease to Poland in February 1831: there were a reported 250,000 cases of cholera and 100,000 deaths in Russia. The cholera brought to Poland and East Prussia by Russian soldiers forced Prussian authorities to close their borders to Russian transports. There were 'cholera riots' in Russia, ignited by the anti-cholera measures undertaken by the tsarist government.

Immigrants took it to Canada and the United States in 1832, whence it spread down to Mexico and Cuba. In mid-1832, 57 Irish immigrants died laying a stretch of railroad called Duffy's Cut, 30 miles west of Philadelphia. The pandemic reached Portugal and Spain by 1833 and then spread across to France and Italy between 1834 and 1836. Through other offshoots of the pandemic, cholera spread to Egypt (130,000 deaths) Syria, Palestine, Mecca, and Cairo, travelling along the trade routes, from port to port, boosted in Europe by the urbanization of the industrial revolution.

The epidemic made its debut in Great Britain in December 1831 in Sunderland, in the shape of keelman William Sproat; it was carried by passengers on a ship from the Baltic. It then spread to Gateshead and Newcastle and riots broke out in Liverpool. In London, the disease claimed 6,536 victims; in Paris, 20,000 died (out of a population of 650,000), with about 100,000 deaths in all of France. In England the pandemic led to the enactment of the landmark Public Health Act and the 1848 Nuisances Removal and Diseases Prevention Act – the 'cholera bill'. Property owners were encouraged to clean their dwellings, to prevent 'atmospheric impurity', and 'Householders of all classes should be warned, that their first means of safety lies in the removal of dung heaps and solid and liquid filth of every description from beneath or about their houses and premises.'[1] The establishment in 1848 of the Metropolitan

---

1. *London Gazette* 20903

Commission of Sewers[2] was to bring its sewer and drainage infrastructure under the control of a single public body.

However, much of this backfired as the cleansing remedy in the case of central London was to effectively dump the contents of cesspools and raw sewage pits into the Thames. The middle classes did not help with the increasing popularity of the flushing water closet adding to the large amounts of sewage slopping in the river.

Sensationalism and fake news did nothing to help. Katrina Navickas, a specialist in 19th-century protest at the University of Hertfordshire, says corpse-related horror stories also added to a climate of fear. 'People didn't trust the doctors, they didn't trust the government, and they were wound up by body snatching stories in the press. On top of this, Mary Shelley's *Frankenstein* was a popular novel at the time, so there was a lot of gothic imagery around bodies and corpses.'

There were stories too where dying victims looked like they were dead and were buried alive, clawing at the coffin lid from the inside. Even the usually sober *Lancet* succumbed to sensationalism and hyperbole when it told us: 'No rank escapes its attack...whole families are exterminated...civilised nations changed to savage hordes... all grades and bonds of social organisation disappear'. *The Times* spoke of 'great panic' and 'complete panic' with riots in thirty towns and cities from Liverpool to Exeter, from Manchester to London, from Glasgow to Leeds, from Dumfries to Bristol. But life did go on despite it all: mass rallies on the 1832 Reform Bill went ahead in York, as did the inviolable Race Week.

Norwegian poet Henrik Wergeland wrote a stage play inspired by the pandemic: in *The Indian Cholera* (*Den indiske Cholera*, 1835), he criticized British colonialism for spreading the pandemic. One good outcome was the development of a major medical advance in the shape of the intravenous saline drip. Dr Thomas Latta of Leith established from blood studies that a saline drip greatly improved the condition of patients and saved many lives by preventing dehydration; sadly he was one of the many medical workers who died in the epidemic.

The miasma theory of transmission still prevailed so in Britain the population was urged to burn...

> '...decayed articles, such as rags, cordage, papers, old clothes, hangings...filth of every description removed, clothing and furniture should be submitted to copious effusions of water, and boiled in a strong ley (lye); drains and privies thoroughly cleansed by streams of water and chloride of lime...free and continued admission of fresh air to all parts of the house and furniture should be enjoined for at least a week.'
> – *The London Gazette*, 21 October 1831. p. 2160

The need for hasty burials caused a lot of anxiety and anger with authorities breaking up wakes; the Irish were particularly upset by this. Special constables refused to collect

---

2. *London Gazette* issue 20895

corpses so, in one case, watermen volunteered to do the job – for 5s each, two or three days' work – the wages of fear.

Based on the reports of two English doctors who had observed the epidemic in St. Petersburg, the English board of health published a detailed description of the disease's symptoms and onset:

'Giddiness, sick stomach, nervous agitation, intermittent, slow, or small pulse, cramps beginning at the tops of the fingers and toes, and rapidly approaching the trunk, give the first warning. Vomiting or purging, or both these evacuations of a liquid like rice-water or whey, or barley-water, come on; the features become sharp and contracted, the eye sinks, the look is expressive of terror and wildness; the lips, face, neck, hands, and feet, and soon after the thighs, arms, and whole surface assume a leaden, blue, purple, black, or deep brown tint according to the complexion of the individual, varying in shade with the intensity of the attack. The fingers and toes are reduced in size, the skin and soft parts covering them are wrinkled, shrivelled and folded. The nails put on a bluish pearly white; the larger superficial veins are marked by flat lines of a deeper black; the pulse becomes either small as a thread, and scarcely vibrating, or else totally extinct. The skin is deadly cold and often damp, the tongue always moist, often white and loaded, but flabby and chilled like a piece of dead flesh. The voice is nearly gone; the respiration quick, irregular, and imperfectly performed. The patient speaks in a whisper. He struggles for breath, and often lays his hand on his heart to point out the seat of his distress. Sometimes there are rigid spasms of the legs, thighs, and loins. The secretion of urine is totally suspended; vomiting and purgings... succeed.'

– *The London Gazette*, 21 October 1831. p.2159

Remedies knew no bounds, as did the cashing in, with Daffey's Elixir, Moxon's Effervescent Magnesium Aperient, and Morrison the Hygienist's Genuine Vegetable Universal Mixture. And all this while the nation was ravaged by a whole host of other infectious diseases such as typhus fever, typhoid, smallpox, scarlet fever, diphtheria and TB.

Barnet, M., 1972. The 1832 cholera outbreak in York, *Medical History* 16

Durey, M., 1974, *The First Spasmodic Cholera Epidemic in York*, 1832, York

Durey, M., 1976, Popular reactions to the 1832 cholera outbreak in Britain. Unpublished paper given at the annual conference of the urban *History Group, Cambridge University* 7-8 April 1976

Johnson, Steven, 2006. *The ghost map: the story of London's most terrifying epidemic – and how it changed science, cities, and the modern world*. New York

Morris, R., 1976, *Cholera 1832: the social response to an epidemic*, New York

Chapter 38

The 1829 Groningen malaria epidemic

The Groninger ziekte (also called 'intermittent fevers') that broke out in 1826 was a malaria epidemic that killed 2,844 people out of a population of 30,000 – nearly 10 per cent of the population of the city of Groningen in the Netherlands. In February 1825 the dykes broke in several places causing widespread flooding in the region. The decay of plants and cattle under swamplike conditions and the flooding in Groningen in the subsequent hot spring and summer of 1826 triggered the epidemic which also struck Friesland and the German Wadden Sea region. The Frisian town of Sneek reported a tripling of the number of deaths in 1826 as compared to previous years.

We should not be surprised that malaria afflicts parts of northern Europe – the mosquitoes are made of stern stuff. Parts of the Netherlands in particular are prone to outbreaks as Groningen shows us; the country had a reputation: in 1824 one Dutch physician wrote that Italy apart 'there is probably no other land where the intermittent fevers are so malignant as in ours,' while Verhave (1988) says 'the Netherlands has always been a fever ridden country'.

Endemic northern malaria reached 68 degrees N latitude in Europe during the 19th century, where the summer mean temperature only irregularly exceeded 16 degrees C, the lower limit needed for sporogony of *Plasmodium vivax*. Groningen lies 53 degrees N. In 1857 there was another malaria outbreak in Zeeland.

Hulden, Lena, 2005, Endemic malaria: An 'indoor' disease in northern Europe. Historical data analysed, *Malaria Journal* 4

Verhave, J., 1988. The Advent of Malaria Research in The Netherlands. *History and Philosophy of the Life Sciences*, 10(1), 121–128.

Chapter 39

The 1837 Great Plains Smallpox Epidemic

'The Mandans & Rees gave us two splendid dances, they say they dance, on account of their not haveing a long time to live, as they expect to all die of the small pox – and as long as they are alive, they will take it out in dancing.'

– Francis Chardon

'Thirty million white men are struggling and scuffling for the goods and luxuries of life over the bones and ashes of twelve million red men, six million of them dead of smallpox...'

– George Catlin

In 1837 an American Fur Company steamboat, the SS *St. Peter*, was carrying more than furs and supplies when it headed into the Missouri Valley. People infected with smallpox were also on board and when they disembarked they proceeded unwittingly to infect and kill more than 17,000 indigenous people along the Missouri River alone, with some tribes reduced to near extinction. Trader Francis Chardon saw the terrible impact of the disease on the Mandan tribe and wrote 'the small-pox had never been known in the civilized world, as it had been among the poor Mandans and other Indians.' Only twenty-seven Mandans were left to tell the tale.

By the 1730s smallpox had made its insidious way west to Canada and the northern United States. The Assiniboine First Nation had controlled much of this territory, but were forced to give it up as their population decreased dramatically. Along the Missouri River the Arikara population was reduced by half by the end of the 1730s. Other communities decimated in the 1730s by smallpox include the Lower Loup, Pawnee of Nebraska, Cherokee and the Kansa. In short, if you were an indigenous community on the Great Plains in the 1730s then smallpox was probably going to get you.

Epidemics of 1781 and 1801 claimed the lives of thousands of Mandans, Hidatsas, and Arikaras and forced them to move north to re-build their villages near the mouth of the Knife River. Then the 1837 epidemic came.

The *St. Peter* steamboat travelled up the Missouri River to Fort Union from St. Louis liberally infecting people along the way. By 29 April she arrived at Leavenworth where a deckhand displayed signs of smallpox before three Arikara women joined the ship on their way back to the Mandan community. The women too showed signs of the infection but astonishingly they were allowed to return to their village where they then, unknowingly, spread smallpox amongst their community. The disease that spread to the Mandan people turned out to be of the most virulent, malignant hemorrhagic form. In July 1837, the Mandan dead numbered about 2,000; by October the tribe had dwindled to 23 or 27 survivors by some accounts, 138 by another account, reflecting a 90 per cent mortality rate. Whatever, the figure was below the genetic survival threshold and the hunters were now too few to maintain a food gathering capability. The result was an increased dependence on traded goods (including furs) and on government aid.

Fort Clark was a key American Fur Company trading post built in 1823 just a few miles south of the mouth of the Knife River on the west bank of the Missouri River. The Yanktonais, Crows, Assiniboines and other tribes routinely visited Fort Clark bringing buffalo hides and furs to trade for tobacco, guns, cloth and other goods. Fort Clark was a busy, densely populated regional entrepôt. On 18 June 1837, the *St. Peter* headed there; on board was Andrew Jackson Chardon, the 2-year-old younger son of Fort Clark's superintendent, Francis Chardon. Chardon met the boat some 30 miles downstream and removed his son when he heard the disconcerting news that passengers were infected with smallpox. Docking at Fort Clark, the *St. Peter* was thronged with the usual frenetic activity and crowds with shiphands and dock workers unloading bales of furs in twenty-four hours amid a 'frolick' of singing and dancing and celebration amongst hands and residents. Once reloaded, the *St. Peter* headed upstream to Fort Union carrying the deadly virus insinuated in its cargoes. Indeed, dancing helped to avert the impending sense of doom, as Chardon records: 'The Mandans & Rees gave us two splendid dances, they say they dance, on account of their not haveing a long time to live, as they expect to all die of the small pox —and as long as they are alive, they will take it out in dancing.'

Within two months, on 11 August, Chardon, a widower who lost his elder son to the disease, wrote, 'I Keep no a/c of the dead, as they die so fast it is impossible,' and by the end of the month, 'the Mandan are all cut off except 23 young and old men.' Scapegoating was the order of the day and survivors swore revenge against Chardon for introducing death to their villages. There were murders and threats of murder as the frantic Mandans tried to avenge the deaths of their families and friends. On 28 July Chardon reports:

> 'This day was very Near being my last — a Young Mandan came to the Fort with his gun cocked, and secreted under his robe, with the intention of Killing me, after hunting me in 3 or 4 of the houses ... Mitchel caught him, and gave him in the hands of two Indians who conducted him to the Village, had not Mitchel perceived him the instant he did, I would not be at the trouble of Makeing this statement — I am upon my guard, . . . I have got 100 Guns ready and 1000 lb Powder, ready to hand out to them when the fun commences.'

Some people, sick with smallpox or desperate from grief over the loss of whole families, committed suicide. Suicide was virtually unknown among the Mandans and Hidatsas before the epidemic.

A longboat was despatched to Fort McKenzie via the Marias River, only for the disease to spread among the Blackfoot and thence into the Great Plains, killing many thousands between 1837 and 1840: it is estimated that two-thirds of the Blackfoot population died, along with half of the Assiniboines and Arikaras, a third of the Crows and a quarter of the Pawnees. A trader at Fort Union reported 'such a stench in the fort that it could be smelt at a distance of 300 yards'. The bodies were buried in large pits, or slung into the river, which may have contributed to the contagion as bodies remained infectious after death.

The survivors needed meat and crops to get through the coming winter, but there were few Mandan women healthy enough to manage the harvest. To add to their plight, the Sioux attacked the weakened villages. As if the ruthless scourge of the disease and the Sioux attacks were not cataclysmic enough there have been, as we shall see, documented cases of smallpox being intentionally spread among the indigenous people of the Americas by white fur traders and settlers: this ineffably atrocious behaviour lies somewhere between bioterrorism on a prodigious scale and ethnic cleansing; according to Esther Wagner Stearn (1945):

'...this disease was the most dreaded of scourges, the most frequent disastrous dictator of destiny and action among the Indians. This fact the white man soon learned, for history records numerous instances of the French, the Spanish, the English, and later on the American, using smallpox as an ignoble means to an end. For smallpox was more feared by the Indian than the bullet: he could be exterminated and subjugated more easily and quickly by the death-bringing virus than by the weapons of the white man.'

An example of this despicable behaviour comes from fur trader James McDougall, who is quoted as saying to a gathering of local chiefs, 'You know the smallpox. Listen: I am the smallpox chief. In this bottle I have it confined. All I have to do is to pull the cork, send it forth among you, and you are dead men. But this is for my enemies and not my friends.'[1] Likewise, another fur trader threatened Pawnee Indians that if they failed to agree to certain conditions, 'he would let the smallpox out of a bottle and destroy them'.

When the time came, not unreasonably all this made native Americans suspicious and nervous of vaccination as observed by artist and writer George Catlin: 'They see white men urging the operation so earnestly they decide that it must be some new mode or trick of the pale face by which they hope to gain some new advantage over them.'[2] So deep was the distrust of the settlers that the Mandan chief Four Bears denounced the white man, whom he had previously treated as a brother, for deliberately imposing the disease on his people. After losing his wife and children to smallpox, and acquiring the disease himself, his final speech to the Arikara and Mandan tribes before dying on 30 July 1837 ended, according to Chardon, with: 'I have Never Called a White Man a Dog, but to day, I do Pronounce them to be a set of Black hearted Dogs'... all that you hold dear, are all Dead, or Dying, with their faces all rotten, caused by those dogs the whites, think of all that My friends, and rise all together and Not leave one of them alive.'

---

1. Stearn, 1945
2. Hopkins, 1983

According to Ramenofsky,[3] '*Variola Major* can be transmitted through contaminated articles such as clothing or blankets. In the nineteenth century, the US Army sent contaminated blankets to Native Americans, especially Plains groups, 'to control the Indian problem.' Ward Churchill claimed in 1837[4] that at Fort Clark the United States Army deliberately infected Mandan Indians by distributing blankets that had been exposed to smallpox, adding that the blankets were taken from a military infirmary in St. Louis, that smallpox vaccine was withheld from the Indians, and that an army doctor had ordered the infected Indians to disperse, further spreading the disease and causing over 100,000 deaths.

Meanwhile the response to the epidemic was pathetically inadequate: Chardon was dispensing Epsom Salts while 'The Rees are Makeing Medicine for their sickness. Some of them have made dreams, that they talked to the Sun, others to the Moon, several articles has been sacrifised to them both'. He tells of a complete breakdown in local society:

> 'The Wife of a young Mandan that caught the disease was suffering from the pain, her husband looked at her, and held down his head, he jumped up, and said to his wife, When you was young, you were hansome, you are now ugly and going to leave me, but no, I will go with you, he took up his gun and shot her dead, and with his Knife ripped open his own belly — two young men (Rees) Killed themselves to day, one of them stabbed himself with a Knife, and the other with an arrow.'

August 29th saw individual attempts at inoculation:

> 'An Indian Vaccinated his child, by cutting two small pieces of flesh out of his arms, and two on the belly – and then takeing a Scab from one, that was getting well of the disease, and rubbing it on the wounded part, three days after, it took effect, and the child is perfectly well.'

But the suicides and murder went on:

> 'A young Mandan that died 4 days ago, his wife haveing the disease also — Killed her two children, one a fine Boy of eight years, and the other six, to complete the affair she hung herself... This Morning two dead bodies, wrapped in a White [bison hide], and laid on a raft passed by the Fort, on their way to the regions below, May success attend them... a young Mandan that was given over for dead, and abandoned by his Father, and left alone in the bushes to die, came to life again, and is now doing well, he is hunting his Father, with the intent to Kill him, for leaveing him alone. . .'

Which brings us back to the *St. Peter*: undoubtedly the unwillingness of Captain Pratte to quarantine those on his ship suspected of infection contributed to thousands of

---

3. 1987, pp. 147–8
4. pp. 11, 35

subsequent deaths. He chose to follow his business plan to deliver goods and pick up furs and return quickly to St. Louis. His commercial choice had deadly consequences for his company's business partners – the peoples of the northern Great Plains. The law deemed Pratte's offence criminal negligence. Despite all the fatalities, the almost complete annihilation of the Mandans, and the general depradation of the region, a judgement of criminal negligence seems somewhat flaccid and forgiving for an action that had such horrific consequences[5] and is a natural consequence of putting commerce above public health. Smallpox returned to the Northern Great plains in 1851, again with devastating effect.

Churchill, Ward, 1994. *Indians Are Us? Culture and Genocide in Native North America.* Monroe, ME: Common Courage Press

Dollar, Clyde D., 1977. 'The High Plains Smallpox Epidemic of 1837–38'. *Western Historical Quarterly.* 8 (1): 15–38.

Robertson, R. G., 2001. *Rotting Face: Smallpox and the American Indian.* Caxton Press.

Stearn, Esther Wagne, 1945, *The Effect of Smallpox on the Destiny of the Amerindian;* University of Minnesota

---

5. Robertson, 2001, pp. 80–83, 298–312

Chapter 40

1847 North American typhus epidemic: coffin ships and fever sheds

'Black Forty-Seven' – a year black with Famine, Disease, Death and Exile

Emigration usually involves transportation of some kind, and in the 19th century this more often than not entailed ships and the sea. The 1847 Great Irish Emigration was no different; however, it was exceptional not just for the number of people involved, but also for the fact that it was accompanied by epidemic typhus. This massive movement of people was in itself triggered partly by the Great Famine. The Irish had died in their droves from starvation and malnutrition; now they were being slaughtered by a virulent epidemic. Between 1841 and 1851 death and mass emigration, mainly to Great Britain and North America, caused Ireland's population to fall by over 2 million. In Connacht alone the population fell by almost 30 per cent.

That the mass emigration from Ireland was a 'flight from famine' is only partly true because the Irish had been coming to build canals and other civil engineering projects in Britain since the 18th century, and emigration did not slow down when the famine was over; indeed in the succeeding years there were more emigrants than during the four years of the blight. The famine was, however, the catalyst for people to move who were on the point of leaving Ireland anyway. What is indisputable was the huge number of people involved and the prodigious death toll of the epidemic.

Apart from Britain, Canada was a major destination. In Canada, more than 20,000 people died in 1847 and 1848, with many quarantined in execrable fever sheds. The story of the 1847 epidemic is the story of the fever sheds and coffin ships. The Reverend John Gallagher (1936) describes these fetid old timber vessels from an eye witness account:

> 'Where there was hardly room for one, three human beings were stalled…There was no light – no ventilation whatever, except what we got from two hatchways. Each immigrant was allowed by law thirty-three inches of room in width, but we didn't get it….The supply of water, hardly enough for cooking and drinking, does not allow washing…I dare not describe further the disgusting condition of these ships wherein four hundred men, women and children were confined together without regard for sex, age or condition. .. The foul pestilential air was the best conductor of germs. Before the ship was a day out at sea, the dread typhus or ship fever was raging in every vessel. Constitutions which were broken down and weakened by famine and its accompanying diseases became the easy prey of ship fever.'

A fever shed (or pest house or plague house) was used for forcibly quarantining anyone afflicted with communicable diseases such as tuberculosis, cholera, smallpox or typhus. Many towns and cities had by now one or more pesthouses along with a cemetery or a waste pond nearby for disposal of the dead. In eastern Canada fever sheds were built to quarantine those sick and dying Irish immigrants, who had contracted typhus on the voyage to the New World during the Great Famine.

On 29 July 1847, Robert Whyte, in his *Famine Ship Diary: The Journey of a Coffin Ship* recorded the neglect of his fellow passengers at Grosse Isle, who 'within reach of help …were to be left enveloped in reeking pestilence, the sick without medicine, medical skill, nourishment, or so much as a drop of pure water'. However, conditions on others were worse still. Two Canadian priests visited the *Ajax* where they had been 'up to their ankles in filth. The wretched emigrants crowded together like cattle and corpses remain[ed] long unburied'. Whyte contrasted this with German immigrants arriving at Grosse Isle who were sickness free, 'comfortably and neatly clad, clean and happy'. *The Times* also remarked on the 'healthy, robust and cheerful' Germans.

Whyte estimated that 5,293 people died at sea. During the crossing itself, bodies were slung overboard, but on arrival at Grosse Isle the deceased were kept in the hold until burial on land was possible. The dead were dragged out of the holds with hooks and 'stacked like cordwood' on the shore.

Robert Whyte's 1847 *Famine Ship Diary: The Journey of an Irish Coffin Ship*, Mercier Press, 1994

Gelston, Arthur, 1977. 'Typhus Fever: The Report of an Epidemic in New York City in 1847'. *Journal of Infectious Diseases*. 136 (6): 813–821.

Jordan, J., 1909, *The Grosse Île Tragedy*

Chapter 41

The Third Cholera Pandemic 1846–1860; John Snow and the Broad Street pump and 'fetid Redcar'

'It is beyond dispute that…a portion of the inhabitants of the metropolis [London] are made to consume, in some form or other, a portion of their own excrement and, moreover, to pay for the privilege.'

– Arthur Hill Hassall, microscopist, 1850

The Third Pandemic began in India and was the most rapacious of the cholera pandemics; it began in the lower Bengal region and spread to Afghanistan in 1839. The disease was conveyed by British troops to China in 1840 and had spread through the Philippines and Burma by 1844. In 1845, the pandemic re-emerged in India and devastated the Middle East killing 15,000 in Mecca. After a brief respite, it spread up the Caspian coast to penetrate Russia – between 1847 and 1851 more than one million people died there – and by 1848, it tore into Europe.

Between 1848 and 1850 52,000 victims died in Britain; in London, it was the worst outbreak in the city's history, claiming 14,137 lives, over twice as many as the 1832 outbreak. Cholera struck Ireland in 1849 and killed many Irish Famine survivors, already vulnerable from starvation and fever. In 1849, cholera claimed 5,308 lives in Liverpool, an embarkation point for immigrants to North America and a disembarkation port for Irish immigrants; 1,834 died in Hull. In 1849, a second major outbreak occurred in Paris; in Spain, over 236,000 died.

In the US cholera spread throughout the Mississippi river system, killing over 4,500 in St. Louis and over 3,000 in New Orleans. Thousands died in New York, a popular destination for those Irish immigrants. During the California Gold Rush, cholera was transmitted along the California, Mormon and Oregon Trails: between 6,000 and 12,000 are believed to have succumbed on their way to Utah and Oregon in 1849–55. Cholera claimed more than 150,000 victims in the United States during the two pandemics between 1832 and 1849; 200,000 died in Mexico. In New York posters recommended treatments, including laudanum (morphine), calomel (mercury) as a binding laxative and camphor as an anaesthetic. High doses sometimes did a lot more harm than good. Poultices of mustard, cayenne pepper and hot vinegar were also applied, as well as opium suppositories and tobacco enemas.

In Russia more than one million people died of cholera. In 1859 an outbreak in Bengal helped transmission of the pernicious disease by travellers and troops to Iran, Iraq, Arabia and Russia. Between 100,000 and 200,000 people died of cholera in Tokyo in an outbreak in 1858–60.

John Snow and the Broad Street pump

In 1854 the physician John Snow from York later called it 'the most terrible outbreak of cholera which ever occurred in this kingdom'; he was working with the poor in Soho when he made one of medical science's greatest discoveries: Snow identified contaminated water as the pathway by which cholera was transmitted. Soho was a mess: filth was everywhere due to the large influx of people and the absence of proper sanitary services since the London sewer system had not reached Soho. Cowsheds, slaughter houses and grease-boiling dens lined the streets and contributed animal droppings, rotting garbage, infected fluids and other contaminants to the foul Soho streets. Many cellars had cesspools swilling around underneath their floorboards, replenished from the sewers and the excrement seeping in from the streets. And so it was decided to dump all this waste into the River Thames, polluting the water supply to unbelievable levels.

Many of the victims in 1854 were taken to the Middlesex Hospital, where their treatment was superintended by Florence Nightingale. According to a letter from Elizabeth Gaskell, 'She herself [Nightingale] was up night and day from Friday afternoon (1 Sept.) to Sunday afternoon, receiving the poor creatures (chiefly fallen women of that neighbourhood – they had it the worst) who were being constantly brought in – undressing them – putting on turpentine stupes, et cetera, doing it herself to as many as she could manage.'

After the 1854 cholera flare up which took 616 people Snow dot-mapped the cases around the Broad Street (now Soho's Broadwick Street) pump and observed a cluster of cases there. To test this theory, he simply convinced the St James parish authorities to disable the pump by removing the handle: the number of cholera cases in the area fell immediately. Snow realised that the disease had nothing to do with miasma; it was, in fact transmitted by germ-contaminated water. 'There was nothing in the air to account for the spread of cholera,' Snow said; cholera was spread by persons ingesting a substance, not through atmospheric transmittal. He cited a case of two sailors, one with cholera and one without. Eventually the second became sick as well from 'accidentally' ingesting bodily fluids of the first.

He also did a statistical analysis to illustrate the connection between the quality of the water source and cholera cases, demonstrating that water was being delivered to the outbreak area from the Thames which was highly contaminated with visible and invisible products. The main culprits were the Southwark & Vauxhall Waterworks Company, and the Lambeth Waterworks Company. Dr Arthur Hassall examined the filtered water and found it contained animal hair, among other foul and fetid substances. Snow's breakthrough helped bring the epidemic under control although he, good scientist as he was, advised caution.[1]

> 'There is no doubt that the mortality was much diminished, as I said before, by the flight of the population, which commenced soon after the outbreak; but the attacks had so far diminished before the use of the water was stopped, that it is impossible to decide whether the well still contained the cholera poison in an active state, or whether, from some cause, the water had become free from it.'

However,

> 'It will be observed that the deaths either very much diminished, or ceased altogether, at every point where it becomes decidedly nearer to send to another pump than to the one in Broad street. It may also be noticed that the deaths are most numerous near to the pump where the water could be more readily obtained.'

Apparently, after the cholera epidemic had subsided, government officials replaced the Broad Street pump handle. They had responded only to the urgent threat posed to the population and afterwards they rejected Snow's theory. To accept his proposal would have meant indirectly accepting the oral-faecal method of transmission of disease, which they deemed too disgusting for most of the public to contemplate.

Snow was a founding member of the Epidemiological Society of London, he is surely one of the fathers of epidemiology. His discovery had a major public health impact around the globe and generated the construction of improved sanitation facilities. Later, the term 'focus of infection' would be used to describe sites, such as the Broad Street pump, in which conditions promote transmission of an infection. John Snow's experimentation caused him to unknowingly create an early double-blind experiment. In 1853–54, London's epidemic had claimed 10,739 lives.

Further north, in seaside Redcar, we get a good example of what can and was done to delimit the disgusting conditions which allowed cholera and other diseases to flourish.

September 1854 saw cholera visit Redcar with twenty cases and eight deaths, seven of which were clustered in squalid Fishermen's Square, owned by the Earl of Zetland. The Earl immediately demolished the houses and built a new street, South Terrace, for the fishermen: twenty-two terraced houses 'with every sanitary improvement to prevent the recurrence of the disease'. Then came typhus with thirty cases and one death in Back Lane; there were also two deaths in North Side.

The resulting Ranger Report concluded that much of Redcar was a dirty, fetid, insanitary place, somewhat at odds with the eulogies found in the contemporary travel guides. Springs and wells were often polluted with seepage from cess pits.

---

1. 1855, p.38 & P.1.

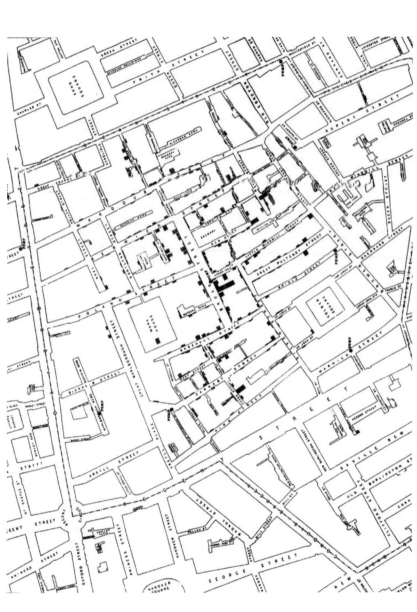

This map was created by John Snow in 1854. London was fighting a deadly cholera epidemic, when Snow tracked the cases on this map. The cholera cases are highlighted in black. Using this map, Snow and other scientists were able to trace the cholera outbreak to a single infected water pump.

There were no scavengers – the men who emptied the privies and ash pits by night; refuse was simply thrown into the road or heaped up.

In June 1855 the Redcar Board of health was set up to remedy this calamitous situation. Enteric fever struck in 1890 and 1891: the filth and squalor from forty years previously had not been eradicated and was the cause: the Kirkleatham Board of Health reported 'large accumulations of filth of every description such as ash pit refuse and human excrement from privies and closets…it is certain that all the filth will be washed into the stream…and carried to the Stockton and Middlesbrough pumping station'. From August 1893 the region took its water supply from the clean water of the reservoir at Lockwood Beck leaving the local Water Board high and dry.

Halliday, S., 2001, Death and miasma in Victorian London: an obstinate belief. *BMJ*, 323:1469–71.

Hempel, Sandra, 2006, *The Medical Detective: John Snow and the mystery of cholera*, London

Snow, John, 1855, *On the mode of communication of cholera* (2nd ed), London

Chapter 42

The 1853 Copenhagen Cholera Outbreak

A part from the 4,737 people who tragically died, this outbreak is notable for the measures taken post-epidemic to remedy those things which had contributed to the spread of the disease. Local medical professionals predicted a disaster when in the 1840s they warned against the wretched sanitary conditions in the city and the rampant overcrowding due to the ban on urban development outside the city walls. A total of 7,219 infections were reported of whom 4,737 (56.7 per cent) died. From Copenhagen the outbreak spread to the provinces where twenty-four towns were hit and 1,951 more people died.

Cholera was a key factor in the decision to decommission Copenhagen's fortifications, the decision to build a new cattle market, the so-called Brown Meat District, in 1878 and the decision to construct a safer municipal water supply. After 1878 all slaughterings at the numerous private open air stockyards around the city were prohibited and had in future to take place in the public slaughterhouses. Mandatory meat control was also introduced, requiring all fresh meat coming into the city to be inspected and stamped.

It also resulted in several housing developments from 1857 built by philanthropic organisations to provide healthy homes outside the city centre for people with lower incomes – Brumleby in Østerbro is a good example. The developments are Denmark's first examples of affordable social housing.

There is a growing consensus that domestic and community water, sanitation and hygiene interventions have had an important role to play in the control of cholera around the world.

D'Mello-Guyett, L., 2020, Prevention and control of cholera with household and community water, sanitation and hygiene (WASH) interventions: A scoping review of current international guidelines. *PLoS One.* 15(1)

Phelps, Matthew et al., 2018, 'Cholera Epidemics of the Past Offer New Insights Into an Old Enemy.' *The Journal of infectious diseases* vol. 217,4: 641-649.

Schleisner, P. A., 1871, 'The Cholera in Copenhagen in 1866; the Precautions There Taken against the Spread of the Disease; and the Frequency of Diarrhœal Complaints in Denmark Generally.' *The British and Foreign Medico-chirugical review* vol. 48,96, 462-476.

Chapter 43

Smallpox in British Columbia –
a case of genocide

W hen European settlers first descended on Canada's Pacific shelf, they liked to think of themselves as harbingers of light, ushering in as they did the glow of the European enlightenment. Natives saw it very differently; what they experienced was an insidious cloak of darkeness which began with settlers intentionally spreading smallpox in a systematic programme to displace the indigenous peoples of what is now British Columbia. Their aim: to 'cleanse' the region of the indigenous population.

It started with a gold rush. On 12 March 1862, the San Francisco steamer *Brother Jonathan* docked at the busy colony of Vancouver Island, a former Hudson Bay Company fur trading post that had witnessed an explosion in population after a mainland gold rush. 'The town was taken completely by surprise,' according to the *British Colonist*, reporting that along with merchandise and mules, the ship carried 350 passengers to Victoria – home to 4,000–5,000 colonists, with slightly more indigenous people from various nations in camps nearby hoping for trade and work.

According to Joshua Ostroff (2017):

> 'Most of the passengers were heading to a new gold strike on the Salmon River. But along with his pickaxe and gold pan, one of these miners brought another piece of cargo: smallpox. The man was quarantined. But the *Colonist* noted that 'the measures the colonial government chose – limited vaccination efforts, and declining to try a general quarantine, which would have kept the crisis localized – wound up leading to an epidemic when police emptied the camps at gunpoint, burned them down, and towed canoes filled with smallpox-infected Indigenous people up the coast. Over the next year, at least 30,000 indigenous people died, representing about 60 per cent of the population – a crisis that left mass graves, deserted villages, traumatized survivors and societal collapse.'

When on 4 July 1862, Francis Poole and eight men from what had begun as a party of forty arrived at Fort Alexandria in the Nuxalk Ancestors' territory, smallpox carriers knowingly left the disease at Nanaimo, Fort Rupert (north Vancouver Island), and at a Heiltsuk community on the approach to Bella Coola. Rumour has it that the disease arrived in blankets that had been infected with smallpox and then repackaged as new for trade. As in other documented cases, such as that of John McLain who admitted taking smallpox-infected blankets to Tatla, those traders were also carriers of the disease. Within thirty days an eye-witness estimated 75 per cent of the Nuxalk at Bella Coola were dead or dying from the disease.

One indigenous nation, though, fought back to defend its land. In 1864, the Tsilhqot'in declared war after being threatened with smallpox by the foreman of a road being built through their territory. This battle, the Chilcotin War, ended with the hanging of five chiefs – the martyrdom of the 'Chilcotin Chiefs'. Over 75 per cent of all the Tsilhqot'in people would be dead before year end – a sign of systematic disease introduction? Events in Nuxalk territory during this 'Smallpox War' connects the violence in Tsilhqot'in territory with similar smallpox epidemics elsewhere in the British Pacific Colonies. Shawn Swankey (2015) tells how:

> 'In the sudden catastrophe flowing from these artificial epidemics, 70 per cent or more of all the Tsilhqot'in died in a year or less. Some other indigenous peoples in B.C. suffered similar death tolls. In the face of this carnage, the Tsilhqot'in held a war council, killed up to 20 settlers implicated in smallpox distribution schemes and closed their territory. B.C. then invaded Tsilhqot'in territory with two settler militias. Unable to find the war party, agents for the Crown invited Tsilhqot'in representatives to a peace conference. The Colony violated the conditions of the conference to ambush the Tsilhqot'in and five, including the 'Head War Chief' were put through show trials and executed.'

'The smallpox epidemic … it changes everything in British Columbia,' says John Lutz, the head of the University of Victoria's history department and an indigenous-settler relations specialist. 'The citizens of Victoria, one could say, panicked. Or, one could say, with a less charitable view, that they deliberately drove the Indigenous people out of town, and that spread the disease back to their home communities up and down the coast.' If they had contained those people who contracted smallpox within the Victoria area, the indigenous population would be much higher today. The government clearly wanted to be able to claim those lands without having to compensate or recognize Indigenous title.

Colonist numbers duly surged as indigenous populations fell by as much as 90 per cent in some areas. Cole Harris reports in *The Resettlement of British Columbia* that by 1863 in southeastern British Columbia large areas were 'almost completely depopulated' and that census-takers on the north coast found the Haida people had fallen from a pre-epidemic count of 6,607 people to only 829 in 1881.

On the 150th anniversary of the hanging in 2014, British Columbia exonerated six Tsilhqot'in leaders hanged in 1864/65; the Premier Christy Clark expressed British Columbia's 'profound sorrow' for this execution of officials who had done no more than seek to protect their people from genocide through the continued intentional introduction of smallpox.

The publication of 'The True Story of Canada's "War" of Extermination on the Pacific,' *by writer and lawyer Tom Swanky, has made avoiding that conclusion that Canada's methods of ethnic cleansing also included the use of smallpox blankets and deliberate exposure to infected individuals increasingly difficult. In fact, the provincial government of British Columbia was so convinced of the authenticity of Swanky's claims of deliberate smallpox infection that they publicly exonerated the six Tsilhqot'in chiefs who were hung for murder in the early 1860s. Swanky's book demonstrates that the chiefs had acted in self-defence and that their trials were a judicial mockery.*

Swanky's search for the true story about smallpox matters to me, not only for its rewriting of colonial history by providing a counter-narrative, but also because it indicates that our ongoing disregard for the health and wellbeing of BC's First Nations has roots in both the racist policies of the federal government and the colonial administration of James Douglas.

– Garry Geddes, 'Medicine Unbundled', Heritage House Publishing Company, 2017.

Ostroff, Joshua, 2017, How a smallpox epidemic forged modern British Columbia
Swankey, Shawn, A Missing Genocide and the Demonization of its Heroes, https://www.macleans.ca/news/canada/how-a-smallpox-epidemic-forged-modern-british-columbia/
Swanky, Shawn, The Smallpox War in Nuxalk Territory
Swankey, Tom, *The True Story of Canada's 'War' of Extermination on the Pacific*

Chapter 44

The third plague pandemic 1855–1960

Yunnan, China was where in 1855 the third plague pandemic began; it spread to all inhabited continents, and ultimately led to more than 12 million deaths in India and China, 10 million of which were in India. According to the World Health Organization, the pandemic was live until 1960, when worldwide casualties dropped to 200 per year.

This pandemic originated from two different sources: the first was mainly bubonic and was carried around the world through ocean-going trade; the second, more virulent strain, was primarily pneumonic with a strong person-to-person contagion. This strain was largely confined to Asia, in particular Manchuria and Mongolia.

The third pandemic of plague originated in west Yunnan after a rapid influx of Han Chinese to exploit the demand for minerals, primarily copper, in the second half of the 19th century; by 1850, the population had exploded to over 7 million people. The plague would have been brought from the interior to the coastal regions by troops returning from battles against the Muslim rebels and by the lucrative opium trade from about 1840.

The plague was introduced from Hong Kong to British India, where it killed about one million; later it buried another 12.5 million there over the next thirty years.

Benedict, Carol, 1996. *Bubonic plague in eighteenth-century China*. Stanford, CA

Orent, Wendy, 2004. *Plague: The Mysterious Past and Terrifying Future of the World's Most Dangerous Disease*. New York

Pryor, E.G., 1970. 'The Great Plague of Hong Kong'. *Journal of the Hong Kong Branch of the Royal Asiatic Society*. 15: 61–70.

Chapter 45

The Fourth Cholera Pandemic 1863–1875: Wales

Religion and war both had major roles to play in the fourth cholera pandemic which originated in the Ganges delta of the Bengal region and travelled with Muslim pilgrims to Mecca. In 1863, the epidemic claimed 30,000 of 90,000 pilgrims. Cholera spread throughout the Middle East and then on to Russia, western Europe, Africa and North America, spreading freely via travellers and cargoes from port cities and along inland waterways.

The pandemic reached northern Africa in 1865 and spread to sub-Saharan Africa, killing 70,000 in Zanzibar in 1869–70. Cholera claimed 90,000 lives in Russia in 1866; it was facilitated by troop movements in the Austro-Prussian War (1866) and is estimated to have taken 165,000 lives in the Austrian Empire, including 30,000 each in Hungary and Belgium, and 20,000 in the Netherlands. There were 115,000 deaths in Germany.

In 1867, Italy lost 113,000 to cholera, and 80,000 died of the disease in Algeria. Outbreaks in North America in the 1870s killed some 50,000 Americans as cholera spread from New Orleans via passenger boats along the Mississippi River and to ports on its tributaries.

In June 1866, an epidemic in the East End of London claimed 5,596 lives, just before the city completed construction of its major sewage and water treatment systems. In the same year, the use of contaminated canal water in local water works caused a minor outbreak at Ystalyfera near Swansea. Workers and their families, were most affected and 119 died.

Merthyr was badly hit too. During August a number of sanitary precautions were instituted there. Here is an extract from the official report: 'The patient was a married woman, aged thirty years, who died after eighteen hours illness. She resided with her husband and three children in a two-roomed, ill-ventilated tenement, underneath the Duffryn Arms, Canal side. The room was excessively dirty. The family lay upon a filthy mattress placed upon a damp sodden floor. The husband is employed in the Plymouth Iron Works, but he spends most of his wages on drink &c....'.

At Dowlais, ... the new visitation prompted the Dowlais Company to open a temporary hospital to deal with the cases. But this proposal... engendered such local antipathy that soon after the first patient was admitted some of the Dowlais workers rioted, burst into the building, and insulted the nurses. When the miners threatened to strike if the hospital continued, the Company had no alternative but to abandon the project... It was during that month, however, that the disease was particularly active in North Wales, coinciding there with a severe epidemic of scarlet fever.

Chapter 46

The 1871 Buenos Aires Yellow Fever Epidemic

'Businesses closed, streets deserted, a shortage of doctors, corpses without assistance, everyone flees if they can...'

All the usual collateral from an epidemic, as recorded on 13 April in the diary of a witness to the 1871 epidemic, Mardoqueo Navarro. Navarro was an Argentine businessman and diarist who was born in the province of Catamarca, in 1824. In the mid-1840s he moved to Buenos Aires and then spent the whole of the following decade in Rosario, where he worked as the manager of a meat-salting plant belonging to General Justo José de Urquiza.

Navarro reveals that the 1871 epidemic, as you would expect, bears all the characteristics we have seen in earlier outbreaks of yellow fever, 'black vomit'. One of the significant peculiarities, though, was the number of outbreaks: it struck in 1852, 1858, 1870 and 1871, the last killing about 8 per cent of Porteños (inhabitants of the city of Buenos Aires); in a city where the usual daily death rate was less than 20, there were some days on which more than 500 people died.

Once again war was the answer to how and why it erupted: the epidemic originated in Asunción, Paraguay, brought home by Argentine troops returning from the war they had just fought there; earlier it had spread in the city of Corrientes, population 11,000 and a military base for the Argentinians. The population of Buenos Aires was reduced by two thirds because of the deaths, compounded by the exodus of those trying to escape the scourge. The Paraguayan War, also known as the War of the Triple Alliance, was fought from 1864 to 1870, between Paraguay and the Triple Alliance of Argentina, the Empire of Brazil, and Uruguay. It was the deadliest and bloodiest inter-state war in Latin America's history. The previous year's epidemic came in from Brazil on board a merchant ship and caused 100 deaths.

The reasons why the disease caught on in 1871 and spread are legion: an inadequate water supply; there was no sewerage system: human waste collected in cesspools, which contaminated the ground water and hence the wells; the Río de la Plata, from which the inhabitants extracted water by carts, was devoid of sanitation; the warm and humid summer climate; stifling overcrowding endured by the black population and, from 1871, further overcrowding caused by the endless stream of European immigrants. Add to this the *saladeros* (manufactures producing salted and dried meat) which polluted the Matanza River while the creeks, full of dumped debris which ran through the city helped the mosquito *Aedes aegypti* to proliferate. The city streets were very narrow while the the the filth and waste were used for levelling those streets. To make matters even worse there were, unsurprisingly, also outbreaks of cholera in 1867 and 1868, which killed hundreds.

Things started to hot up on 27 January 1871 when three cases of yellow fever were diagnosed in Buenos Aires – in the dense tenement-filled San Telmo neighbourhood. Doctors Tamini, Salvador Larrosa and Montes de Oca warned the City Commission but the Commission, under Narciso Martínez de Hoz, ignored their warnings and refused any public health measures. Instead the Municipality proceeded with preparations for the official carnival. March began with over 40 deaths a day, rising to 100 a day. Dances were banned; one third of the inhabitants abandoned the city. The three main hospitals were swamped, as was the orphanage; emergency clinics were set up, the port was quarantined and the provinces closed their borders to people or goods coming from Buenos Aires.

The municipality could not cope so a People's Commission of Public Health was set up to take control of the streets and of those who lived in places affected by the fever; in some cases they burnt their belongings. The Italians, who formed the majority of the foreigners, were unjustly blamed by the rest of the population for having brought the pestilence from Europe. The black population, by virtue of its wretched living conditions, was worst hit: the army surrounded the areas where they lived to prevent any escape from what was in effect a ghetto: they died in huge numbers and were buried in mass graves.

While the national and provincial authorities were fleeing the city, including the president, the secular and regular clergy stuck by their posts and complied with their evangelical mandate, to help the sick and dying in their homes; the Sisters of Charity suspended their teaching in order to work in the hospitals; seven died. Of the 292 city priests, 60 or so died. The demand for burials created the usual problems: the city's forty funeral carriages were insufficient so coffins were piled up waiting for the carriages to pick them up; they were reinforced by the Plaza carriages, which charged extortionate fees. The same was true with ever rising daily prices of ineffective medicines. Carpenters were dying so they stopped making coffins from wood and started wrapping the corpses in curtains instead. Refuse carts were deployed in funeral service and mass graves proliferated; twelve gravediggers at La Chacarita Cemetery died leaving 630 corpses without graves, with others dumped on the roadside. Such was the carnage and the chaos that people had to be rescued from mass graves when they showed signs of life. Looting and assaults increased with cases of thieves disguising themselves as invalids to inveigle their way into hospitals.

Between 9–11 April over 500 deaths were registered daily, reaching the peak on 10 April with 583 deaths. The Buenos Aires Western Railway extended a line from Bermejo down to the cemetery and started running trains just for the dead, with two journeys a day; there were two other corpse pick-up points after Bermejo.

June 2nd was the first day when not a single case was registered. The scourge of 'black vomit' never came back to the city. *The Revista Médico Quirúrgica* puts the official toll at 13,641 deaths including 60 priests, 12 doctors, 7 nuns, 22 members of the Commission of Hygiene and 4 of the heroic People's Commission. Nationalities of the dead were: 3,397 Argentinians, 6,201 Italians, 1,608 Spanish, 1,384 French, 220 English, 233 Germans, 571 unidentified. The epidemic was one of the main causes of the reduction of the black population in Buenos Aires. A torrent of lawsuits began, many related to wills suspected of being forged by criminals looking to make their fortune from the dead.

The establishment of a pure water system and sanitation became a priority. In 1869, English engineer John F. La Trobe Bateman had presented a project of running water, sewers and drains, building on a previous proposal of the engineer John Coghlan. These were accepted and in 1874 Batement started construction of the network, which by 1880 provided water to a quarter of the city. In 1873 he began construction of the sewage works. In 1875, the collection of waste was centralised with the creation of rubbish dumps.

Fiquepron, Maximiliano. 2017. The people of Buenos Aires and their reaction to cholera and yellow fever epidemics (1856–1886). *Quinto Sol.* 21. 1–22. 10.19137/qs.v21i3.1230.

Meik, Kindon T., 2011, 'Disease and Hygiene in the Construction of a Nation: The Public Sphere, Public Space, and the Private Domain in Buenos Aires, 1871–1910' *FIU Electronic Theses and Dissertations.* Paper 547.

http://digitalcommons.fiu.edu/etd/547

Chapter 47

The Fiji measles pandemic: 1875

'Given that this was one of the first acts of British rule there, rumours started to circulate that this was a deliberate attempt by the British to pollute the country with the virus and thus drastically reduce the native population.'

Britain annexed Fiji in 1874 when the Fijian warlord, Ratu Seru Epenisa Cakobau (c. 1815- 1883) who had established a united Fijian kingdom, signed the Deed of Cession. Thus the Colony of Fiji was founded making way for 96 years of British rule. To celebrate this momentous event Hercules Robertson, soon to become the British Governor of Fiji, took Cakobau and his two sons to Sydney. Never can such a well-meaning gesture have ended in so much tragedy. There happened to be a measles outbreak in the city and the three Fijians all came down with the disease. When the ship on which the patients were convalescing returned to Fiji, the colonial administrators, amazingly, decided not to quarantine the vessel despite the British having a extensive knowledge of the horrendous effect of infectious disease on a previously unexposed population. The decision was to have cataclysmic effects when in 1875–76, the resulting epidemic of measles killed over 40,000 Fijians, about one-third of the population.

Given that this was one of the first acts of British rule there, rumours started to circulate that this was a deliberate attempt by the British to pollute the country with the virus and thus drastically reduce the native population. Whatever the case, gross negligence, incompetence and British arrogance it certainly was.[1]

One of the chiefs who died in the epidemic was Ratu Meli; Tui Colo, his dog, was a status symbol for the chief. The dog was buried alive with his master in his grave mound at Navunitavola-Navaulele – probably a Christian concession to the burial rite where in former times, the high chief's wives would have been strangled so as to accompany him to the underworld.

Gravelle, Kim, 1983. Fiji's Times. Suva: *Fiji Times*. pp. 139–143

---

1. Gravelle 1983

Chapter 48

The Fifth cholera pandemic 1881–1896: the Hamburg Riots

'The [sanitary] officer in the hands of the mob was struck on the head with a large stone and knocked to the ground. Then the mob jumped on him and kicked him about the head and body until life was extinct. In the meantime the crowd had succeeded in knocking a policeman down, and he, too, soon met his death, the rioters kicking his face until it was a pulp. Even after he was dead some of the mob danced upon his body.'

– *The New York Times* October 10 1893
reporting the Hamburg riots

Another horrific death toll: from 1883–87 it cost 250,000 lives in Europe and at least 50,000 in the Americas. In 1892 cholera claimed 267,890 lives in Russia, 120,000 in Spain, 90,000 in Japan, 8,600 in Hamburg, the only major European outbreak to be accompanied by cholera riots in 1893; there were over 60,000 deaths in Persia (Iran) and more than 58,000 lives lost in Egypt. Pope Leo XIII authorized the construction of a hospice inside the Vatican for afflicted residents of nearby neighbourhoods. In western Europe this was the last serious cholera outbreak, as cities gradually improved their sanitation and water systems.

Mark Twain, an inveterate traveller, visited Hamburg during the cholera outbreak, and he described his experience in a short, uncollected piece dated '1891–1892'. He was alarmed to note the lack of information in the Hamburg press about the cholera, particularly death totals. He also criticized the treatment of the poor, as many, Twain says, were getting 'snatched from their homes to the pest houses', where 'a good many of them ... die unknown and are buried so'. Twain concluded by lamenting the lack of awareness worldwide, especially in America.

The New York Times locates the riots in the St Pauli district of Hamburg, 'inhabited entirely by the poor and ignorant classes'. The paper goes on to describe how troops had to be called in who fixed bayonets and charged the baying mob. The crowd finally dispersed. We also hear of a riot in Grimsby where two died. The Lisbon authorities declared Blyth in Northumberland a no-go area.

Thomas, Amanda J., 2020, *Cholera: the Victorian Plague*, Barnsley

Chapter 49

The flu pandemic: 1889–1890:
the Russian Influenza

I n Persia, the first established evidence of influenza dates back to 1833, when it erupted violently in Tehran. The epidemic, thought to have arrived there via trade routes from Syria and Constantinople, was part of a larger global pandemic that had killed thousands throughout Asia and Europe. The high number of sick people among the British diplomatic corps convinced Sir Robert Campbell, the British minister in Persia, to relocate his mission from its summer camp in the foothills of Šamirān to Tehran where the dead and dying lay on every street corner.

A new pandemic of influenza arrived in 1889. Beginning in Siberia and spreading westward through Russia, hence the name, influenza eventually overtook the whole of western Europe, and by September of that year reached Persia in the northern city of Rašt. Soon cases broke out in Tabriz, and by the end of November Tehran was again in its clutches. On 14 March 1890 the epidemic struck the southern port-city of Bušehr, and at least one-half of Persia's population contracted the disease.[1] Persian physicians who encountered influenza for the most part initially mis-diagnosed the illness as a common-cold distemper and as a result were wrong-footed in the face of mounting fatalities.

The flu was especially lethal among the young: over 6,000 children died as a result of associated illnesses such as severe throat ailments and measles. Persian physicians could only advise the people to keep their homes warm and to avoid the cold. The consumption of purgatives was recommended as a means of depleting the body of its various 'poisons'. Finally, as a last resort for lowering fevers and chills, the doctors prescribed quinine and camphor. The influenza epidemic lasted through the spring of 1890 and fizzled out with the advent of summer.

But in 1918 it returned with a vengeance. War, once again, was pestilence's companion as Russian troops returning to Ashkhabad brought the flu with them; they had themselves contracted the disease from the American expeditionary force, which had landed infected troops in October at the Baltic port of Archangel. Having contracted the disease from the Americans, the Tsarist troops, in retreat from the Bolsheviks, unwittingly transmitted the disease southwards along their retreating lines into Persia. The flu reached the northeastern city of Mašhad by the third week

---

1. Tholozan, p. 251

of August. Mašhad, a pilgrimage centre on the supply route for the White Russian and the British armies, served as a focal point for the spreading of the disease throughout the country, not only because of all the soldiers, but also on account of the ubiquitous crowds of pilgrims from all parts of the Shi'ite world.

British and Indian troops who had embarked at Bombay as part of the British expeditionary force in the Middle East introduced the disease to the Persian Gulf ports of Bandar-e 'Abbās and Bušehr. The second, more virulent form of influenza followed and struck Kermānšāh and Hamadān: the huge number of Armenian and Assyrian Christian refugees who had escaped Turkish persecution in the Caucasus following the retreat of British troops from Baku, thronged the cities. During the last two weeks of September, Kermānšāh alone had received 60,000 hungry and diseased refugees, a number equal to the native population of the city.

Mortality was considerably higher among those with chronic malaria and, furthermore, cases of the flu were much more prevalent among indigenous Persians than among Europeans residing there. Estimates would indicate that Persia could have lost from 902,400 to 2,431,000 inhabitants indicating that Persia's losses were anywhere from 8.0 per cent to 21.7 per cent of its population placing it near the top of the 1918–19 influenza pandemic's international mortality ladder.

King, Anthony, 2020, 'An uncommon cold.' *New Scientist* vol. 246,3280 32–35.

Parsons, Henry Franklin, 1893. Further Report and Papers on Epidemic Influenza, 1889–92. *Local Government Board.*

Ziegler, Michell, 2011, '*Epidemiology of the Russian flu, 1889–1890*'. Contagions: Thoughts on Historic Infectious Disease.

THE 20TH CENTURY

Chapter 50

Plague in the 20th century

'*Often there appears to be no forewarning of a pandemic, which may move rapidly and give little time to prepare. By analysing past events we can gain insights into how and why diseases have spread. The successes and failures of the past can help us plan for the future and should inform current public health policy. There is so much we can learn from what happened before – we ignore history at our peril. One thing that all plague experts are certain about is that plague has a future.*'

–Dr Robert Peckam, History of Medicine and Health, University of Hong Kong

Bombay plague epidemic 1896–1905 riots

'*The anti-plague activities measures included squads of soldiers and local volunteers forcibly entering homes of victims, burning bedding and personal belongings, smashing the roofs and sanitising. The house was then marked UHH (unfit for human habitation).*'

The epidemic of 1896 paralyzed the city. Bombay was not just the financial capital of British India but also a thriving international port and a major manufacturing centre for cotton yarn and textiles. The revenue that the city generated made up a significant part of the annual home payments sent back to Great Britain. Rapid commercial growth attracted a large influx of workers but with not even the most basic of facilities to accommodate them, 70 per cent of the immigrant workers ended up living in the *chawls*, low-rent tenements. Plague hit in September 1896 arriving on board the ship *Mandarin* from British Hong Kong, spreading rapidly to create a death toll estimated at 2,624 people per week through the rest of the year. At this time from September 1896 to March 1897, 33,161 people fled Bombay, as reflected in the census of 1901, which showed the population to have fallen to 780,000.

The man who identified the contagion as plague, Dr. Acacio Gabriel Viegas, a Goan doctor, discovered the disease first in Manvi, an area close to the Bombay docks and home to warehouses, grain merchants and dense, crowded dwellings. He then launched a highly vocal campaign to clean up slums and exterminate rats; the British Colonial Government pressed W.M. Haffkine, a Jewish doctor from Odessa who had earlier developed a vaccine for cholera, to work the same magic for plague. After three months of effort with a limited, stressed staff, Haffkine successfully grew plague cultures in a high-fat broth made using ghee and created a vaccine out of the weakened bacteria. On 10 January 1897 Haffkine injected himself with the vaccine after tests on rabbits were successful. Volunteers at the Byculla jail were then used in a control test; all inoculated prisoners survived the epidemics, while seven inmates of the control group died. Like other early vaccines, the Haffkine formulation had nasty side effects, and did not provide complete protection, though it was said to have reduced risk by up to 50 per cent.[1] By the turn of the century, the number of inoculees in India alone reached four million. Haffkine was appointed the Director of the Plague Laboratory (now called Haffkine Institute) in Bombay.

The anti-plague measures included squads of soldiers and local volunteers forcibly entering homes of victims, burning bedding and personal belongings, smashing the roofs and sanitising. The house was then marked UHH (unfit for human habitation). The victim, usually very ill, was forcibly carried away to a plague hospital to contend with their low survival rates – all of this was widely regarded by the locals as offensive, intrusive and alarming, triggering a backlash and the murder of W.C. Rand, British chairman of the Special Plague Committee, and his military escort. Often the victims were dying by the time they got to hospital so it is hardly surprising that the death tolls in the hospitals were very high, prompting misinformation that the hospitals were killing the patients. This in fact led to an attack on the Arthur Road Hospital on 29 October 1896 by 800 or so people – essentially an attack on medical personnel. On 9 March 1898, riots erupted in Madanpura when a medical team and plague officer were refused admission to a house to examine a suspected plague case. The crowds attacked them, the police started shooting and five people were killed.

The unpopular controls and the panic prompted a mass exodus of migrant labour out of the city back to their villages. They carried the infection with them throughout India as did the freight trains carrying goods. In 1896, Bombay had 133 cotton mills: the departure of its mill operatives and dock workers severely impacted the city's economy. In order to keep the mills humming, there was frequent open and cut-throat bidding by mill agents for labour on street corners.

In 1900, the mortality rate from plague was about 22 per 1,000. In the same year, the corresponding rates from tuberculosis were 12 per 1,000, from cholera about 14 per 1,000, and about 22 per 1,000 from various other illnesses classified as 'fevers'. All of these were blamed on the unsanitary conditions endured by the local population.

One of the more innovative measures taken by the British Bombay City Improvement Trust was the building of roads which would channel the sea air into the crowded parts of the town. How else did the plague change Bombay? Underneath these roads they laid drainage and sewage pipes. However, in doing so they were at the same time demolishing homes and displacing people, people who were never rehoused. They also, after ten years, created planned suburbs for the middle classes. They took areas that were previously 'plague camps' and put in sewage lines, roads, public transport, amenities. This period also saw more banks, jobs, colleges, parks, religious spaces and railway lines created.

---

1. Echenberg, 2002

Catanach, I.N., 2001, The Globalization of Disease? India and the Plague, *Journal of World History* (University of Hawaii Press), Volume 12. 1

Echenberg, Myron, 2007. *Plague ports: the global urban impact of bubonic plague, 1894–1901.* New York

Echenberg, Myron, 2002. Pestis redux: the initial years of the third bubonic plague pandemic, 1894–1901. *Journal of World History.* 429(21) Vol. 13

Ramanna, Mridula, 2010, Coping with Epidemics: Indian Responses, Bombay Presidency, 1900–1919, in Bandyopadhyay, Arun, ed, *Science & Society 1750–2000* New Delhi, 2010

1899 Porto plague outbreak

This outbreak which killed 132 people is significant on account of the the controversial decision to surround the city by a military-enforced *cordon sanitaire* for four months, imposed by Portugal's Prime Minister José Luciano de Castro. Eminent bacteriologist Luís da Câmara Pestana contracted the disease after receiving a small scratch while examining a plague corpse and died shortly afterwards.

The plague outbreak had considerable political, social and economic repercussions: it exacerbated class divisions and tensions between republicans in Porto and the royalist government in Lisbon: the centuries-old Portuguese monarchy would be replaced by the Portuguese First Republic in a revolution in 1909 and Portugal's public health legislation was modernised in the years following the crisis; the Directorate-General of Health was established.

San Francisco plague of 1900–1904

> 'The Health Board then 'attempted to sidestep the decision by instituting a quarantine order that avoided mention of race, but which was precisely drafted so as to encompass all of the Chinatown area … while excluding white-owned businesses on the periphery of that area'. This was rejected with the court noting that the boundaries of the quarantine corresponded with the ethnicity of building occupants rather than the presence of the disease.'
>
> – Brian Dean Abramson, *Vaccine, Vaccination, and Immunization Law,* 2019

The plague focused on San Francisco's Chinatown and was the first plague epidemic to hit the continental United States. The epidemic was recognized in March 1900, but its existence was covered up for more than two years by California's Governor Henry Gage acting for commercial reasons, to protect the reputations of San Francisco and California and to prevent the inevitable loss of revenue due to quarantine. Gage was also clearly influenced by his powerful railroad and city business interests. He accused federal authorities, particularly Dr. Joseph J. Kinyoun, the doctor who first identified the plague, of injecting plague bacteria into cadavers to falsify evidence.

Gage lost the governorship in the 1902 elections. The new Governor, George Pardee, implemented a medical programme and the epidemic was stopped in 1904. There were 121 cases identified, including 119 deaths.

Before all that, though, on 7 February 1900, Wong Chut King, the owner of a lumber yard, became infected with what the Chinese doctors thought was typhus or gonorrhoea; he passed away after suffering for four weeks. In the morning, the body was taken to a Chinese undertaker where it was examined by San Francisco police surgeon Frank P. Wilson. Wilson called for A.P. O'Brien, a city health department officer, after finding suspiciously swollen lymph glands. Wilson and O'Brien then summoned Wilfred H. Kellogg, San Francisco's city bacteriologist, and the three men performed a post mortem. Looking through his microscope, Kellogg thought he saw plague bacilli. Wilson and O'Brien insisted that Chinatown be quarantined immediately.

The Chinese got the blame. Chinatown was encircled by ropes and surrounded by policemen preventing anyone going in or out, unless they were white. Approximately 25,000–35,000 residents were unable to leave. Chinese Consul General Ho Yow felt that the quarantine was based on false assumptions and that it was prejudiced against the Chinese people; he determined to seek an injunction to lift the quarantine. However, San Francisco mayor James D. Phelan wanted to keep the Chinese-speaking residents separated from the Anglo-Americans – claiming that Chinese-Americans were unclean, filthy, and 'a constant menace to the public health'.

The Board of Health lifted the quarantine on 9 March after it had been in force for only 2½ days. As noted, the scientist who confirmed the existence of plague in California, Dr. Joseph J. Kinyoun was subjected to a defamation and hate campaign. The Health Board shrouded all information regarding the outbreak in a cloak of secrecy by implementing strict regulations on what physicians could write on official death certificates.

On 11 March Kinyoun's lab presented its results. Two guinea pigs and one rat died after being exposed to samples from the first victim, proving the plague was indeed in Chinatown. Without restoring the quarantine, the Board of Health inspected every building in Chinatown, and disinfected the neighbourhood. Property was taken and burned if it was suspected of contamination. Using physical violence, policemen enforced compliance with the Board of Health's directives. Angry and worried Chinese communities reacted by hiding those that were sick. Physicians were banned from entering Chinatown to identify and help the infected.

The plan was to inoculate the Chinese residents with Haffkine's vaccine, a prophylactic anti-plague vaccine that was intended to provide some protection against the plague for a six month period. No one mentioned the side effects and that the vaccine had not been approved for humans. Accordingly, most Chinese refused and demanded the vaccine be tested in rats first. The vaccination programme was halted. However, by then hundreds of Chinese, Japanese, and other residents had already been vaccinated and were exhibiting horrific side effects.[2]

---

2. Risse 2012

Racism towards Chinese immigrants was the norm during the Chinatown plague. Basic rights and privileges were denied to the Chinese people, as exemplified in the way American landlords would refuse to maintain the properties they had rented to Chinese immigrants. Housing for the majority of Chinatown Chinese immigrants was not fit for human habitation. The extended quarantine of Chinatown was motivated more by racist perceptions of Chinese Americans as carriers of disease than by any clinical evidence. The Health Board then 'attempted to sidestep the decision by instituting a quarantine order that avoided mention of race, but which was precisely drafted so as to encompass all of the Chinatown area... while excluding white-owned businesses on the periphery of that area'.[3] This was rejected with the court noting that the boundaries of the quarantine corresponded with the ethnicity of building occupants rather than the presence of the disease.

Clearly San Francisco's quarantine measures were explicitly discriminatory and segregatory, allowing European Americans to leave the affected area, but Chinese and Japanese Americans required a health certificate to depart the city. Residents were initially angered as those with jobs outside of San Francisco were prevented from earning a living.

In the wake of the 1906 San Francisco earthquake rebuilding began immediately; with reconstruction in full swing, a second plague epidemic hit San Francisco in May and August 1907 with cases throughout the city. Approximately $2 million was spent between 1907 and 1911 to kill as many rats as possible in the city. In June 1908, there were 78 deaths; all of the infected people were European, and the California ground squirrel was identified as another vector of the disease. Some xenophobic American experts held the mistaken belief that a rice-based diet left Asians with a lower resistance to plague, and that a diet of meat kept Europeans free from the disease.

Abramson, Brian Dean, 2019, *Vaccine, Vaccination, and Immunization Law*, Bloomberg Law

Haas, Victor H., 1959. 'When Bubonic Plague Came to Chinatown'. *The American Journal of Tropical Medicine and Hygiene.* 8 (2): 141–147.

Kalisch, Philip A., 1972. 'The Black Death in Chinatown: Plague and Politics in San Francisco 1900–1904'. *Arizona and the West.* 14 (2): 113–136

Risse, Guenter B., 2012. *Plague, fear, and politics in San Francisco's Chinatown.* Baltimore

The 1900 Glasgow outbreak: don't blame the rat fleas

'The Glasgow bubonic plague may have also spread between people through human ectoparasite vectors such as body lice (Pediculus humanus humanus) or human fleas (Pulex irritans).'

– From a 1901 report on the Glasgow plague

In August 1900 bubonic plague erupted in Glasgow for the first time during the Third Pandemic. A team of researchers at the University of Oslo Centre for

---

3. Abramson 2019

Ecological and Evolutionary Synthesis has made some remarkable discoveries relating to the outbreak published by the Royal Society.

On 25 August the Glasgow sanitary authorities were notified of several suspected cases of bubonic plague, despite no known cases of plague in Britain at the time. The local authorities robustly tracked the spread of the disease and on 25 August they confirmed their initial diagnosis of *Y. pestis* infection by a doctor in Belvidere Hospital. The Medical Officer of Health in Glasgow opened an immediate investigation into the spread of the disease. This led to the identification of the index case, a Mrs Bogie, a fish hawker, who fell ill and died along with her granddaughter, on 3 August (Day 0 of the outbreak). She lived in Rose Street, Gorbals, with her docker husband. The sanitary authorities searched for contacts associated with Mrs B. or the 100 or so attendees at her wake, leading to the examination and quarantine of more than 100 people in a 'reception house' for observation. They found that nearly all of the 35 cases could be linked by contact with a previous case. There was a high rate of secondary transmissions within households.

As well as contact tracing and quarantining, the sanitary authorities put into place a number of other measures to control the spread of plague including: removal of cases to the hospital; stopping wakes for deaths attributed to plague; fumigation of infected homes with liquid sulfur dioxide and disinfection with a formalin solution; removal and treatment of victims' clothing and sheets; disinfection of all homes and communal areas in infected tenements with chloride of lime (chlorine powder) solution; emptying of ashpits and publishing information about the disease to the public and health professionals.

In 1898, two years before the outbreak in Glasgow, Paul-Louis Simond had discovered that rats and their fleas could transmit plague to humans. The sanitary authorities in Glasgow were, therefore, particularly interested in the role of their rats in spreading the disease. We all know, thanks to Simond, that in the past large scale epidemics of plague were caused by infected rat-flea vectors looking for alternative mammalian hosts. However, there is now some evidence, from an official government report of the plague published in 1901, that in Glasgow bubonic plague may have also spread between people through human ectoparasite vectors such as body lice (*Pediculus humanus humanus*) or human fleas (*Pulex irritans*). Experimental and epidemiological studies have shown that human ectoparasites are potential vectors for plague and have been found infected during modern outbreaks in Africa.

Despite trapping and testing 326 rats in the area, there was, unusually, no evidence of plague in the rat population at any time during the outbreak, leading them to conclude that plague may have spread directly between humans through clothing or other means, and possibly by 'the suctorial parasites of mankind' – fleas and lice.

In the official report the local authorities identified 37 cases of plague in and around Glasgow between 3 August and 24 September 1900, mainly located in the densely populated Gorbals area. Most of the cases after notification were identified as a primary bubonic or septicaemic plague by the presence of external buboes.

Some data: 31 (88 per cent) suspected cases of plague in Glasgow were diagnosed by the presence of external buboes. The case-fatality rate was 42.8 per cent for both men and women; 21 (60 per cent) of the cases were female and 14 (40 per cent) were male. From the 15 fatal cases, the median symptomatic period was six days. In addition, the unusually high figure of 62.5 per cent of infections occurred between household contacts. The reproduction number decreased after notification of the disease with an estimate of 1.6 before notification. The small size and short duration of the outbreak suggests that quarantining and sanitation were effective in stopping the spread of plague, which is also reflected in the drop in R # below 1 after the implementation of control measures.

Initially the outbreak was believed to be typhoid: the people of Glasgow demanded the disinfecting of all the trams and ferries, and coins in case they carried the contagion. Foreign sailors and prostitutes were blamed.

Dean, Katharine R., (2019) Epidemiology of a bubonic plague outbreak in Glasgow, Scotland in 1900; *Royal Society Open Science* January 2, 2019

The 1900 Sydney plague epidemic

'Captain Thomas Dudley, who also worked at the wharves as a sailmaker, exhibited symptoms: he had been living near east Darling Harbour where he noticed scores of dead rats; moreover, he had been pulling dead rats from his toilet before falling ill.'

Plague came knocking on Australia's door in 1900; before that the Australian colonial government was concerned that, since the 1894 outbreak in Hong Kong, it was a probably only a matter of time before it hit Australia via shipping trade routes. Sure enough, when it did make landfall panic and terror filled the air as the disease's reputation had preceded its arrival. The scientific community still largely believed the pestilence to be a human infection spread through human contact with the infected. However, there was building evidence that plague epidemics were an epizootic infection in rats: the Australians began to formulate preventative strategies to stop its entry through the ports.

All to no avail: in Sydney on 19 January 1900 Arthur Payne was Australia's first victim to come down with the disease (patient zero): he was a 33-year-old carter working for Sydney's Central Wharf Company. Apparently, when he got home that evening to 10 Ferry Lane, Millers Point he took castor oil, vomited and passed out in bed. The next day, he was officially diagnosed with bubonic plague and he and his family were quarantined. The authorities did not know it at the time but later investigations showed that Payne may well have been bitten by a flea – a flea which probably started its journey in Mauritius. About a month later, Captain Thomas Dudley, who also worked at the wharves as a sailmaker, exhibited symptoms: he had been living near east Darling Harbour where he noticed scores of dead rats; moreover, he had been pulling dead rats from his toilet before falling ill. Dudley was the city's first plague fatality: his death unleashed a wave of panic. For the next eight months Sydney was a city under siege.

Subsequently there were twelve major plague outbreaks in Australia between 1900 and 1925 as ships delivered wave after wave of infection. Government archives record 1,371 infections and 535 deaths. Sydney was hit hardest, but the disease also spread to North Queensland, Melbourne, Adelaide and Fremantle. A fledgling public health department was established: they went on to produce ground-breaking research on plague and are credited with developing 20th century scientific understandings of the disease, in particular that *Yersinia pestis* is spread to humans by fleas from infected rats – a revolution in Australian social medicine.

Those who could afford to fled the city while estate agents were inundated with calls for suburban properties. Fear bred the usual blame game and hostility: people were marched off in the middle of the night to be quarantined and the names of those infected or deceased were published daily. Xenophobic attacks also emerged in the press, with Italian and Chinese migrants among those blamed for importing the plague through poor hygiene. Squads of ratcatchers were formed: tens of thousands of vermin were killed and burned in a custom-built rat incinerator; some councils payed 6d a rat, making rat catching extremely lucrative.

The infected were quarantined, the dead buried with quicklime supposedly to expedite their decomposition and by year's end, more than 1,700 people had been sent to the quarantine station.

The plague had far-reaching socio-economic effects for Sydney, then a city with a population nearing half a million. It paved the way for significant urban renewal of waterfront precincts such as The Rocks and Millers Point, where 100 years of unregulated building had created shanty towns, reservoirs of disease.

Government inspectors undertook a programme of photographing buildings to reveal just how squalid the conditions were for the poor in the city. These are held in the State Library of New South Wales. By the end of August 1900, the outbreak had run its course: Australia got off comparatively lightly: a total of 303 cases were reported with 103 deaths. A coordinated response from health authorities and government obviously helped.

1903 Kashmir plague epidemic

> 'The report says that the policeman and his brother, who was the hospital attendant, had come in close contact with the deceased servant while trying to steal his belongings from the tent after he passed away. The hospital attendant is said to have tried to remove a ring from the corpse with his teeth.'
>
> – Extract from a report by A Mittal, then Chief Medical Officer of Kashmir, who traced the origin and spread of the plague.

The plague epidemic, 19 November 1903 to 31 July 1904, in Kashmir illustrates the potential consequences when sufferers conceal their infection and when the authorities rob the bodies under their supervision.

The disease did not originate here, but all efforts to keep Kashmir safe were ruined when three travellers – a veiled and influential Kashmiri-origin woman, Mrs Bailey, travelled from plague-ridden Rawalpindi along with her two servants on 13 November 1903. They came in a tonga and passed two screening points undetected on the Srinagar-Muzaffarabad road, then known as the Jhelum Valley cart road. At the health screening on the border the travellers lied about where they had come from and did not disclose that one of the servants was unwell.

A report by A. Mittal published in *The Indian Medical Gazette* – he was then Chief Medical Officer of Kashmir and had traced the origin and spread of the plague – noted that one person from Rawalpindi had died of plague in Uri on 8 October 1903, and was cremated there. It adds that elaborate arrangements for the decontamination of the area were made. But on 13 November 1903, a 'veiled native Kashmiri woman, in a horse cart, with two servants crossed the Uri examination point, where the temperature of each traveller was being taken. In this case, the inspectors failed to detect the disease. Subsequent investigation revealed that they had taken the temperature of the tonga travellers but their temperature was normal at that time,' the report adds.

The three had reached Srinagar on 13 November and checked into a houseboat at Shiekhbagh near Lal Chowk. The report says they had left for Kralpora in Budgam on 16 November where they stayed at the house of Subhan Bhat, the woman's relative. Five days later, one of her servants, Ghulam Mohammed, was found at the gate of State Hospital in Srinagar. 'The symptoms at once suggested (to doctors) plague and he was removed to an isolated tent away from the city in an open place, where a policeman was kept as a guard, 500 metres away.' However, the servant died on the night of 19 November, becoming the first imported case of plague in the Kashmir valley, the report notes. He was buried in a 10-foot-deep grave with 2-feet of carbonate of lime surrounding it to further prevent the spread of disease. 'Only two persons helped in the burial,' the report says.

As a precautionary measure, Subhan Bhat's house, along with all its belongings and the grains stored in the compound of the house by various dealers, was torched by the authorities. Track and trace clicked in when the deceased's close contacts, including the woman and the second servant, the policeman who guarded his tent and a hospital attendant were isolated and quarantined. 'However the woman, servants and other contacts at Subhan Bhat's house did not develop plague symptoms.' But on the night of 25 November 1903, the policeman on guard at the tent of the plague-hit servant also died. He was buried in a 10-foot deep grave.

The report says that the policeman and his brother, who was the hospital attendant, had come in close contact with the deceased servant while trying to steal his belongings from the tent after he passed away. The hospital attendant is said to have tried to remove a ring from the corpse with his teeth; he was put in quarantine but went missing from the camp on 28 November 1903; he had somehow reached the village of Geru. He soon died there, but not before becoming a super-spreader of infection.

Shortly after the policeman's death, there was an outbreak of plague in Srinagar on 11 December 1903. Five sudden deaths were reported in two houses in the Karfali

Mohallah and Kralgund locality of Srinagar; they were all relatives of the policeman and his brother.

The disease maintained its grip until July 1904 after over eight months. It had taken thousands of lives the length and breadth of Kashmir.

Mitra, A. The Plague in Kashmir, *Ind Med Gaz*. 1907 Apr; 42(4): 133–138

1910–1911 Manchurian plague

'Gérald Mesny disputed Wu Lien-Teh's recommendation to wear masks; a few days later, he died after catching the plague when visiting patients without wearing a mask.'

A tarbagan marmot infected with bacterial pneumonia is thought to be the origin: tarbagan marmots were hunted for their fur in Manchuria. The spread was amplified by marmot hunters gathering together in the bitter winter months. Manchuria's extensive railway network further facilitated the rapid transmission of the disease by helping the movement of large numbers of migrant workers returning home for the Chinese New Year. Mortality estimates suggest around 60,000 people, including many doctors and nurses, died. It had an unprecedented mortality rate of 100 per cent.

As the German chemical industry developed new dyes, cheap marmot fur could be manufactured into imitation sable, mink and otter fur. Consequently, the value of marmot fur rose from a 'few kopecks a skin to a rouble', acting as a magnet for migrant hunters. The only trouble was that these migrants were inexperienced; whereas local hunters could identify and avoid diseased marmots, the migrant hunters collected unhealthy marmots, infecting themselves with the plague bacilli.

Cambridge-trained doctor Wu Lien-Teh (Wu Liande) led the Chinese fight against the plague and promoted quarantine and the wearing of cloth face masks. Track and trace, particularly for passengers on the trains, was deployed. Wu Lien-Teh received Qing imperial permission to burn the dead bodies of victims, thus thousands of corpses were safely disposed of. Similarly, Russian C.E.R. authorities organised sanitary zones, monitored the population and burned lodgings which plague might have contaminated. As a result of these measures and the end of the cold winter, the epidemic was over by the end of April 1911.

Wu Lien-Teh convened the International Plague Conference in Mukden in April 1911, the first major event of its kind and firmly established Chinese scientists as members of the international scientific community. The conference also initiated the creation of the North Manchurian Plague Prevention Service (1912) in the first year of the Chinese Republic, whose object was to promote public health by 'means of illustrated letters, lantern demonstrations and popular pamphlets'. The plague also resulted in a Presidential mandate legalising human dissection, in addition to the earlier Imperial mandate permitting cremation. Thus, by instigating changes that removed 'a great deal of the superstition surrounding ancestor worship', the plague facilitated the advancement of Chinese science and disease control.

The Chinese government enlisted the support of foreign doctors, a number of whom died in service, highlighting the importance of a multi-national, coordinated medical response and paving the way for later consortiums such as the World Health Organization. Wu Lien-teh's promotion of cloth plague mask-wearing by doctors, nurses, patients, contacts, and (to the degree that it was possible) the population at large, was the first time such an epidemic containment measure had been attempted. The event was also influential in establishing the use of personal protective equipment and is credited for the origins of the modern hazmat suit.

Nevertheless trade and commerce – especially the fur and food trades – were hit badly. The *South China Morning Post*, 27 February 1911 commenting on the soybean trade, reported that 'the plague caused a loss estimated at $7,000,000'. Furthermore, the plague brought additional economic consequences. *The Economist*, 4 February 1911, documented the depressing influence of the plague on Chinese stock prices and government bond prices, demonstrating its impact on China's economy.

Knab, Cornelia, 2011, 'Plague Times: Scientific Internationalism and the Manchurian Plague of 1910/11', *Itinerario* 35:03 87–105

Lynteris, Christos, 2018. 'Plague Masks: The Visual Emergence of Anti-Epidemic Personal Protection Equipment'. *Medical Anthropology*. 37 (6): 442–457

Summers, William C., 2012, *The Great Manchurian Plague 1910–11: The Geopolitics of an Epidemic Disease*, London

Yu-lin, Wu, 1995, Memories Of Dr Wu Lien-teh, Plague Fighter. *World Scientific*.

Chapter 51

The sixth cholera pandemic, 1910–1911

In Europe, advances in public health were starting to have a significant impact which accounts for the fact that the region was less affected than others in the sixth cholera pandemic. However, major Russian cities and the Ottoman Empire were still particularly hard hit: more than 500,000 died of cholera in Russia from 1900 to 1925, not helped by the upheaval caused by revolution and warfare.

The epidemic also claimed 200,000 lives in the Philippines including their revolutionary hero and first prime minister Apolinario Mabini. Cholera broke out twenty-seven times during the Hajj at Mecca from the later 19th century to 1930. The sixth pandemic killed more than 800,000 in India.

The blame game, xenophobia and racism reached their respective ugly zeniths: because immigrants and travellers often carried cholera from infected areas, infectious disease became associated with the marginalised in each society. The Italians blamed the Jews and gypsies, the British accused the 'dirty natives', and the Americans put cholera down to the Philippines.

In 1911, *The Boston Medical and Surgical Journal* of the Massachusetts Medical Society reported that 'in New York, up to July 22, there were eleven deaths from cholera, one of the victims being an employee at the hospital on Swinburne Island, who had been discharged. The tenth was a lad, 17 years of age, who had been a steerage passenger on the steamship, *Moltke*. The plan has been adopted of taking cultures from the intestinal tracts of all persons held under observation at Quarantine, and in this way it was discovered that five of the 500 passengers of the *Moltke* and *Perugia*, although in excellent health at the time, were harboring cholera microbes.'

In 1913, the Romanian Army, during its invasion of Bulgaria during the Second Balkan War, suffered a cholera outbreak that caused 1,600 deaths.

Azizi, Mohammad-Hossein, 2010, 'History of Cholera Outbreaks in Iran during the 19th and 20th Centuries'. *Middle East Journal of Digestive Diseases.* 2 (1): 51–55.

Moraña, Mabel, 'Modernity and Marginality in Love in the Time of Cholera'. *Studies in Twentieth Century Literature* 14:27–43

Smallman-Raynor, M., 2000, The Epidemiological Legacy of War: The Philippine—American War and the Diffusion of Cholera in Batangas and La Laguna, South-West Luzón, 1902–1904. *War in History*, 7(1), 29–64.

Chapter 52

1915–1926 *Encephalitis Lethargica* Pandemic

*E*ncephalitis lethargica is an atypical form of encephalitis which also goes by the names of 'sleeping sickness' or 'sleepy sickness' (as distinct from the tsetse fly-transmitted sleeping sickness). The disease attacks the brain, leaving some victims in a statue-like condition, speechless and motionless. Between 1915 and 1926, an epidemic of *encephalitis lethargica* spread around the globe afflicting nearly five million people, a third of whom died in the acute stages. Many of those who survived never regained their pre-morbid vigour.

Patients would be conscious and aware – yet not quite fully awake sitting motionless and speechless all day long in their chairs, devoid of energy, emotion, initiative, motive, appetite or desire; they register what is going on about them but without active recognition and with complete indifference. In short, they were listless, as insubstantial as ghosts and as passive as zombies.

There has been no recurrence of the epidemic, though isolated cases continue to occur. Signs and symptoms are many and numerous. It is characterized by high fever, sore throat, headache, lethargy, double vision, delayed physical and mental response, sleep inversion and catatonia. In severe cases, patients may enter a coma-like state (akinetic mutism); they may also experience abnormal eye movements ('oculogyric crises'), Parkinsonism, upper body weakness, muscular pains, tremors, neck rigidity and behavioural changes including psychosis. Klazomania (a vocal tic) is sometimes present.

Before the 1915 pandemic there were a number of episodes which may have been manifestations of *Encephalitis lethargica*:

- In 1580, parts of Europe were afflicted by a serious febrile and lethargic illness, which led to Parkinsonian and other neurological sequelae.
- In 1673–1675, a similar serious epidemic occurred in London, which Thomas Sydenham described as '*febris comatosa*'.
- In 1695, a 20-year-old woman in Germany experienced oculogyric crises, Parkinsonism, diplopia, strabismus and other symptoms following an attack of somnolent brain fever, as described by Dr. Albrecht of Hildesheim.
- In 1712–13, a severe epidemic of *Schlafkrankheit* (*encephalitis lethargica*) broke out in Tübingen, Germany, followed in many cases by persistent slowness of movement and lack of initiative (aboulia).

- Between 1750 and 1800, France and Germany experienced minor epidemics of '*coma somnolentum*' with Parkinsonian features, including hyperkinetic hiccough, myoclonus, chorea, and tics.
- Between 1848 and 1882, Paris-based neurologist Jean-Martin Charcot documented numerous isolated cases of juvenile Parkinsonism, associated with diplopia, oculogyria, tachypnoea (hyperventilation), retropulsion, tics, and obsessional disorders, which were almost certainly post-encephalitic in origin.
- In 1890 in Italy, following the influenza epidemic of 1889–90, a severe epidemic of somnolent illnesses (nicknamed the 'Nona') appeared. For the few survivors of the Nona, Parkinsonism and other sequelae developed in almost all cases.

So, when the epidemic started to spread there was significant data available to tell clinicians and scientists what they were dealing with? Unfortunately this was not the case. The winter of 1916–17 saw a 'novel' illness suddenly emerge in Vienna and other cities and, over the next three years, rapidly spread around the globe. Variable symptoms and a world war did not help with the result that international communication about the disease was slow and chaotic. The confusion is reflected in the hit and miss naming and attribution of this protean disease; it persisted until neurologist Constantin von Economo identified in 1917 a unique pattern of damage among the brains of deceased patients and established the name *encephalitis lethargica*; they included botulism, toxic ophthalmoplegia, epidemic stupor, epidemic lethargic encephalitis, acute polioencephalitis, Heine-Medin disease, bulbar paralysis, hystero-epilepsy, acute dementia, and sometimes just 'an obscure disease with cerebral symptoms'. Ten days before von Economo's breakthrough pathologist Jean-René Cruchet described forty cases of '*subacute encephalomyelitis*' in France.

The damage worldwide was terrible: in the ten years that the pandemic raged, nearly five million people succumbed. It disappeared in 1927 as abruptly and mysteriously as it came. The great encephalitis pandemic coincided, of course, with the 1918 influenza pandemic; the influenza virus seriously potentiated the effects of the encephalitis virus or lowered resistance to it in a truly destructive way.

Many surviving patients of the pandemic seemed to make a complete recovery and return to normal life. However, the majority of survivors subsequently developed neurological or psychiatric disorders, often after years or decades of seemingly perfect health. Today the cause of the *encephalitis lethargica* epidemic remains uncertain. Some believe that the co-occurrence of the encephalitis and the 1918 influenza pandemic was no coincidence, and that the influenza virus somehow affected the brain in some cases, causing *encephalitis lethargica*. Others believe that a virus related to the polio virus was the cause.

In a timely November 2020 blog Kate McAllister of the Department of Medical Humanities at the University of Sheffield, 'reflects on parallels between COVID-19 and the early twentieth century epidemic of Encephalitis Lethargica'.

Badrfam, Rahim, 2020, 'From encephalitis lethargica to COVID-19: Is there another epidemic ahead?.' *Clinical neurology and neurosurgery* vol. 196

Hoffman, L.A., 2017, Encephalitis lethargica: 100 years after the epidemic. *Brain* 140

Koch, Christof, 2016. 'Sleep without End'. *Scientific American Mind*. 27 (2): 22–25.

McAllister, Kate (November 2020), https://thepolyphony.org/2020/11/17/look-out-for-changes-in-behaviour-encephalitis-lethargica-and-covid-19/

Reid, A.H.; 2001. 'Experimenting on the Past: The Enigma of von Economo's Encephalitis Lethargica'. *J. Neuropathol. Exp. Neurol.* 60 (7): 663–670.

Sacks, Oliver, 1990. *Awakenings*. London

Sacks, Oliver, 1983. 'The origin of 'Awakenings'. *Br. Med. J. (Clin. Res. Ed.)*. 287 (6409): 1968–1969.

Chapter 53

The American Polio Epidemic: 1916 –
'The Crippler'.

'In 1953, a survey of what frightened Americans most put polio in second place, just below nuclear annihilation.'

– Gareth Williams, 2013

W hile the *Encephalitis lethargica* pandemic was taking its deadly toll, the USA was simultaneously assailed by a polio (acute poliomyelitis or infantile paralysis) epidemic which was officially announced on 17 June 1916 in Brooklyn, New York. That year there were over 27,000 cases and more than 6,000 deaths due to polio in the United States, with over 2,000 deaths in New York City alone, centred in the borough of Brooklyn. By 1 July 1916 there were 259 confirmed cases of polio in New York City with 59 deaths; the outbreak appeared to be confined to infants and young children, less than 10 per cent of the cases occurring in children over the age of 5. The peak came in early August, by which time the total number afflicted was in the tens of thousands, and the number of deaths exceeded 1,000. The disease then began a slow decline for much of the rest of the year. The first outbreak of polio in epidemic form in the US had occured in Vermont, with 132 cases in 1894.

New York reacted quickly although 'the public health authorities were blindsided from the start. The Commissioner of Public Health (who was nicknamed 'the last of the Puritans') made many mistakes'.[1] Nevertheless, a special field force was assembled under Dr. Simon R. Blatteis of the New York City Health Department's Bureau of Preventable Diseases, with authority to quarantine those infected with polio and institute hygiene measures thought to slow the transmission of the disease. A team of medical inspectors, sanitary inspectors, nurses, and sanitary police, were recruited to assist Blatteis, visiting all cases daily, seeing that strict quarantine was maintained and that all the premises where a case of infantile paralysis exists were placarded.

The Department of Health set up a special pavilion at Kingston Avenue Hospital for patients to be cared for by specialists in children's diseases, orthopaedic specialists

---

1. Williams 2013

and neurologists. The Department ruled that a patient, in order to be allowed to remain at home, should have a separate room, separate toilet, a nominated person for nursing and facilities for the proper disposal of all waste. Where these could not be guaranteed, the Health Department would hospitalize the patient at no charge. By 8 July 1916, Blatteis had established six clinics in Brooklyn specifically set up to receive polio victims.

Polio was still poorly understood at this time so public health measures generally consisted mainly of quarantines, the closure of public places and the use of chemical disinfectants to cleanse areas where the disease had been recognised. Public hygiene measures began with hand washing and sewage disposal, and when those failed, the city's roads were scrubbed with four million gallons of water each day. Possible vectors were eliminated as far as possible, notably flies and cats; 50,000 cats were allegedly shot during that summer. Special polio clinics were established at various points in the city for the treatment and quarantine of patients.

For weeks more than 1,000 children left New York City every day with their medical certificates that confirmed freedom from symptoms, but inevitably this missed many asymptomatic and highly infectious cases. Many fled to nearby mountain resorts while the city closed down theatres, swimming pools, beaches and amusement parks. Children were warned not to drink from fountains. Every day the press published names and addresses of people confirmed with polio; their houses were identified with placards and their families were quarantined. Neighbouring cities barred New Yorkers with Hoboken, New Jersey deploying police officers to intercept children under 16 arriving from Brooklyn by ferry, rail or private boat and escorting them back to Brooklyn. Pennsylvania did the same. Predictably the Italians took the blame and were ostracised, vilified and assaulted even though their infection rates were low.

Less official were the many popular remedies or preventative measures tried by an anxious and frightened population; quackery apart, some of these were dangerous. In John Haven Emerson's *A Monograph on the Epidemic of Poliomyelitis (Infantile Paralysis) in New York City in 1916* one remedy recommends:

> 'Give oxygen through the lower extremities, by positive electricity. Frequent baths using almond meal, or oxidising the water. Applications of poultices of Roman chamomile, slippery elm, arnica, mustard, cantharis, amygdalae dulcis oil, and of special merit, spikenard oil and Xanthoxolinum. Internally use caffeine, Fl. Kola, dry muriate of quinine, elixir of cinchone, radium water, chloride of gold, liquor calcis and wine of pepsin.'

Medieval? Pagan? Witchcraft? all spring to mind.

The heart-wrenching enforced separation of families during the early, acute phase of the disease contributed to the intense dread and fear that polio aroused. Children and parents were not allowed any contact for ten to fourteen days and then only limited visiting for weeks afterward. When the patient returned home weeks or months later, adjustment to changed circumstances brought more stress.

Here is one father's tragic experience:

> 'Unable to obtain a physician, he put the boy into an automobile and drove to the Smith Infirmary, but the child died on the way and the doctors at the hospital would not receive the body.... He drove around Staten Island with the boy's body for hours looking for some one who would receive it.'
>
> – *New York Times*, July 26, 1916

Many subscribed to the belief that there was a relation between polio and the stable fly, so a survey was conducted to determine whether the cases were in the vicinity of stables; the Sanitary Bureau saw to it that the manure in all of the stables in the affected districts was properly disposed of to prevent flies breeding.

Arita, I., 2006. Is polio eradication realistic? *Science* 312: 852–855.

Oshinsky, David, 2005, *Polio: An American Story*, Oxford

Paul, John, 1971, *A History of Poliomyelitis*, New Haven CT

Roberts, L., 2006. Polio eradication: Is it time to give up? *Science* 312: 832–835

Rogers, Naomi, 1992, Dirt and Disease: Polio before FDR, Health and Medicine in American Society New Brunswick, NJ

Williams, Gareth, 2013, *Paralysed with Fear: The Story of Polio*, Basingstoke

Chapter 54

Influenza in the 20th Century

T here are four types of influenza viruses: A, B, C and D. Human influenza A and B viruses trigger the annual seasonal epidemics of disease we know as the flu season almost every winter. Influenza A viruses are the only influenza viruses to cause flu pandemics, in other words, global epidemics of flu disease. A pandemic can occur when a new and very different influenza A virus emerges with the ability to infect people and can spread efficiently between people. Influenza type C infections usually cause mild illness and are not thought to cause human flu epidemics. Influenza D viruses mainly affect cattle and are not known to infect or cause illness in people.

Influenza A virus causes influenza in birds and some mammals. Strains of all subtypes of influenza A virus have been isolated from wild birds, although disease is uncommon. Some isolates of influenza A virus cause severe disease both in domestic poultry and, rarely, in humans. Occasionally, viruses are transmitted from wild aquatic birds to domestic poultry, and this may cause an outbreak or give rise to human influenza pandemics. Influenza A viruses are divided into subtypes based on two proteins on the surface of the virus: hemagglutinin (H) and neuraminidase (N). While there are potentially 198 different influenza A subtype combinations, only 131 subtypes have been detected in nature. Current subtypes of influenza A viruses that routinely circulate in people include: A(H1N1) and A(H3N2).

Currently circulating influenza A(H1N1) viruses are related to the pandemic 2009 H1N1 virus that emerged in 2009 and caused a flu pandemic (see Swine flu below). This virus, called '2009 H1N1', has continued to circulate seasonally since then. These H1N1 viruses have undergone relatively small genetic changes and changes to their antigenic properties (the properties of the virus that affect immunity) over time.

The influenza A virus subtypes that have been confirmed in humans in order of the number of known human pandemic deaths, are:

H1N1 caused 'Spanish flu' in 1918 and the 2009 swine flu pandemic

H2N2 caused 'Asian flu' in the late 1950s

H3N2 caused 'Hong Kong flu' in the late 1960s

H5N1 considered a global influenza pandemic threat through its spread in the mid-2000s.

H7N9 is responsible for a 2013 epidemic in China and considered by Dr. Michael Greger, author of *How Not to Die*, to have the greatest pandemic threat of the influenza A viruses.

H7N7 has some zoonotic potential: it has rarely caused disease in humans.

H1N2 is currently endemic in pigs but not in humans.
H9N2, H7N2, H7N3, H5N2, and H10N7.

Barry J.M., 2004, *The great influenza: the epic story of the deadliest plague in history*. New York

Brown, J., 2018, Influenza: The Hundred Year Hunt to Cure the Deadliest Disease in History. New York Emerging Infectious Diseases. 12 (1): 9–1

Fergus, R., et al. 2006. Migratory birds and avian flu. *Science* 312: 845.

Gust, I. D., 2001. Planning for the next pandemic of influenza. Review in *Medical Virology* 11: 59–70.

Kilbourne, E.D., 2006. Influenza pandemics of the 20th century. Emerging Infectious Diseases 12: 9–14.

Johnson, N.P., 2002. Updating the accounts: Global mortality of the 1918–1920 "Spanish" influenza pandemic. *Bulletin of the History of Medicine* 76: 105–115.

Snacken, R., et al. 1999. The next influenza pandemic: Lessons from Hong Kong, 1997. Emerging Infectious Diseases 5: 195–203.

Taubenberger, J.K., 1997. Initial genetic characterization of the 1918 "Spanish" influenza virus. *Science* 275: 1793–1796.

Webster, R.G., 1997. Predictions for future human influenza pandemics. *Journal of Infectious Diseases* 176: S14–S19.

'The next pandemic and how to head it off: eat a plant-based diet.' *South China Morning Post*. 19 October 2020.

Spanish Flu: 1918–1920

'It stalked into camp when the day was damp And chilly and cold. It crept by the guards And murdered my pards With a hand that was clammy and bony and bold; And its breath was icy and mouldy and dank, And it killed so speedy And gloatingly greedy That it took away men from each company rank.'

– From *The Flu* by Private Josh Lee, 1919

The First World War is remembered as being the war to end all wars, supposedly. Likewise the Spanish flu pandemic, which coincided with the final months of the Great War, has been dubbed as the pandemic to end all pandemics. If only both were true: the idealism and hope which spawned both sound bites quickly turned into irony and cynicism and illustrate how we continually underestimate the processes which govern war and disease and their manifold legacies. War and disease cannot be compartmentalised and archived in a tidy historical pigeonhole; they are both much bigger and pervasive than that and so deserve due attention and respect because all wars and all pandemics have lasting consequences; they leave a hinterland which we must acknowledge and deal with.

The Spanish flu was an unusually deadly influenza pandemic caused by the H1N1 influenza A virus. Lasting from February 1918 to April 1920, it infected 500 million people – about a third of the world's population at the time – in four successive waves.

An article by Peter C. Wever and Leo van Bergen (2014) gives an interesting perspective on the effects of the pandemic on First World War combat.

The setting is the Meuse-Argonne offensive, a decisive battle during the war, which remains the largest frontline commitment in American military history involving 1.2 million US troops. With over 26,000 deaths among American soldiers, the offensive is considered 'America's deadliest battle'. Despite these prodigious numbers the authors remind us that 'It has been stated, however, that more Americans were buried in France because of 1918 pandemic influenza than of enemy fire.'[1] The offensive coincided with the highly fatal second wave of the influenza pandemic which ran its deadly course over about eight weeks, from 15 September to 15 November 1918. Wever and van Bergen reveal how:

> 'In Europe and in US Army training camps, 1918 pandemic influenza killed around 45,000 American soldiers making it questionable which battle should be regarded 'America's deadliest'. The origin of the influenza pandemic has been inextricably linked with the men who occupied the military camps and trenches during the First World War. The disease had a profound impact, both for the military apparatus and for the individual soldier. It struck all the armies and might have claimed toward 100,000 fatalities among soldiers overall during the conflict while rendering millions ineffective.'

Indeed, the highest morbidity rate was found among the Americans as the disease infected 26 per cent of the U.S. army, over one million men. In comparison, the German army recorded over 700,000 cases of influenza, while the British Expeditionary Forces (BEF) listed 313,000 cases in 1918 in France[2].

There are a number of claims as to its origin.

Some contend that it started in a British military base at Étaples, a base crowded with soldiers near sea marshes with lots of migratory birds, many farms nearby with pigs, ducks, and geese reserved as food for soldiers, and a storage facility for mutagenic war gasses. These conditions might have contributed to an outbreak of acute respiratory infection between December 1916 and March 1917 which clinically resembled 1918 pandemic influenza.

Others say that the origin can be traced to Indochinese soldiers from Vietnam, Laos, and Cambodia fighting in France among which several epidemics of acute respiratory infections were noted (Annamite pneumonia).

The best candidate for this dubious privilege is Camp Funston, a US Army training camp in Kansas where in March 1918, Chinese contract workers at the

---

1. van Bergen 2009
2. Byerly 2005

camp presented with influenza. Soon, the disease spread across the camp requiring hospitalization of over 1,100 soldiers within three weeks besides thousands more receiving treatment at infirmaries around the camp. Between early March and the summer, five consecutive outbreaks occurred in the camp, coinciding with the arrival of large numbers of new recruits. From Camp Funston the influenza jumped to other US Army training camps and travelled to Europe aboard troop ships. In all, 11·8 per cent (143,986) of over 1.2 million men in US. Army training camps were hospitalized for respiratory illness in March-May 1918, although death rates from respiratory illness showed only a limited increase in that period.

How did such numbers of the debilitated affect the protagonists? Wever explains:

'In France, influenza appeared in the BEF in April 1918. In the First Army, the total number of admissions to casualty clearing stations for influenza between 18 May and 2 July was 36,473, although a low case mortality rate illustrated the mild character of the first wave. In the Second Army, the highest number of cases admitted to casualty clearing stations for one day was reached on 25 June with 683 admissions. Correspondingly, the French Army was evacuating 1,500–2,000 cases per day in May 1918.

Siegfried Sassoon described the impact of the disease: 'The influenza epidemic defied all operation orders of the Divisional staff, and during the latter part of June more than half the men in our brigade were too ill to leave their billets.' Likewise, German General Erich Ludendorff said: 'Influenza was rampant ... It was a grievous business having to listen every morning to the chiefs of staffs' recital of the number of influenza cases, and their complaints about the weakness of their troops if the English attacked again.'

The super lethal second wave struck in August and September 1918 when on 6 October:

'Influenza and pneumonia... increased by thousands of cases. Case mortality of pneumonia, 32 per cent,' even further increasing to 45·3 per cent in the week of 11 October. In that week, during the height of the Meuse-Argonne offensive, the highest number of deaths from influenza in the AEF was reached with 1,451 reported fatalities.'[3]

By 23 October, there were 20,000 more patients than normal bed capacity in the AEF. Captain Geoffrey Keynes of the Royal Army Medical Corps (RAMC) would never forget the sight of the mortuary tents at Bohain, France: 'There were rows of corpses, absolutely *rows* of them, hundreds of them, dying from something quite different. It was a ghastly sight, to see them lying there dead of something I didn't have the treatment for.' Back at Camp Devens near Boston 'By the end of September, over 14,000 cases of influenza had been noted... approximately one quarter of its population, resulting in 757 deaths and a case-fatality rate exceeding 5 per cent.

---

3. Byerly 2005

During the second wave, 27.5 per cent (437,224) of over 1.5 million men in US Army training camps were hospitalized for respiratory illness, with a case-fatality rate that peaked at 5.1 per cent in September, while in the week of 4 October the highest number of deaths from influenza was reached with 6,160 fatalities.

According to Wever and van Bergen:

> 'Still, even until this day, virological and bacteriological analysis of preserved archived remains of soldiers that succumbed to 1918 pandemic influenza has important implications for preparedness for future pandemics.'

Yet, it remains unclear whether 1918 pandemic influenza had an impact on the course of the First World War.

After the war, one military medical historian even went so far as to state that 'in World War I the American Expeditionary Forces suffered no major epidemic problems', which is illustrative of the dismissal of the influenza epidemic as unimportant or even to ignore it altogether.[4]

Breitnauer, Jaime, 2020, *The Spanish flu epidemic and its influence on history*, Barnsley

Byerly, C.R., 2005, *Fever of War. The Influenza Epidemic in the U.S. Army during World War I*. New York.

Byerly, C.R., 2005, The U.S. military and the influenza pandemic of 1918–1919. *Public Health Rep.* 2010;125 (Suppl 3):82–91

van Bergen, L., 2009, *Before My Helpless Sight. Suffering, Dying and Military Medicine on the Western Front, 1914–1918*. Farnham

Wever, P.C., 2014, Death from 1914–1918 pandemic influenza during the First World War: a perspective from personal and anecdotal evidence. Influenza Other Respir Viruses. 5:538–46

---

4. Byerly 2005

Although we have had 30 years [after the 1918 outbreak] to prepare for what should be done in the event of an[other] influenza pandemic, I think we have all been rushing around trying to improvise investigations with insufficient time to do it properly. We can only hope that people will have taken advantage of their opportunities and at the end it may be possible to construct an adequate explanation of what happened.

So said J. Corbett McDonald of the Public Health Laboratory Service to Ian Watson, Director of the College of General Practitioners' Epidemic Observation Unit in the autumn of 1957. In the event, neither the Unit nor the PHLS undertook any large scale research projects during the outbreak and later studies were limited.

After the influenza pandemic of 1918–20, influenza reverted to its usual seasonal pattern – until the pandemic of 1957. This first came to light with the news that an epidemic in Hong Kong had affected 250,000 people in a very short period. It originated in Guizhou, China. A 2016 study estimated the number of deaths caused by the 1957–58 pandemic at 1.1 million worldwide despite the availability of a vaccine by late 1957. It was a unique event in the history of influenza, as for the first time the rapid global spread of the virus could be studied by laboratory investigation. The virus was quickly identified as influenza A virus subtype H2N2, a recombination of avian influenza, probably from geese, and human influenza viruses.

On 17 April 1956, *The Times* reported that 'an influenza epidemic has affected thousands of Hong Kong residents'. By the end of the month, Singapore was hit in an epidemic which peaked in mid-May with 680 deaths. In Taiwan, 100,000 were affected by mid-May, and India suffered a million cases by June. In late June, the pandemic reached the United Kingdom. At about the same time it got to the United States; some of the first people affected were US Navy personnel at Newport Naval Station, Rhode Island and new military recruits elsewhere. The first wave peaked in October and affected mainly children who had recently returned to school after the summer holiday. The second wave, in January and February 1958, was more pronounced among elderly people and so had a higher mortality rate.

In the UK the week ending 17 October saw the number of deaths peak with 600 reported in England and Wales. The first vaccines were not distributed until October in the UK, and then on an extremely limited basis.

Except for people over 70, who may have been exposed to an influenza pandemic in 1898 – also probably a H2N2 pandemic – the human population was again confronted by a virus that found it to be virgin prey, and again, the virus could develop into lethal pneumonia. However, underlying health conditions – chronic heart or lung disease for example – were soon found to be present in most of these patients; women in the third trimester of pregnancy were also vulnerable. One GP recalled 'we were amazed at the extraordinary infectivity of the disease, overawed by the suddenness of its outset and surprised at the protean nature of its symptomatology'. Not much learnt there then from the 1918 experience.

The 1957 pandemic was also the first opportunity medical researchers had to observe the vaccination response in the majority of people who had not previously been exposed to the novel virus. By 1960 as the virus kept coming back as a seasonal infection, immunity levels in the general population increased and vaccine responses were better, due to 'priming' of the response by natural infection or first immunisation.

As Claire Jackson (2009) puts it:

> 'Despite Watson's early prediction that "in the end, and in spite of the scare stuff in the lay press, we will have our epidemic of influenza, of a type not very different from what we know already, with complications in the usual age groups," the core group of main sufferers was aged 5 to 39 years with 49 per cent between 5–14 years. In London, 110,000 children were off school suspected of having influenza. With adults there was usually a connection to children; for example, parents, teachers, doctors, or a closed group such as the armed forces and football teams.'

Jackson continues: 'Patients were often able to pinpoint the start of Asian flu to the very minute with wobbly legs and a chill followed by prostration, sore throats, running nose, and coughs; together with achy limbs (adults), head (children), and a high fever following. Young children, particularly boys, suffered nose bleeds.' Symptoms were mostly mild and there were complications in 3 per cent of cases with 0.3 per cent mortality. Pneumonia and bronchitis accounted for half of these, the rest being cerebro- and cardiovascular disease brought on by the flu.

Communication, or the lack of it, was a problem; Jackson asks: 'was a clear message being given to the public as to what to expect and to do in the event of illness? Was there a leadership role for medical organisations such as the BMA or the College [of GPs] that was not taken up? Some members of the College of General Practitioners called for the UK Government to issue a warning about the dangers presented by the virus and coordinate a national response. The Ministry of Health dithered allowing the virus to run its course and wreak carnage in the form of 20,000 UK deaths. By late September, the *BMJ* correspondence column was full of complaints: 'It is time the BMA took urgent steps to counteract the ... exaggerated publicity in the press ... One woman in the best of health had obeyed instructions given her in a woman's magazine.'

The new H2N2 virus completely replaced the previous H1N1 type, and became the new seasonal influenza type. H2N2 influenza virus continued to be transmitted until 1968, when it transformed via antigenic shift into influenza A virus subtype H3N2, the cause of the 1968 influenza pandemic.

In the US the Dow Jones Industrial Average shrank by 15 per cent in the second half of 1957.

> 'By early 1958 it was estimated that "not less than 9 million people in Great Britain had ... Asian influenza during the 1957 epidemic. Of these, more than 5.5 million were attended by their doctors. About 14,000 people died of the immediate effects of their attack." Not only was £10,000,000 spent on sickness benefit, but also with factories, offices and mines closed the economy was hit.'

'Setback in Production — Recession through Influenza'
Manchester Guardian, 29 November, 1958.

Jackson, Claire, 2009. 'History lessons: the Asian Flu pandemic'. *British Journal of General Practice*. 59 (565): 622–623.
Viboud, Cécile, 2016. 'Global Mortality Impact of the 1957–1959 Influenza Pandemic'. *The Journal of Infectious Diseases*. 213 (5): 738–745

The 'Hong Kong Flu' of 1968–69

'When hysteria is rife, we might try some history' – Simon Jenkins in *The Guardian*

The subsequent 1968 influenza pandemic – or 'Hong Kong flu' or 'Mao flu' as it was dubbed – would have an even more dramatic impact, killing more than 30,000 individuals in the UK and 100,000 people in the USA, with half the deaths among individuals under 65 years. Yet, while at the height of the outbreak in December 1968 *The New York Times* described the pandemic as 'one of the worst in the nation's history', there were few school closures and most businesses continued to operate as normal.

It started in mid-1968 in Hong Kong, and spread ferociously in a few months via ships, aeroplanes and trains to India, the Philippines, Australia, Europe and the USA. In the US the virus came to California carried by troops returning from the Vietnam War. By 1969, it had extended its reach to Japan, Africa and South America. Worldwide, the death toll peaked between December at around one million.

In Berlin, the high number of deaths led to corpses being stored in subway tunnels, and in West Germany, rubbish collectors had to bury the dead because of a lack of undertakers. In total, East and West Germany registered 60,000 estimated deaths. In some areas of France, half of the workforce was bedridden, causing major disruption in manufacturing due to absenteeism. British postal and train services were also adversely affected.

Nevertheless mortality was lower than in 1957–58; there are a number of reasons for this which include: the virus was similar in some respects to the Asian Flu variant which conferred partial immunity; the more widespread availability of antibiotics meant secondary bacterial infections were less of a problem; the pandemic did not gain momentum until near the winter school holidays, thus limiting the infection's spread; and a vaccine specific to the new virus was available a month after the epidemic peaked in the USA.

Soon after, it was discovered that waterfowl are the natural hosts of all influenza A viruses – and that there was a greater diversity of viruses in birds than in humans.

Though largely forgotten, the world did learn key lessons such as the need for proactive vaccine development, and the effective and rigorous deployment of vaccination programs. But the lessons we forgot, such as the need for frequent hand-washing, have helped keep the flu alive season after season.

Charles Graves, the brother of Robert Graves, reveals that his publishers, Icon, delayed publication of his 1969 book *Invasion by Virus: Can it Happen Again?*, citing concerns about 'frightening the public'. In the book Graves compared the 1957 and 1968 pandemics to that of the 1918–19 influenza pandemic, posing the question in his subtitle: could it happen again? His answer was yes and that the UK had been lucky that the recent pandemics had been of a 'mild type' of influenza. He closed by reassuring readers that history was unlikely to repeat itself before 1998, 'by which time the medical profession will know a great deal more about immunisation than it did in 1918 – or does now.'

Graves was right on both counts, but wrong to think that better medical knowledge of vaccines and statistical modelling would reduce public anxiety about pandemics.

Graves, Charles, 1969, Invasion By Virus: Can it Happen Again? London

Honigsbaum, M.A., 2020, *The Pandemic Century: A History of Global Contagion from the Spanish Flu to Covid 19*, London

Honigsbaum, M.A., 2020, *A history of the great influenza pandemics: death, panic and hysteria, 1830–1920*. London

Kilbourne, E.D., 2006, Influenza pandemics of the 20th century. *Emerg Infect Dis.* 12(1):9–14.

The 'Red Flu' of 1977

Between May and November of 1977, an epidemic of influenza made its way out of north-eastern China and the former Soviet Union. The disease was, however, limited to people under the age of 25 – and was generally mild. It was soon found that the virus responsible was effectively identical to the H1N1 that had circulated from 1918 through to 1958, and which had been replaced by the Asian flu, which was in turn supplanted by the Hong Kong flu. This was decidedly odd, given that it was already known that influenza A viruses mutated rapidly as they multiplied – and it had been twenty years since the Spanish or H1N1 flu had been seen in humans. It also explained why infections were limited to young people: anyone who had caught the seasonal flu prior to 1958 was protected.

There has been speculation that the pandemic was due to an inadequately-inactivated or attenuated vaccine released in a trial; there has even been mention of escape from a freezer in a biological warfare lab raising fears of bioterrorism. Firm evidence for either possibility continues to elude.

Chapter 55

1929–30 The great parrot fever pandemic

'Parrots were all the rage and itinerant peddlers went door-to-door with "lovebirds" for widows and bored housewives, the idea that one's pet parrot or parakeet might be harbouring a deadly pathogen from the Amazon was the stuff of domestic nightmares and a story few newspaper editors could resist.'

– Mark Honigsbaum, 2019

In 1880, physician Jakob Ritter described a cluster of seven people with atypical pneumonia with connections to his brother's house. No one at the time linked this to sick exotic birds in that house: twelve finches and parrots confined in the study in Uster, near Zürich, Switzerland. Three of the seven affected people died, including Ritter's brother and the metal-worker who visited the home to fix the bird cage.

Ritter detailed the natural history of the disease, and, noting its similar features to typhoid and typhus, he called it 'pneumotyphus' proposing that the birds might be the vectors; those twelve birds had recently been imported from Hamburg. This was followed, in 1882, by a second outbreak in Bern, in which two people died; sick parrots from London were blamed. Subsequently, further similar outbreaks with a coincidence of exposure to birds appeared in other parts of Europe, including in Paris in 1892, centred on the homes of two bird fanciers who had recently imported 500 parrots from Buenos Aires. During the crossing, 300 of the birds had died, and people coming into contact with the survivors had developed symptoms of influenza.

The disease was named psittacosis (ψιττακός, ancient Greek for parrot) in 1895 by Antonin Morange. Before the 1929 outbreak in the United States, the last known cases were in 1917, found in captive birds in the basement of a department store in Pennsylvania. The causative pathogen, *C. psittaci*, was not discovered until the 1960s. Infected people typically experienced headache, poor sleep, fatigue and a cough following several days of fever. Some subsequently became delirious and semi-conscious, after which some died, while others recovered with a long convalescence.

The 1929–30 parrot fever pandemic was a series of simultaneous outbreaks of psittacosis or parrot fever, accelerated by the breeding and transportation of birds in crowded, insanitary containers for purposes of trade. It was initially found to have spread from various species of birds from several countries worldwide to humans between mid 1929 and early 1930. Indeed, despite its name, parrot fever is not confined only to parrot-like birds but has been isolated from some 450 other bird species, including canaries, finches, pigeons, doves and kestrels. In non-psittacine birds, the infection is known as ornithosis.

The disease affected 750 to 800 people around the globe, with a mortality rate of 15 per cent (so, up to 120) and with 33 deaths recorded in the United States between November 1929 and May 1930. Of the 167 cases where the sex of the victim was known, 105, or two-thirds, were women. Germany too was badly hit with 215 cases and 45 deaths. Berlin Zoo had to close its gates to frightened parrot owners desperately abandoning their birds.

In the UK cases were reported in Birmingham in mid 1929. In December 1929, a ship's carpenter presented at The London Hospital with a typhoid-like illness. He had previously purchased two parrots that had come from from Buenos Aires, which had died en route to London; the carpenter died. By March 1930, 100 suspected cases were reported across England and Wales. Although most cases seemed to involve sustained exposure to live birds, British researchers observed that this was not always the case, citing one example where a man went into a pub for a pint; a (sick) parrot was also in the pub and transmitted the disease to the man with no close contact involved. The 'Parrots (Prohibition of Import) Regulations, 1930' was enacted; it prohibited the trade of parrots unless for research. By January 1930, outbreaks were also being reported in Germany, Italy, Switzerland, France, Denmark, Algeria, the Netherlands, Egypt and Honolulu.

How did the disease transmit to humans? No one knew at the time but it was by mouth-to-beak contact or by inhaling dried bird secretions and droppings. The cause, *Chlamydia psittaci*, from the same family of bacteria that transmits chlamydia, a common infection in humans of the eye and genital tract, was only discovered after the pandemic subsided. It usually remains dormant in birds but is activated by shortage of food, and stress and fear of capture and confinement. The most common symptom is diarrhoea: the birds' faeces pose the principal threat to humans, especially when they become dry and dessicated and are circulated in the air after, for example, a mere flap of the wings. Even though in many cases patients had not touched sick birds or handled their faecal matter it was enough just to have been in the same room as them with no mask or other protection.

How did the pandemic start? The origin of the outbreak in the Argentine city of Córdoba was traced to an import of 5,000 parrots from Brazil confined in unsanitary and crowded containers. Although the Argentine parrot trade was outlawed, passengers on cruise ships calling at Buenos Aires were mostly unaware of the ban, creating an opportunity for unscrupulous dealers to offload their sickly birds on gullible tourists. It was this that most probably led to the introduction of psittacosis to the United States, Germany and the United Kingdom.

In January 1930 parrots took centre stage when reports of cases among an Argentine theatrical group in Córdoba, after they had purchased an Amazon parrot in Buenos Aires, made it into the 5th January edition of the *American Weekly* under the unhelpful, sensationalist headline 'Killed By A Pet Parrot'. Two of the actors died from the illness. A doctor at the hospital spotted the link. He learnt from the troupe's prop man that the actors had been directed to pet the parrot on stage and that the bird had since died. As a result, an alert was issued by the Argentine National Health Board, and soon reports of similar outbreaks connected to sickly parrots, but wrongly diagnosed as typhoid or influenza started to emerge. In Córdoba, fifty cases were traced back to a parrot dealer who had set up shop in a local boarding house. His birds were slaughtered but too late to prevent infection to other suspect psittacines. The outbreaks in Argentina were entirely avoidable and would not have occurred had dealers observed some simple precautions, precautions which were familiar to and routinely observed by indigenous forest peoples accustomed to living alongside wild birds in their natural habitat.

Following further cases, bans on parrot trafficking were implemented, and subsequently cases were reported in several other countries, including Germany, France and Australia. Later, it was discovered that the main source in the US was domestic lovebirds raised in hundreds of independent Californian backyard aviaries by breeders intent on boosting their incomes following the recent Wall Street Crash. Mark Honigsbaum[1] puts the situation into context:

> 'Today few people recall the hysteria surrounding the great parrot fever pandemic of 1929–30, but in an era when parrots were all the rage and itinerant peddlers went door-to-door with 'lovebirds' for widows and bored housewives, the idea that one's pet parrot or parakeet might be harbouring a deadly pathogen from the Amazon was the stuff of domestic nightmares and a story few newspaper editors could resist.'

The result, as we have seen, was that most victims in the US were women; women were probably more likely to kiss their birds and to look after them when they were ill. The situation was exacerbated in the winter of 1929 by an influenza epidemic and there were fears of a rebound of Spanish Flu.

A report in the *New York Times* ('30,000 Parrots Here; Amazon Best Talker,' 29 January 1930) declaring New York City alone to be habitat for some 30,000 parrots, was taken up by the *National Geographic* who nicknamed Amazons and African grays 'the ballyhoo barkers of birddom, the noisy, clever, side-show performers of the tropical forest.' Honigsbaum adds (p.72)

> 'Their pint-sized cousin, the parakeet or lovebird (genus Agapornis), had a reputation for similarly buffoonish behaviour, and with their talent for hanging upside down or dancing on their owners' shoulders were a source of endless amusement for children and an entertainment for house guests. Little wonder then that in 1929 nearly 50,000 parrots, parakeets and lovebirds, and some 500,000 canaries, were imported to the United States.'

---

1. 2019, p.69

From early January 1930 the press gradually whipped up parrot fever into a frenzy, paving the way for what has been termed the 'killer germ genre of journalism'.[2] Honigsbaum (p.75) elaborates:

> '...this genre played on the dangers that lurked in everyday objects, such as coins, library books, or drinking cups. Dust and insects were targets of similar scaremongering, hence the advertisements urging housewives to mop regularly with disinfectants and spray their homes with insecticides. By the 1920s, as Americans adopted new germ-conscious regimes, even handshaking and kissing babies came to be frowned upon.'

An outbreak of 'mysterious pneumonias' came to media attention when cases in three members of one Maryland family – Lillian, Edith and Lee Martin – were traced to the previous Christmas importation of parrots from South America. Ten days before that Christmas, Simon Martin, secretary of the Chamber of Commerce in Annapolis, Maryland, had bought a parrot from a pet shop in Baltimore which Edith and Lee, his daughter and son-in-law, had kept at their home – the plan being to give the bird to Lillian as a surprise on Christmas Day. Lillian, his wife along with their daughter and son-in-law, became seriously ill. On Christmas Day the parrot died.

In January 1930, when the syndicated story of the Córdoba cases reached the Maryland family doctor a link was made back to the theatrical group, and 'parrot fever' erupted in the American press. At the same time Martin's doctor sent a telegram to the United States Public Health Service (PHS) in Washington DC, requesting advice on parrot fever. The story came to the attention of Surgeon General Hugh S. Cumming, who received a deluge of similar messages and urgent telegrams from Baltimore, New York, Ohio and California. The task of solving the cause of parrot fever was assigned to George W. McCoy, the director of PHS's Hygienic Laboratory (known as the Hygienic) and a renowned bacteriologist and to his deputy, Charlie Armstrong, neither of whom had ever heard of parrot fever. No one can accuse Armstrong of not living for his work; over his illustrious career he survived infections of malaria, Dengue fever, encephalitis, Q fever and tularaemia. Just the man you needed at this worrying time and 'definitely not the sort of man who would own a parrot let alone kiss it'.

But, by 8 January Lillian and her daughter and son-in-law were not the only ones believed to have contracted parrot fever. Four employees of the pet store at North Eutaw Street were also ill, as was a woman who had bought a parrot at another store in southeast Baltimore. Then, on 10 January, people started dying: the first victim was a Baltimore woman, Louise Schaeffer, whose death was originally attributed to pneumonia but it emerged she had been in contact with a parrot several days earlier. The second death was, worryingy, in Toledo, Ohio, nearly 500 miles to the northwest of Baltimore. The victim was Mrs Percy Q. Williams. She had died at Toledo's Mercy Hospital three weeks after her husband had returned from Cuba with a gift

---

2. Tomes, 2000

of three parrots; one of the parrots had died shortly after his return. It was the first sign of the true range and extent of the epidemic and the challenge facing state and federal health officials.

Cumming warned the nation to avoid imported parrots; he 'did not fear an epidemic,' he said, as it was generally believed that psittacosis was transmitted 'only from bird to human being, and not from person to person.' He made things worse when he announced: 'We do not consider it practical to place an embargo on importation before making sure where the sick parrots are coming from,' thus losing invaluable time in the suppression of the disease. In the meantime Baltimore officials had visited seven pet stores in the city and the homes of 38 people who had recently purchased parrots. Of these, 36 were ill; the reaction clearly proved the efficacy, indeed absolute need for of a track and trace system.

Sailors at sea were ordered by a US Navy admiral to throw their parrots overboard. One health commissioner encouraged people to kill their pet parrots, and some just released them on the streets – (disease) carrier parrots.

The director of the Bureau of Communicable Diseases, Daniel S. Hatfield, ordered the confiscation of all birds at Baltimore pet stores. The six major US pet dealers stood to make a loss of $5 million per year as a result of an executive order issued by President Herbert Hoover on 24 January prohibiting 'the immediate importation of parrots into the United States, its possessions and dependencies from any foreign port', until research could find the cause and mode of transmission. The newly formed Bird Dealers Association of America denied the connection between the disease and parrot imports: 'no bird dealers whose hourly contact with feathered pets presumably would render them likely to contract psittacosis if it is communicable to humans, have been affected.'

Two of the 16 people who developed the illness from exposure at the National Hygiene Laboratory died. Bacteriologist William Royal Stokes succumbed only weeks after beginning research on the parrot dropping samples given to him by Charlie Armstrong, despite warnings from Armstrong that the agent may be a contagious virus and not a bacterium. They had failed to isolate the causative agent, and McCoy was subsequently forced to kill the birds and fumigate the Hygienic Laboratory.

The establishment of the National Institutes of Health is a result of the outbreak that occurred in Maryland.

The failure to isolate the causative agent resulted in a scramble by laboratories around the world to succeed where the National Hygiene Laboratory and other US facilities had not. The first was a team led by Samuel Bedson at the London Hospital who concluded that 'the aetiological agent of psittacosis in parrots is a virus which cannot be cultivated on ordinary bacteriological media, and which is capable of passing through some of the more porous filters.' Soon after, Charles Krumwiede at the New York Board of Health, demonstrated that the virus could be readily transferred from parakeets to white mice, thus facilitating safer laboratory research. When Krumwiede fell ill the mantle was taken up by Thomas Rivers, bacteriologist and virologist – the 'father of modern virology' – at the Rockefeller Institute for Medical Research. Rivers was only too aware that psittacosis was highly infectious, so he insisted his team wear full body suits, with glass goggles in the helmets and rubber gloves attached to the sleeves – personal protective equipment (PPE) that would become standard in biosafety for anyone working in biomedical research or treating patients with contagious diseases. Rivers also demonstrated that psittacosis could be transferred to rabbits, guinea pigs and monkeys and established that the principal transmission route in humans was via the respiratory tract, and not through scratches or parrot bites.

Today, psittacosis has largely receded from public view: this is for the most part due to the work of Karl Friedrich Meyer (1884–1974), the 'Pasteur of the 20th century' and one of the most prominent scientists in infectious diseases in man and animals. Following the development of chlortetracycline (Aureomycin), by Lederle Laboratories, a tetracycline antibiotic in 1948, Meyer went to the Hartz Mountain Distribution Company, then the largest supplier of milled bird seed in the United States, to develop a line of medicated millet. By the middle 1950s chlortetracycline-impregnated seed had become standard in the bird breeding industry. There are still isolated outbreaks, mainly on turkey farms or in poultry processing plants, where exposure to psittacosis was, and still is, an occupational hazard. In most cases, all it takes is a course of tetracycline to eradicate human infections and return a flock to health.

Honigsbaum, Mark, 31 May 2014. 'In search of sick parrots: Karl Friedrich Meyer, disease detective'. *The Lancet*. 383 (9932): 1880–1881.

Honigsbaum, Mark, 2019. '*The Great Parrot Fever Pandemic*'. *The Pandemic Century: One Hundred Years of Panic, Hysteria and Hubris*'. London

Lepore, Jill, 1 June 2009. 'The Spread; Outbreaks, media scares, and the parrot panic of 1930'. *The New Yorker*.

Ramsay, Edward C., 2003. 'The Psittacosis Outbreak of 1929–1930'. *Journal of Avian Medicine and Surgery*. 17 (4): 235–237

Chapter 56

Seventh cholera pandemic 1961–1975

Ominously, the strain involved, El Tor, in the seventh pandemic persists to this day. The first record of the new lineage comes from a laboratory in El Tor, Egypt, in 1897 and by this time, the 'El Tor' strain differed from its relatives by 30 per cent. According to David Schulz (2016):

> 'The next decade was pivotal for the bacterium's evolution. It bounced around the Middle East, picking up a key gene called tcpA, which encodes a hairlike structure on its surface that clings to the wall of the small intestine. This change alone didn't make the strain pathogenic, but it may have helped it live longer in the guts of religious pilgrims travelling to and from Mecca. Then, sometime between 1903 and 1908, the El Tor strain picked up a crucial piece of hitchhiking DNA that likely triggered its ability to cause disease in humans.'

This strain of El Tor started life in Makassar, Indonesia where it adopted new genes which probably increased transmissibility. It then spread to Bangladesh by 1963 whence it hit India in 1964, followed by the Soviet Union in 1966. In July 1970, there was an outbreak in Odessa and in 1972 reports of outbreaks in Baku, but this information was suppressed by the Soviet Union. It reached Italy in 1973 from North Africa. Japan and the South Pacific saw outbreaks by the late 1970s. In 1991, the number of cases reported worldwide was 570,000. Mortality rates, however, plummeted as governments began modern curative and preventive measures. The usual mortality rate of 50 per cent dropped to 10 per cent by the 1980s and less than 3 per cent by the 1990s.

Ryan, E.T., January 2011. 'The cholera pandemic, still with us after half a century: time to rethink'. *PLoS Neglected Tropical Diseases.* 5 (1): e1003

Schultz, David, How today's cholera pandemic was born. Nov. 18, 2016, *Science* AAAS

Chapter 57

Legionnaires' Disease, 1976

'Windscreen wiper water may be the cause of 20% of cases of Legionnaires' disease in England and Wales. The Health Protection Agency (HPA) has said that simply adding screenwash to wiper fluid kills the bacteria and could save lives.'

Legionnaires' disease, legionellosis, is a form of atypical pneumonia caused by any type of Legionella bacteria although over 90 per cent of cases of Legionnaires' disease are caused by Legionella pneumophila. Signs and symptoms include cough, shortness of breath, high fever, muscle pains and headaches. There may also be nausea, vomiting and diarrhoea. Most people catch Legionnaires' disease by inhaling the bacteria from water or soil. The bacterium is found naturally in fresh water. It can contaminate shower heads, hot water tanks, hot tubs, and cooling towers of large air conditioners. It is usually spread by breathing in mist that contains the bacteria. Dr Isabel Oliver, regional director of the HPA South West, said people may want to check they have screenwash in their cars as they usually contain agents which would stop the growth of bacteria. A report published in the *Journal of Epidemiology* found that there was high risk from not adding screenwash to windscreen wiper water.

It typically does not spread directly between people and most of those who are exposed do not become infected. There is no vaccine. The disease got its name after the outbreak where it was first identified, at a 1976 American Legion convention at the Bellevue-Stratford Hotel in Philadelphia, although cases of legionellosis have occurred all over the world. Of the 182 Philadelphia reported cases, mostly men, 29, died. In 1977, the causative agent was identified as a previously unknown strain of bacteria, subsequently named Legionella. The negative publicity from the outbreak caused occupancy at the Bellevue-Stratford to plummet to 4 per cent and the hotel finally closed on 18 November 1976. After a $25 million restoration the hotel reopened in 1979 as the Fairmont Hotel; it is now the Park Hyatt.

Between 1995 and 2005, over 32,000 cases of Legionnaires' disease and more than 600 outbreaks were reported to the European Working Group for Legionella Infections. In 2002, Barrow-in-Furness suffered an outbreak when six women and one man died as a result of the illness; another 172 people also contracted the disease. The cause was found to be a contaminated cooling tower at the town's Forum 28 arts centre. Barrow Borough Council later became the first public body in the UK to be charged with corporate manslaughter but was cleared. They were, however, along with architect Gillian Beckingham, fined for breaches of Health and Safety regulations in 2006. In 2012 nineteen people were infected in a warehouse hot tub at Fenton near Stoke-on-Trent. One person died.

The fatality rate of Legionnaires' disease has ranged from 5 to 30 per cent during various outbreaks and approaches 50 per cent for nosocomial infections, especially when treatment with antibiotics is delayed. Hospital-acquired Legionella pneumonia has a fatality rate of 28 per cent: the principal source of infection in such cases is the drinking-water distribution system.

Altman, L.K., 1 August 2006. In Philadelphia 30 Years Ago, an Eruption of Illness and Fear'. *The New York Times*.

Tsai, T.F., 1979. 'Legionnaires' disease: clinical features of the epidemic in Philadelphia'. Annals of Internal Medicine. 90 (4): 509–17.

Wilkinson, E. 'Windscreen water infection risk'. BBC News 13/6/2010.

Chapter 58

HIV/AIDS pandemic and epidemic: 1981–

'It's alarming to see just how many people believe you can get HIV from kissing, sneezing, or coughing. Lack of understanding leads to stigma and discrimination towards people living with HIV.'
– National Aids Trust, 2014, 'British public still in the dark about HIV 30 years on'

'If you look at three diseases. The three major killers. HIV, tuberculosis and malaria, the only disease for which we have really good drugs is HIV. And it's very simple, because there's a market in the United States and Europe.'
– Jim Yong Kim, MD, President, World Bank 2012–2019

Anyone born just before or in the years since 1990 will remember with some anxiety how HIV and AIDS tore through the United Kingdom and the rest of the world from 1981 although, as we will show, there is significant evidence to show that it was around in the 1970s in certain demographics. According to the World Health Organization more than 70 million people have so far been infected with HIV and about 35 million (50 per cent) have died from AIDS since this brutal pandemic took hold. AIDS is still prevalent in Africa.

Statistics from Public Health England and published by the National Aids Trust reveal that the United Kingdom had an estimated 101,600 people living with HIV in 2017 which translates into an HIV prevalence of 1.7 per 1,000 people of all ages or 2.2 per 1,000 of people aged 15–74 years. In the same year, 4,363 people were newly diagnosed with HIV, a number that is steadily declining each year, falling by 17 per cent between 2016 and 2017 alone largely due to the decrease in new diagnoses among gay and bisexual men, the group most affected by HIV in the UK, which fell by almost a third (31 per cent) between 2015 and 2017. Despite this, half of all new HIV diagnoses (53 per cent) in 2017 in the UK occurred among gay, bisexual men and other men who have sex with men, while 18 per cent and 24 per cent of diagnoses occurred among heterosexual men and women respectively. In 2017, black African men and women comprised 38 per cent of heterosexual adults with a new HIV diagnosis, although these groups account for a relatively small proportion of the overall UK population.

The human immunodeficiency virus, or HIV, attacks the immune system, specifically CD4 cells (or T cells) and is transmitted through bodily fluids such as blood, semen, vaginal fluids, anal fluids and breast milk. Historically, HIV has most often been caught through unprotected sex, the sharing of needles for drug use and through childbirth.

In due course, HIV is able to destroy so many CD4 cells that the body is left defenceless against infections and diseases, eventually leading to the most severe form of an HIV infection: acquired immunodeficiency syndrome, or AIDS. Anyone with AIDS is highly vulnerable to cancers and to life-threatening infections such as pneumonia. There is no cure for HIV or AIDS, but the good news now is that, given early enough treatment, a person with HIV can live nearly as long as someone free of the virus. A study in 2019 in *The Lancet*, showed how an anti-viral treatment effectively halted the spread of HIV in trial patients.

We know that HIV derives from simian immunodeficiency virus (SIV), an HIV-like virus that attacks the immune system of monkeys and apes, and in 1999, researchers identified a strain of chimpanzee SIV called SIVcpz, which was very similar to HIV. Chimps, it was later discovered, feed on two smaller species of monkeys – sooty mangabey and greater spot-nosed monkeys – these two both carry, and infect, the chimps with two strains of SIV which probably combined to form SIVcpz, which in turn began to infect chimpanzees and humans during the late 19th or early 20th century.

SIVcpz would have jumped to humans in a kind of zoonosis when African hunters ate infected chimps, either that or the chimps' infected blood was introduced when a hunter or bushmeat vendor was bitten or cut while hunting or butchering the animal. The first transmission of SIV to HIV in 1910 was in Kinshasa (formerly Léopoldville, Belgian Congo), now the capital and largest city in the Democratic Republic of Congo. We can, therefore link the HIV epidemic with the contemporary rise of colonialism, the Scramble for Africa, and the consequent growth of large colonial African urban centres. This led to social changes such as rapid population growth, crowded and less than sanitary urbanisation, the use of unsterilized needles in health clinics, an explosion of casual sexual activity, an unusual number of unmarried girls and women, some divorced, enjoying the comparative freedom of release from tribal society, a predomimantly unaccompanied male influx fuelled by labour forces, plantation workers and administratative posts, the growth in supply and demand for prostitution, and the corresponding increasing frequency of genital ulcer diseases such as syphilis, chancroid, lymphogranuloma venereum and genital herpes in early colonial cities.

These diseases increase the probability of HIV transmission dramatically, from around 0.01–0.1 per cent to 4–43 per cent per heterosexual act, because the genital ulcers provide a portal of viral entry, and contain many activated T cells, the main cell targets of HIV. Many of the male workforces would have been fed on bushmeat, a proven source of infection, the availability and provision of which would have increased dramatically, facilitated by easier access to firearms.

A compromised or laboured immune system would have expedited the spread as well. Desperate living conditions, hard labour, infected, unsterilized needles used in multiple injections for smallpox, trypanosomiasis (sleeping sickness), leprosy, yaws and other communicable disease vaccinations between 1910–1940 (just around the time the HIV-1 groups started to spread), along with sexually transmitted infections

– they all had a role to play in depressing resistance to the HIV virus and facilitating its adaptation and serial passage to the human host.

From Kinshasa it would, as viruses usually do, have spread along roads, railways and rivers via migrants, travellers and the sex trade. A 2014 study from the Universities of Oxford and Leuven in Belgium, revealed that because approximately one million people every year would surge through Kinshasa, passengers riding on the region's Belgian railway trains were able to spread the virus to larger areas with ease.

In the 1960s, HIV spread from Africa to Haiti and the Caribbean when Haitians in Congo returned home. The virus then migrated from the Caribbean to New York City around 1970 and then on to San Francisco. The virus eventually percolated into male gay communities in other large United States cities, where a combination of casual, multi-partner sexual activity with individuals averaging over eleven unprotected sexual partners per year and relatively high transmission rates associated with anal intercourse allowed it to spread explosively enough to finally be noticed. International travel did the rest, assisting the virus to spread across the rest of the globe.

Because of the long incubation period of HIV – up to a decade or longer – before symptoms of AIDS appear, and because of the initially low incidence, nothing much appeared to be happening: but HIV was working insidiously and covertly. By the time the first reported cases of AIDS were found in large United States cities, the prevalence of HIV infection in some communities had passed 5 per cent. Worldwide, HIV infection had spread from urban to rural areas and began appearing in regions such as China and India.

Still nothing much happened until in 1981, the Centers for Disease Control and Prevention (CDC) published a report in its *Morbidity and Mortality Weekly Report* about five previously healthy homosexual men infected with Pneumocystis pneumonia, which is caused by the normally harmless fungus *Pneumocystis jirovecii*. This type of pneumonia, the CDC noted, almost never affects people with uncompromised immune systems. The report marked the official start of the HIV/AIDS pandemic. Over the next eighteen months, more PCP clusters were discovered among otherwise healthy men in cities throughout the country, along with other opportunistic diseases such as Kaposi's sarcoma and persistent, generalized lymphadenopathy, common in immunosuppressed patients.

The first news story on 'an exotic new disease' appeared on 18 May 1981 in the gay newspaper *New York Native*. In 1982 alarm bells started to ring loudly when the *New York Times* published a piece about a new immune system disorder, which had infected 335 people, killing 136 of them (41 per cent) – a high mortality rate by any measure. At this point the disease appeared to target mostly homosexual men – it was initially called, somewhat dismissively and perjoratively, gay-related immune deficiency, or GRID. However, health authorities soon realized their gaffe when they worked out that nearly half of the people identified with the syndrome were not homosexual men. The same opportunistic infections were also reported among haemophiliacs, users of intravenous drugs and Haitian immigrants – leading some researchers to call it the '4H' disease. By August 1982, the disease was being referred to by its new CDC-coined name: Acquired Immune Deficiency Syndrome (AIDS).

By the end of the year, AIDS cases were also reported in some European countries. Despite the fact that the CDC had discovered a number of major routes of transmission – as well as the game-changing discovery in 1983 that female partners of AIDS-positive men could be infected – the public (helped by the media) persisted in thinking of AIDS as a gay disease and was, unhelpfully, given the derogatory name, the 'gay plague' for many years after.

June 5th 1981 is the day on which the HIV/AIDS pandemic is officially said to have started; however, there is a significant body of evidence to suggest that it was thriving in certain communities in the previous decade when it was variously called junkie flu, the dwindles, disco fever or junkie pneumonia. In 1984, researchers finally identified the cause of AIDS – the HIV virus – enabling the Food and Drug Administration (FDA) to license the first commercial blood test for HIV in 1985. Today, numerous tests can identify HIV, usually by detecting HIV antibodies. These tests can be done on blood, saliva, or urine, though blood tests detect HIV sooner after infection due to higher levels of antibodies.

The pernicious virus continued apace: by the end of 1985, there were more than 20,000 reported cases of AIDS, which had penetrated every region of the world. The year 1987 was a good year for the battle against AIDS – because this was when the first antiretroviral medication for HIV, azidothymidine (AZT), became available. This has been joined by many other drugs which are typically used in combination in what is known as antiretroviral therapy (ART) or highly active antiretroviral treatment (HAART). How do they work? By inhibiting the virus from multiplying, giving the immune system breathing space to fight off infections and HIV-related cancers. The therapy also helps reduce the risk of HIV transmission, not least between an infected mother and her unborn child.

In 1991 basketball player Magic Johnson announced he had HIV, helping to bring high profile awareness to the issue and diminish the stereotype of it being a gay disease. In 1994, the FDA approved the first oral (and non-blood) HIV test followed two years later by the first home testing kit and the first urine test.

In 2001, generic drug manufacturers began selling much cheaper copies of patent protected HIV drugs to developing countries, forcing several major global pharmaceutical manufacturers to reduce their prices on their HIV drugs. In 2006, researchers discovered that penile circumcision can reduce the risk of female-to-male HIV transmission by 60 per cent. Uli Linke has argued that female genital mutilation, either or both clitoridectomy and infibulations, is responsible for the high incidence of AIDS in Africa, since intercourse with a female who has undergone clitoridectomy is conducive to exchange of blood.

In 2009, then President Barack Obama rescinded a 1987 US ban on HIV-positive people from entering the country. The FDA approved pre-exposure prophylaxis, or PrEP, for HIV-negative people in 2012: according to the CDC a daily dose of PrEP can reduce the risk of HIV from sex by more than 90 per cent and from intravenous drug use by 70 per cent. More welcome news came in 2019 when a major study demonstrated that over 750 gay men on an anti-viral treatment failed to transmit the virus to their partners. 'Our findings provide conclusive evidence that the risk of HIV transmission through anal sex when HIV viral load is suppressed is effectively zero,' the paper, published in *The Lancet*, stated.

HIV and AIDS have, it seems, dropped off the media radar to some extent in recent years – not surprising given the emergence and topicality of new disease pandemics in the last two decades: SARS, Ebola, Zika, MERS and of course COVID-19. This neglect is a shame because the therapies developed in treating HIV and AIDS are one of global medicine's success stories, on a par at least with the accelerated vaccine development programmes for COVID-19. On the downside HIV has not gone away, by any means. Here are some sobering statistics compiled by UNAID in Geneva which will disabuse anyone of the notion that the world is now AIDs free.

Global HIV & AIDS statistics — 2020 fact sheet

GLOBAL HIV STATISTICS

26 million [25.1 million–26.2 million] people were accessing antiretroviral therapy as of the end of June 2020.

38.0 million [31.6 million–44.5 million] people globally were living with HIV in 2019.
1.7 million [1.2 million–2.2 million] people became newly infected with HIV in 2019.
690,000 [500,000–970,000] people died from AIDS-related illnesses in 2019.
75.7 million [55.9 million–100 million] people have become infected with HIV since the start of the epidemic (end 2019).
32.7 million [24.8 million–42.2 million] people have died from AIDS-related illnesses since the start of the epidemic (end 2019).

People living with HIV accessing antiretroviral therapy

As of the end of June 2020, 26.0 million [25.1 million–26.2 million] people were accessing antiretroviral therapy.

85% [63–100%] of pregnant women living with HIV had access to antiretroviral medicines to prevent transmission of HIV to their child in 2019.

Women

Every week, around 5,500 young women aged 15–24 years become infected with HIV.

In sub-Saharan Africa, five in six new infections among adolescents aged 15–19 years are among girls. Young women aged 15–24 years are twice as likely to be living with HIV than men.

More than one third (35%) of women around the world have experienced physical and/or sexual violence by an intimate partner or sexual violence by a non-partner at some time in their lives.

In some regions, women who have experienced physical or sexual intimate partner violence are 1.5 times more likely to acquire HIV than women who have not experienced such violence.

Women and girls accounted for about 48% of all new HIV infections in 2019. In sub-Saharan Africa, women and girls accounted for 59% of all new HIV infections.

The risk of acquiring HIV is:
26 times higher among gay men and other men who have sex with men.

29 times higher among people who inject drugs.

30 times higher for sex workers.

13 times higher for transgender people.

TB remains the leading cause of death among people living with HIV, accounting for around one in three AIDS-related deaths.

It is estimated that 44% of people living with HIV and TB are unaware of their coinfection and are therefore not receiving care.

https://www.unaids.org/sites/default/files/media_asset/UNAIDS_FactSheet_en.pdf

Cohen, Myron S., 15 June 2019, Successful treatment of HIV eliminates sexual transmission. *The Lancet* 393, 2366–2367

Crimp, Douglas 1987. 'How to Have Promiscuity in an Epidemic'. October Vol. 43, AIDS: Cultural Analysis/Cultural Activism pp. 237–271

Davies, Russell, T., January 2021, It's A Sin, Channel 4

Fowler, Norman 2014. *AIDS: Don't Die of Prejudice*. Biteback Publishing

Pépin, Jacques 2011. *The Origins of AIDS*. Cambridge

Shilts, Randy 1987. *And the band played on: politics, people, and the AIDS epidemic*. New York

Sontag, Susan, 2002. *Illness as Metaphor & AIDS and its Metaphors*. London

Watney, S., 1996. Policing Desire: Pornography, AIDS, and the Media. University of Minnesota Press

TWO OLD FRIENDS:
Leprosy (Hansen's Disease)... and Tuberculosis

Chapter 59

Two Old Friends: leprosy (Hansen's Disease)

'Girls and women affected by Hansen's disease face the added issue of gender and social discrimination, which may also delay detection of the disease. In some countries, the law allows a person to legally divorce a spouse if they are affected by the disease. Unfortunately, this sometimes leaves many women destitute, homeless, and unable to care for their children.'
World Leprosy Day: Bust the Myths, Learn the Facts;
National Center for Emerging and Zoonotic Infectious Diseases,
Division of High Consequence Pathogens and Pathology, 2018

Leprosy is an infectious disease caused by a bacillus, *Mycobacterium leprae*. *M. leprae* develops slowly with an average incubation period of five years. Symptoms can occur between one year or as long as twenty years after infection. It is increasingly known by the name Hansen's Disease after the Norwegian scientist Gerhard Henrik Armauer Hansen, who in 1873 discovered the slow-growing bacterium as the cause of the illness. It was also the first bacterium to be identified as causing disease in humans.

The disease chiefly affects the skin, the peripheral nerves, mucosa of the upper respiratory tract, and the eyes. It is, however, curable with multidrug therapy. It seems likely that it is transmitted via droplets, through coughing and sneezing, during close and frequent contact with untreated cases. Leprosy does not spread during pregnancy to the unborn child, or through sexual contact. Untreated, leprosy can cause progressive and permanent damage to the skin, nerves, limbs, and eyes while treatment in the early stages can prevent disability.

There are two main types of the disease – paucibacillary and multibacillary, which differ in the number of bacteria present. There were 208,619 new leprosy cases registered around the world in 2018, down from 5.2 million in the 1980s. According to WHO figures. New cases routinely occur in 14 countries, with India accounting for more than half (60 per cent) followed by Indonesia (8 per cent). In the 20 years from 1994 to 2014, 16 million people worldwide were cured of leprosy.

Clinical issues apart, throughout history people afflicted have often been ostracized and marginalised by their communities and families. Mythology surrounding the disease and innate stereotyping are usually to blame.

The first modern breakthrough in treatment was in the 1940s when Novartis developed Dapsone; however Dapsone must be taken over a very long time to be effective, making compliance difficult. In the 1960s, *M. leprae* started to develop resistance to Dapsone; fortunately Rifampicin and Clofazimine were discovered by Novartis and added to the treatment regimen as multidrug therapy (MDT). This treatment lasts for six months for pauci-bacillary and twelve months for multi-bacillary cases. MDT acts by killing the pathogen and curing the patient. Rifampicin, or rifampin, is an antibiotic used to treat bacterial infections including tuberculosis, M. avium complex, leprosy, and Legionnaires' disease.

Since 1995 WHO has provided MDT free of charge. Free MDT was initially funded by The Nippon Foundation, and since 2000 it is donated through an agreement with Novartis. Since 2000, Novartis has been providing MDT free of charge to all leprosy patients through the WHO, donating more than 56 million MDT blister packs valued at over $ 90 million, helping to treat over 6 million leprosy patients worldwide. In 2015, as part of its commitment to the London Declaration on Neglected Tropical Diseases (NTDs), Novartis announced the extension of this MDT donation through to 2020. This five-year agreement includes treatments worth more than $40 million and up to $2.5 million to support the WHO in handling the donation and logistics. Overall the programme will reach an estimated 1.3 million patients during the five-year period. Elimination of leprosy as a public health problem (defined as a registered prevalence of less than 1 case per 10,000 population) was achieved globally in 2000.

Since 1981, more than 16 million people have been treated for leprosy through MDT, reducing the global burden by 99 per cent – a public health success story by any measure. The case detection rate for leprosy has plateaued at about 200,000–250,000 over the past 10 years, but the disease remains endemic in many countries in Asia, Africa and Latin America; even countries with low overall endemicity may have localized high-burden pockets. Approximately 10 per cent of newly diagnosed leprosy patients are children. The challenge is still how to interrupt transmission of leprosy.

The Bacillus Calmette–Guérin (BCG) vaccine offers some protection against leprosy in addition to its usual indication for tuberculosis. The WHO concluded in 2018 that the BCG vaccine at birth reduces leprosy risk and is recommended in countries with high incidence of TB and leprosy. Development of a more effective vaccine is ongoing.

Today Hansen's Disease mainly affects people in poorer countries who live in crowded conditions and for whom accessing health care is difficult due to the often long distances to clinics which are au fait with the disease, and to the expense of going to the doctor. Because of this many patients fail to report their illness or don't complete their treatment plan, or don't even get one. In addition, due to the persistent stigma against people with Hansen's Disease, they may not seek help when first symptoms appear, causing delay in diagnosis and the development of disabilities.

Leprosy Stigma

The disease takes its name from the Greek word λέπρα (léprā), from λεπίς (lepís; 'scale'). The barbaric practice of quarantining people affected by leprosy by placing them in leper colonies still happens in some areas of India, China, Africa, and Thailand.

Most colonies have closed since leprosy is not particularly contagious. British India enacted the Leprosy Act of 1898 which institutionalized those affected and segregated them by sex to prevent reproduction. The Act was difficult to enforce and was finally repealed in 1983 but only after multidrug therapy had become widely available.

The word 'leper' is now usually considered offensive due to its negative connotations. The phrase 'person affected with leprosy' does the job just as well without the derogatory connotoations of 'leper'; Leprosy Mission International advocates for the end of the use of the term 'leper'. World Leprosy Day started in 1954 to draw awareness to those affected by leprosy.

Barret, Ronald 2005. 'Self-Mortification and the Stigma of Leprosy in Northern India'. *Medical Anthropology Quarterly*. 19 (2), 216–230.

Jopling, William, 1991, 'Leprosy stigma', *Leprosy Review* 62, 1–12.

Leprosy Mission, Don't call me a leper – Campaign With Us – Join with us – The Leprosy Mission. www.leprosymission.org.uk.

White, Cassandra, 2017. 'Clinical and Social Aspects of Leprosy (Hansen's Disease) and Contemporary Challenges to Elimination', *Journal of Dermatology and Clinical Research*. 5: 1097 https://www.nippon-foundation.or.jp/app/uploads/2019/01/en_wha_pro_lep_03.pdf

History

Skeletal remains from around 2000 BC, discovered in 2009, are the oldest documented evidence for leprosy, located at Balathal, in Rajasthan, northwest India. A proven human case was verified by DNA taken from the shrouded remains of a man discovered in a tomb at the Old City of Jerusalem dated by radiocarbon methods to AD 1–50.

Descriptions of leprosy, or what was thought to be leprosy go back many thousands of years. Various dermatological diseases translated as leprosy appear in the ancient Indian text, the *Atharava Veda* in 600 BC. The *Manusmriti* (200 BC), prohibited contact with those infected with the disease and made marriage to a person infected with leprosy a crime. The Sanskrit medical treatises, the Susrata and the Charaka mention leprosy, as *maha kustha*. According to the former *kustha* is a contagious disease transmitted either through sexual activity, by touch and respiration or by handling objects previously handled by an infectious person. This remarkably precise description of leprosy's infectivity by the Hindu physicians is a landmark in disease diagnosis indicating that leprosy was rampant in India during the first millennium BC.

For ancient Egypt two Coptic mummies from near Aswan were described in 1910 as dating from around 500 BC, one male and one female. The man exhibited the tell-tale bone destruction on the hands and feet while the woman displayed *facies leprosa*. *Facies leprosa* is characterized by a combination of nasal change and resorption of nasal bone, anterior nasal spine, supra-incisive alveolar region and anterior alveolar process of the maxillae, associated with the loss of upper incisors. Danish paleopathologist Vilhelm Møller-Christensen confirmed these to be cases of leprosy.

For the Pharaonic period Polish researcher T. Dzierzykray-Rogalski discovered 31 skulls in a second century necropolis in the Daklah Oasis of which four had leprous stigmata. Was this a deportation station for leprosy victims during the reign of Lagides? In ancient France a skull from the Merovingian era (6th century) has been discovered with leprous stigmata while five cases from Britain have been described from around AD 550–600.

In the Bible, any progressive skin disease, for example, a whitening or splotchy bleaching of skin, raised manifestations of scales, scabs, infections, rashes as well as generalized moulds and surface discoloration of any clothing, leather, or discoloration on walls or surfaces throughout homes – all of these came under the 'law of leprosy' (Leviticus 14:54–57). The *Talmud* (Sifra 63) makes it clear that tsara or tzaraat (צ.ר.ע– tsaw-rah' – to be struck with leprosy, to be leprous) refers to various types of lesions or stains associated with ritual impurity and occurring on cloth, leather, or houses, as well as skin.

The New Testament describes Jesus healing people with leprosy in Luke 17:11, although the relationship between this disease, tzaraath, and Hansen's Disease is not clear. The biblical view that people with leprosy were unclean is in a passage from Leviticus 13: 44–46: 'But if the bright spot is white on the skin of his body, and it does not appear to be deeper than the skin, and the hair on it has not turned white, then the priest shall isolate him who has the infection for seven days.' Some early Christians believed that those affected by leprosy were being punished by God for sinful behaviour. Moral associations have persisted throughout history. Pope Gregory the Great (540–604) and Isidor of Seville (560–636) considered people with the disease to be heretics.

Leprosy was covered by Hippocrates in 460 BC while in 1846, Francis Adams published *The Seven Books of Paulus Aegineta* which included a commentary on all medical and surgical knowledge and descriptions and remedies related to leprosy by the Romans, Greeks and Arabs. Soldiers of Pompey's army, returning to Italy in 62 BC, brought leprosy with them, probably as a new disease, according to Pliny the Elder. The Epicurean philosopher Lucretius (98–55 BC) calls leprosy the elephant disease, confusing it with elephantiasis; Celsus (fl. AD 25) declares that leprosy was rare in Italy, but gives an excellent description of it nevertheless. Excavations, 1966 to 1973, at the 4th century AD Romano-British cemetery at Poundbury Camp in Dorset has yielded a skeleton bearing the distinctive marks of the disease (*The Times* 8 November, 1974). The first hospital for the relief of lepers was founded early in the fourth century in Rome during the reign of Constantine and in AD 372 St Basil established a leper hospital in Cesarna.

Anglo-Saxon England saw several so-called leper-houses established notably by Lanfranc, Archbishop of Canterbury. He organized charitable relief in his see, and in 1084 endowed a hospital for leprosy at Herbaldown in the woods of Blean. Later a hospital was established for 25 leprous sisters at Tannington outside Canterbury. One for leprous monks was built in 1137, called St Lawrence's. Other leper houses were at Nottingham (625), York (936), London and Beverley (both before the Conquest), Chatham (1078) and Northampton (during the reign of William I). The return of the

Crusaders from lands where leprosy was endemic will not have helped. The Crusades presented the church with a huge theological paradox as the church sent victims on their way with its blessing and a promise of inviolability, but taught that leprosy was a punishment by God for wrong-doing. This invested leprous Crusaders with a kind of holy aura. Sufferers from leprosy even came to be called Christ's poor. High born ladies, even royalty like Queen Matilda, wife of Henry I, washed and kissed the feet of those afflicted by leprosy, as an act of compassion and charity, and probably with the tacit hope of gaining favourable treatment on the day of judgement.

In the Middle Ages it would seem that there was a rise in leprosy in Western Europe based on the increased number of hospitals established to treat people with leprosy in the 12th and 13th centuries. France alone had nearly 2,000 leprosariums.

Generally speaking, medieval communities were fearful of people infected with the disease whom they considered to be unclean, duplicitous and and morally corrupt. Segregation from mainstream society was the norm, and people with leprosy were often, humiliatingly, required to wear clothing that identified them as such or to carry a bell announcing their presence. On the plus side, though, the bell was useful for attracting charity. The Third Lateran Council of 1179 and a 1346 edict by Edward III expelled lepers from city limits. More humiliation came with the primitive and crude testing techniques which were conducted on those suspected of having the disease: these were administered by a motley committee of unqualified village elders and other sufferers. They involved seeing how long it took for grains of salt to dissolve in their blood, examining hair and urine, jabbing their extremities with needles and observing facial characteristics through a charcoal flame. On a less scientific level diagnoses were made on the strength of whether the patient 'looked loathsome' or 'satyr-like'.

Norway led the way in taking an enlightened stance on leprosy tracking and treatment and played an influential role in European understanding of the disease. In 1832, Dr. J.J. Hjort conducted the first leprosy survey, thus establishing a basis for future epidemiological surveys. Subsequent surveys resulted in the establishment of a national leprosy registry to study the causes of leprosy and for tracking of the rate of infection.

Other early leprosy research was conducted by Norwegian scientists Daniel Cornelius Danielssen and Carl Wilhelm Boeck whose work led to the establishment of the National Leprosy Research and Treatment Center. Danielssen and Boeck believed the cause of leprosy transmission to be hereditary which was a persuasive factor in advocating for the isolation of those infected by sex to prevent reproduction.

The British presence in India brought Britain into contact with a country which was all too familiar with the scourge of leprosy. Isolation treatment methods were championed by Surgeon-Major Henry Vandyke Carter of the British Colony in India with the financial and logistical assistance of religious missionaries. Colonial and religious influence and associated stigma continued to be a major factor in the treatment and public perception of leprosy in endemic developing countries until the mid-twentieth century.

Leprosy stigma continues to be a major problem in developing countries where the disease is endemic. Leprosy is most common amongst impoverished or marginalized populations where social stigma is likely to be compounded by other associated social inequities. As noted fears of ostracism, loss of employment, or expulsion from family and society may contribute to a delayed diagnosis and treatment. Some who have suffered from Hansen's Disease describe the impact of social stigma as far worse than the physical manifestations despite it being only mildly contagious and curable.

Mythology

Here are just some of the daft myths that still circulate and need to be exploded: fake news by another name stoking the blame culture and prejudice that has dogged Hansen's Disease patients since time immemorial.

Some of the above content comes from the National Center for Emerging and Zoonotic Infectious Diseases, Division of High Consequence Pathogens and Pathology, Centres for Disease Control and Prevention.

Table 5: Myths surrounding leprosy

Myth *Leprosy is very contagious and easy to catch.*

Fact No. Leprosy is difficult to catch, and in fact, 95% of adults don't catch it because their immune system can fight off the bacteria that causes HD. Leprosy was once believed to be highly contagious and was treated with mercury, as was syphilis, which was first described in 1530. Many early cases thought to be leprosy could actually have been syphilis.

Myth *Leprosy causes the fingers and toes to fall off.*

Fact No, it certainly does not. The digits do not 'fall off' due to leprosy. What actually happens is the bacteria that causes leprosy attacks the nerves of the fingers and toes and causes them to become numb. Burns and cuts on numb parts may therefore go unnoticed, which may lead to infection and permanent damage, and eventually the body may reabsorb the digit. This happens in advanced stages of untreated disease.

Myth *The leprosy described in historical and religious texts is the same leprosy we know today.*

Fact Historical leprosy is not the same as modern leprosy. The 'leprosy' found in historical and religious texts described a variety of skin conditions from rashes and patchy skin to swelling. They were noted to be very contagious, which is not true for Hansen's disease and also did not have some of the most obvious signs of Hansen's Disease, like disfigurement, blindness, and loss of pain sensation. The term was also used for mildew on a person's clothes, possessions or living quarters.

Myth *Leprosy is the result of a sin or curse.*

Fact No it is not. Leprosy is caused by *Mycobacterium leprae*.

Myth *People who have leprosy need to live in special houses (leper colonies) isolated from healthy people.*

Fact People with leprosy who are being treated with antibiotics can live a normal life among their family and friends and can continue to attend work or school.

Myth *You can get leprosy when sitting next to someone who has the disease.*

Fact You cannot get leprosy through casual contact such as shaking hands, sitting next to or talking to someone who has the disease. The vast majority (95 per cent) of people who are exposed to *M. Leprae* do not develop leprosy

---

Myth *Once you catch leprosy, you will die.*
Fact Leprosy can be and is cured with antibiotic treatment.
Myth *You are contagious until your treatment is complete.*
Fact A person ceases to be contagious within 72 hours of starting the treatment with
    antibiotics. However, the treatment must be finished as prescribed (which may take up to 2
    years) to make sure the infection doesn't come back.

Folk beliefs, poor education, and stigmatic connotations of the disease continue to influence social perceptions of those afflicted in many parts of the world. In Brazil, for example, folklore maintains that leprosy is transmitted by dogs, it is a disease associated with sexual promiscuity, and is sometimes thought to be a punishment for sins committed or moral transgressions, as distinct from other diseases being accorded to the will of God. Lower-class domestic workers often find their employment in jeopardy when dermatological manifestations of the disease become apparent. In northern India, leprosy is sometimes equated with, according to Ronald Barrett, an 'untouchable' status that 'often persists long after individuals with leprosy have been cured of the disease, creating lifelong prospects of divorce, eviction, loss of employment, and ostracism from family and social networks.'

The last case of leprosy in Britain was in the late 18th century in the Shetland Isles. Girls and women affected by Hansen's Disease face the added issue of gender and social discrimination, which may also delay detection of the disease. In some countries, the law allows a person to legally divorce a spouse if they are proven to have the disease. Unfortunately, this sometimes leaves many women destitute, homeless, and unable to care for their children.

Persecution

In the Middle Ages in Europe leprosy was something of a paradox. For example Bernard of Clairvaux saw leprosy as a divine gift inculcating repentance in the sufferer. French surgeon Guy de Chauliac (d. 1368) similarly believed leprosy not to be a curse but a manifestation of divine election, shortening the obligatory stay in purgatory because of the torments endured in life. Others saw the disease as a punishment for sexual sin and as a STI. Growing fear in the community surrounding lepers prompted the church to legislate for the separation of lepers from society around 1220. They were banned from the streets of London in 1200 and 1273.

Covey, Herbert C., 2001. 'People with leprosy (Hansen's disease) during the Middle Ages'
    Social Science Journal. 38 (2): 315–321.
Grzybowski, Andrzej, 2016, 'Leprosy in the Bible'. *Clinics in Dermatology*. 34 (1): 3–7.
Inskip, S; Taylor, 2017. 'Leprosy in pre-Norman Suffolk, UK: biomolecular and
    geochemical analysis of the woman from Hoxne' *Journal of Medical Microbiology*.
    66 (11): 1640–1649.
Rawcliffe, Carole, 2009, *Leprosy in Medieval England*, Woodbridge
Worobec, S.M., 2008. 'Treatment of leprosy/Hansen's disease in the early 21st century'.
    Dermatologic Therapy. 22 (6): 518–37.

Chapter 60

... tuberculosis

'We are facing an unprecedented pandemic. A quarter of the world's population is infected and, between 2020 and 2021, it is predicted that 10 million people will have fallen ill, 3 million will not have been diagnosed or received care, and more than 1 million – mainly the most vulnerable – will have died.'
'This pandemic is not COVID-19 but tuberculosis.'
– Lancet Respiratory Medicine 8, (6), 536–538, June 1, 2020

This prescient and sobering article goes on to tell us 'both diseases have considerable social impact – including stigma, discrimination, and isolation – in addition to the economic impact from country productivity losses and catastrophic costs to individuals and households... COVID-19, like tuberculosis, will almost certainly be associated with the medical poverty trap, in which poorer people have a higher likelihood of infection, disease, and adverse outcomes. Moreover, unemployed populations and informal or so-called zero-hours contract workers will experience further impoverishment, which increases risk of tuberculosis'.

Tuberculosis (TB) is an infectious disease most often caused by *Mycobacterium tuberculosis* (MTB) bacteria which usually affects the lungs, but can also affect other parts of the body. Most infections are asymptomatic when it is known as latent tuberculosis. About 10 per cent of latent infections progress to active disease which, if left untreated, kills about half of those affected. The classic symptoms of active TB are a chronic cough with blood-containing mucus, fever, night sweats, and weight loss. Infection of other organs cause a wide range of symptoms.

Tuberculosis is spread from person to person through the air when people with active TB in their lungs cough, spit, speak, or sneeze. People with latent TB do not spread the disease. Active infection occurs more often in people with HIV/AIDS and in smokers. People infected with TB bacteria have a 5–15% lifetime risk of falling ill with TB. Treatment requires the use of multiple antibiotics over a long period of time. Antibiotic resistance is a growing problem with increasing rates of multiple drug-resistant tuberculosis (MDR-TB) and extensively drug-resistant tuberculosis (XDR-TB).

The statistics are shocking and astonishing:

- As of 2018 one quarter of the world's population is thought to have latent infection with TB. New infections occur in about 1 per cent of the population each year.

- A total of 1.4 million people died from TB in 2019 (including 208 000 people with HIV). This makes it the number one cause of death from an infectious disease.
- Worldwide, TB is one of the top 10 causes of all deaths.
- People with active TB can infect 5–15 other people through close contact over the course of a year. Without proper treatment, 45 per cent of HIV-negative people with TB on average and nearly all HIV-positive people with TB will die.
- In 2019, an estimated 10 million people fell ill with tuberculosis worldwide resulting in 1.5 million deaths: 5.6 million men, 3.2 million women and 1.2 million children. Child and adolescent TB is often missed by health providers and can be difficult to diagnose and treat.
- People with HIV are 18 times more likely to develop active TB. The risk of active TB is also greater in persons suffering from other conditions that impair the immune system. Malnourished people are 3 times more at risk. Globally in 2019, there were 2.2 million new TB cases in 2018 that were attributable to malnutrition .
- Alcohol abuse and tobacco smoking increase the risk of TB disease by a factor of 3.3 and 1.6, respectively. In 2019, 0.72 million new TB cases worldwide were attributable to alcohol abuse and 0.70 million were attributable to smoking.
- TB is present in all countries and age groups. The good news is that TB is curable and preventable.
- In 2019, the 30 high TB burden countries accounted for 87 per cent of new TB cases. Eight countries account for two thirds of the total, with India the most, followed by Indonesia, China, the Philippines, Pakistan, Nigeria, Bangladesh and South Africa. About half of the global burden of MDR-TB is in three countries – India, China and the Russian Federation. (60 per cent of reported cases), followed by Brazil (13 per cent) and Indonesia (8 per cent)
- Multidrug-resistant TB (MDR-TB) remains a public health crisis and a health security threat. A global total of 206,030 people with multidrug or rifampicin-resistant TB (MDR/RR-TB) were detected and notified in 2019, a 10 per cent increase from 186,883 in 2018.
- Globally, TB incidence is falling at about 2 per cent per year and between 2015 and 2019 the cumulative reduction was 9 per cent. This was less than half way to the End TB Strategy milestone of 20 per cent reduction between 2015 and 2020.
- An estimated 60 million lives were saved through TB diagnosis and treatment between 2000 and 2019.

Ending the TB epidemic by 2030 is among the health targets of the United Nations Sustainable Development Goals (SDGs).
Source: WHO https://www.who.int/news-room/fact-sheets/detail/tuberculosis

Tuberculosis has assumed many names over the centuries. The ancient Greeks called it phthisis (Φθίσις), their word for consumption. Hippocrates described phthisis as a disease of dry seasons. The abbreviation 'TB' is short for tubercle bacillus. 'Consumption' was the most common nineteenth century English word for the disease. The Latin root 'con' meaning 'completely' is linked to 'sumere' meaning 'to take up from under'.

In *The Life and Death of Mr Badman* by John Bunyan, the author calls consumption 'the captain of all these men of death.' 'Great white plague' has also had its day.

Results of a 2014 genome study from the University of Tübingen suggest that tuberculosis is more recent than previously thought. Scientists were able to recreate the genome of the bacteria from remains of 1,000-year-old skeletons excavated in southern Peru. In dating the DNA, they found it was less than 6,000 years old. However there is evidence that the first tuberculosis infection happened about 9,000 years ago in the Neolithic age in Atlit Yam, a settlement in the eastern Mediterranean, when it spread to other humans along trade routes. It also infected domesticated animals in Africa, such as goats and cows. Seals and sea lions breeding on African beaches are believed to have acquired the disease and carried it across the Atlantic to South America. Infected skeletons have been found in a cave at Arma dell'Aqjuila in Liguria dating around 5800 BC. Before the Tübingen study the first evidence of the disease in South America was detected in remains of the Arawak culture around 1050 BC. The most significant finding belongs to the mummy of an 8 to 10-year-old Nascan child from Hacienda Agua Sala, dated AD 700. Scientists were able to isolate evidence of the bacillus.

Traces of the disease have also been found in Egyptian mummies dated between 3000 and 2400 BC., the most convincing of which was found in the mummy of priest Nesperehen, discovered by Grebart in 1881, which exhibited evidence of spinal tuberculosis with the characteristic psoas abscesses. Similar features were discovered on other mummies such as that of the priest Philoc and throughout the cemeteries of Thebes. It appears likely that Akhenaten and his wife Nefertiti both died from tuberculosis, and evidence indicates that hospitals for tuberculosis existed in Egypt as early as 1500 BC. The Ebers papyrus, that important Egyptian medical treatise from around 1550 BC, describes a pulmonary consumption associated with the cervical lymph nodes. It recommended that it be treated with the surgical lancing of the cyst and the application of a ground mixture of acacia seyal, peas, fruits, animal blood, insect blood, honey and salt. A 2700 BC Chinese text refers to the disease.

Deuteronomy 28:22 mentions a consumptive illness that would afflict the Jewish people if they stray from God. It is listed in the section of curses given before they enter the land of Canaan. In ancient India the earliest reference is in the *Rigved*a, 1500 BC, which calls the disease yaksma. *Sushruta Samhita*, written around 600 BC, recommends that the disease be treated with breast milk, various meats, alcohol and rest. The *Yajurveda* advises sufferers to move to higher altitudes.

China can boast numerous references, including the c. 400 BC – 260 BC *Huangdi Neijing* classic Chinese medical text which describes a disease believed to be tuberculosis, called xulao bing (虛癆病 'weak consumptive disease'); the *Huangdi Neijing* describes an incurable disease called huaifu 壞府 'bad palace' (meaning chest) - the text states: 'poisonous drugs bring no cure; it cannot be seized with short needles'. Song dynasty (920–1279) Daoist priest-doctors first recorded that tuberculosis, called shīzhài 尸瘵 (literally 'corpse disease') changes a living being into a corpse.

In the classical era the first reference is in Herodotus' *Histories* 7 in which he relates how a Persian general, Pharnouches in 481 BC, was left behind in Sardis, because he was clearly very ill. He had been thrown from his horse and was vomiting blood due to consumption. His servants cut off the horse's legs at the knees and Pharnouches was discharged from his command, abandoning Xerxes' campaign against the Spartans. Hippocrates, in Book 1, 1,2 of his *Of the Epidemics*, describes the characteristics of the disease: fever, colourless urine, cough resulting in a thick sputa, and loss of thirst and appetite. He notes that most of the sufferers became delirious before they succumbed to the disease. Hippocrates and many other at the time believed phthisis to be hereditary in nature. Aristotle disagreed, believing the disease was contagious.

In Rome one of Pliny the Younger's letters is to Priscus in which he details the symptoms of phthisis presented in Fannia: 'The attacks of fever stick to her, her cough grows upon her, she is in the highest degree emaciated and enfeebled.[1] Galen proposed a series of therapeutic treatments for the disease, including: opium as a sleeping agent and painkiller; blood letting; a diet of barley water, fish, and fruit. He also described the phyma (tumor) of the lungs. Vitruvius, the architect, noted in his *De Architectura* (16,3), that 'cold in the windpipe, cough, pleurisy, phthisis, [and] spitting blood', were common diseases in regions where the wind blew from north to northwest, and advised that walls be so built as to shelter individuals from the winds. Aretaeus was the first to rigorously describe the symptoms of the disease in his text *De causis et signis diuturnorum morborum* ending his description with: 'otherwise of cadaverous aspect...' In his *De curatione diuturnorum morborum*, he recommends that sufferers travel to high altitudes, travel by sea, eat a good diet and drink plenty of milk.

In the 1020s AD Ibn Sina (Avicenna) gave us the first study of TB in his *Canon of Medicine*. He it was who first identified TB as an infectious disease and made the association with its spread through soil and water. He also pioneered quarantine for TB patients.

The *Breviary of St Batholomew* recommended treatment with white wine, liquorice and river crabs, and occasionally sharing a bath with boiled animals.

Medieval Hungary is interesting: during the Inquisition pagans were put on trial: a 12th century document recorded a description of tuberculosis which the pagans claimed was produced when a dog-shaped demon occupied the person's body and started to eat his lungs. When the possessed person coughed, the demon was barking and gearing up to kill the victim.

It was Girolamo Fracastoro who was the first to propose, in his *De contagione* in 1546, that phthisis was transmitted by an invisible virus. Among his claims were that the virus could survive between two or three years on the clothes of those with the disease and that it was usually transmitted through direct contact or the discharged fluids of the infected (fomes).

The incidence of tuberculosis grew steadily during the Middle Ages and Renaissance, displacing leprosy as the most prevalent of diseases and peaking between the 18th and 19th century as workers moved from the fields to the cities for work. In 1808,

---

1. Pliny the Younger, *Letters* 7,19

William Woolcombe was astounded at the prevalence of tuberculosis in 18th-century England: of the 1,571 deaths in Bristol between 1790 and 1796, 683 were due to tuberculosis. Even remote towns slowly succumbed. Consumption deaths in the village of Holycross in Shropshire between 1750 and 1759 were one in six; ten years later, one in three. In London, one in seven died from consumption in the early 18th century, which by 1750 had grown to one in five and to one in four by the start of the 19th century. The Industrial Revolution along with overcrowding, poverty and squalor just made things worse.

TB gained the dubious reputation for being 'the Romantic' disease due to the number of victims from the arts. The poets Keats, Shelley, and Edgar Allan Poe had it as did Chopin, Chekhov, Kafka, Katherine Mansfield, Emily, Anne, Charlotte and Branwell Brontë, Dostoevsky, Thomas Mann, W. Somerset Maugham, George Orwell, and Robert Louis Stevenson, and the artists Watteau, Edvard Munch, Aubrey Beardsley and Amedeo Modigliani either had the disease or mixed with people who did.

Interestingly all three of the Brontë sisters write of consumptive characters: Helen Burns in *Jane Eyre*; Frances Hindley in *Wuthering Heights* and labourer Mark Wood in *Agnes Grey*.

Tuberculosis also haunts Thomas Mann's The Magic Mountain, set in a sanatorium; in popular music it appears, as in Van Morrison's 'T.B. Sheets'; in opera, as in Puccini's *La Bohème* and Verdi's *La Traviata*; in art, as in Monet's painting of his first wife Camille on her deathbed; and in film, such as the 1945 The Bells of St. Mary's starring Ingrid Bergman as a nun with tuberculosis.

Tuberculosis caused alarm in the 19th and early 20th centuries as the disease flourished among the increasing number of urban poor. In 1815 one in four deaths in England was due to 'consumption'. By 1918, TB still caused one in six deaths in France. Hermann Brehmer opened the first TB sanatorium in 1859 in Görbersdorf (now Sokołowsko) in Silesia. After TB was found to be contagious, in the 1880s, it was put on the notifiable disease list in Britain; campaigns started to stop people from spitting in public places, and the infected poor were 'encouraged' to enter sanatoria. Unfortunately these resembled prisons, although the sanatoria for the middle and upper classes offered excellent care and medical attention. Whatever, even under the best conditions, 50 per cent of those who were admitted died within five years around 1916. When the Medical Research Council formed in Britain in 1913, it initially focused on tuberculosis research.

Azher, M., 2013, The next Pandemic - Tuberculosis: The oldest disease of mankind rising one more time. *Br J Med Pract*.6: a615

Comstock, G.W., 1994. 'The International Tuberculosis Campaign: a pioneering venture in mass vaccination and research'. *Clinical Infectious Diseases*. 19 (3): 528–40.

Karamanou, Marianna, 2012, The Masterful Description of Pulmonary Tuberculosis by Soranus of Ephesus (c. 98–138 A.D.), *American Journal of Respiratory and Critical Care Medicine* 186

Morens, D.M., 2002. 'At the deathbed of consumptive art'. *Emerging Infectious Diseases*. 8 (11): 1353–8.

Wilsey, A.M., 2012. 'Half in Love with Easeful Death': Tuberculosis in Literature. Humanities Capstone Projects (PhD thesis). Pacific University.

Wingfield, T., 2018, Addressing social determinants to end tuberculosis. *Lancet* 391: 1129–1132

Chapter 61

Severe acute respiratory syndrome (SARS), 2002

'Scientists were close to a coronavirus vaccine years ago. Then the money dried up "we just could not generate much interest," a researcher [Dr. Peter Hotez] said of the difficulty in getting funding to test the vaccine in humans.'
— Mike Hixenbaugh, *New York Times*, 5 March 2020

The disturbing article continues:

'That was a big missed opportunity, according to Hotez and other vaccine scientists, who argue that SARS, and ... MERS, of 2012, should have triggered major federal and global investments to develop vaccines in anticipation of future epidemics. Instead, the SARS vaccine that Hotez's team created...is sitting in a freezer, no closer to commercial production than it was four years ago.'

Peter Hotez is co-director of the Center for Vaccine Development at Texas Children's Hospital and dean of the National School of Tropical Medicine at the Baylor College of Medicine in Houston.

SARS is an airborne virus and can spread through small droplets of saliva in a similar way to colds and influenza. SARS can also be spread indirectly via surfaces that have been touched by someone who is infected with the virus and subsequently transferred to the mucous membranes, and through human faeces. It was the 21st century's first severe and readily transmissible new disease and exhibited a clear facility to spread along the routes of international air travel and other lines of communication. This how the WHO introduces SARS – https://www.who.int/health-topics/severe-acute-respiratory-syndrome#tab=tab_1

Severe acute respiratory syndrome (SARS) is a viral respiratory disease of zoonotic origin caused by severe acute respiratory syndrome coronavirus (SARS-CoV or SARS-CoV-1). It was first identified at the end of February 2003 during an outbreak in China and spread to four other countries. SARS-CoV is thought to be an animal virus – probably implicating Asian palm civets and a colony of cave-dwelling horseshoe bats in Yunnan. It then mutated and first infected humans in the Guangdong province of southern China in November 2002 where the first case was reported the same month in a farmer from Shunde, Foshan,

Guangdong who was treated in the First People's Hospital of Foshan. The patient died soon after, but no definite diagnosis was made on cause of death. Despite efforts to control it, China did not inform the World Health Organization of the outbreak until February 2003, three months later. Obviously this lack of transparency caused delays in efforts to control the epidemic, with very serious consequences. The area is today considered as a potential zone of re-emergence of SARS-CoV.

The first the international medical community knew about the outbreak was on 27 November 2002, when Canada's Global Public Health Intelligence Network (GPHIN) picked up reports of a 'flu outbreak' in China and sent them to the WHO. An English report was not generated until 21 January 2003; ten days later the first 'super-spreader' was admitted to the Sun Yat-sen Memorial Hospital in Guangzhou, which soon infected nearby hospitals. The WHO requested information from Chinese authorities on 5 and 11 December but it did not receive intelligence reports unti several months after the outbreak. By the time the WHO took action, over 500 deaths and an additional 2,000 cases had already occurred worldwide.

Tragedy followed tragedy when in February 2003 an American businessman travelling from China, Johnny Chen, went down with pneumonia-like symptoms while on a flight to Singapore. The plane stopped over in Hanoi, Vietnam, where Chen died in Hanoi French Hospital. Several of the medical staff who treated him soon developed the disease despite basic hospital cross-infection procedures. Italian doctor Carlo Urbani identified the threat and communicated it to the WHO and the Vietnamese Health Ministry whom he persuaded to begin isolating patients and screening travellers, thus slowing the early pace of the epidemic; Urbani later succumbed in March 2003. On 12 March 2003, the WHO issued a global alert, followed by a health alert by the United States Centers for Disease Control and Prevention. Local transmission of SARS was now happening in Toronto, Ottawa, San Francisco, Ulaanbaatar, Manila, Singapore, Taiwan, Hanoi and Hong Kong, and within China.

The disease spread in Hong Kong from Liu Jianlun, a Guangdong doctor who was treating patients at Sun Yat-Sen Memorial Hospital. He arrived in February and stayed on the ninth floor of the Metropole Hotel in Kowloon, infecting sixteen of the hotel guests. Those guests travelled on to Canada, Singapore, Taiwan and Vietnam, taking SARS with them. In Hong Kong its spread was probably exacerbated by defects in the bathroom drainage system at the Amoy Gardens housing estate; this allowed sewer gases including virus particles to vent into the bathrooms. Fans expelled the gases and wind carried the contagion to adjacent houses downwind.

In Toronto the first case came on 23 February 2003: an elderly woman, Kwan Sui-Chu, who had just returned from Hong Kong died on 5 March. Her son Tse Chi Kwai inadvertently infected other patients at the Scarborough Grace Hospital and died on 13 March. A second major wave of cases was centered on accidental exposure among patients, visitors, and staff in the North York General Hospital.

The official response by the Ontario provincial government and Canadian federal government has been described as 'very, very basic and minimal at best' with poorly outlined and enforced protocol for protecting healthcare workers and identifying infected patients, described as a major contributing factor to the continued spread of the virus. The climate of fear and uncertainty surrounding the outbreak resulted in healthcare workers resigning rather than risk exposure to SARS.

In late May 2003, studies conducted on samples of wild animals sold as food in the local market in Guangdong found that the SARS coronavirus could be isolated from masked palm civets even if the animals were asymptomatic. The conclusion was that the SARS virus crossed the xenographic barrier from palm civets to humans: more than 10,000 palm civets were exterminated in Guangdong Province. The virus was also later found in raccoon dogs, ferret badgers and domestic cats. In 2005, two studies identified a number of SARS-like coronaviruses in Chinese bats. In late 2006, scientists from Hong Kong University and the Guangzhou Centre for Disease Control and Prevention established a genetic link between the SARS coronavirus appearing in civets and humans, substantiating claims that the disease had jumped across species. In December 2017, 'after years of searching across China, where the disease first emerged, researchers reported ... that they had found a remote cave in Yunnan province, which is home to horseshoe bats that carry a strain of a particular virus known as a coronavirus. This strain has all the genetic building blocks of the type that triggered the global outbreak of SARS in 2002.'

The research was undertaken by Shi Zhengli, Cui Jie with co-workers at the Wuhan Institute of Virology, China, and published in *PLOS Pathogens*. The authors offer us a stark warning that 'another deadly outbreak of SARS could emerge at any time. The cave where they discovered their strain is only a kilometre from the nearest village.' The virus is seasonal in bats.

In 2019, the related virus strain severe acute respiratory syndrome coronavirus 2 (SARS-CoV-2) was discovered. This causes COVID-19, a disease responsible for the COVID-19 pandemic which emerged at the end of 2019.

In the end SARS affected twenty-six countries and resulted in 8,098 cases in 2003 and 774 deaths (9.56 per cent). People over the age of 65 were particularly at risk, with over half of those who died from the infection being in this age group. Most patients who contracted SARS were previously healthy adults aged between 25 and 70 years. Only a few suspected cases of SARS have been reported among children under 15. Patients under 24 were least likely to die (less than 1 per cent); those 65 and older were most likely to die (over 55 per cent). As with MERS and COVID-19, SARS caused many more deaths of males than females.

Since the end of the global epidemic in July 2003, SARS has reappeared four times – three times from laboratory accidents in Singapore and Taipei, and once in southern China where the source of infection remains undetermined although there is circumstantial evidence of animal-to-human transmission.The majority of human-to-human transmission cases occurred in the health care setting, where adequate infection control precautions were lacking. The subsequent implementation of appropriate infection control practices put an end to the global outbreak.

The incubation period is usually 2–7 days but may be as long as 10 days. The first symptom of the illness is generally fever (>38°C) sometimes associated with

Table 6: Probable cases > 100 of SARS by country 1 November 2002 – 31 July 2003

COUNTRY	CASES	DEATHS	FATALITY %
CHINA	5,327	349	6.6
HONG KONG	1,755	299	17.0
TAIWAN	346	73	21.1
CANADA	251	43	17.1
SINGAPORE	238	33	13.9

chills and rigors. It may also be accompanied by other symptoms including headache, general malaise and muscle pain. At the onset of illness, some cases have mild respiratory symptoms. Typically, rash and neurologic or gastrointestinal findings are absent, although a few patients have reported diarrhoea during the early febrile stage. After 3–7 days, a lower respiratory phase begins with the onset of a dry, non-productive cough or shortness of breath that may be accompanied by, or progress to, hypoxemia (low blood oxygen levels). In 10–20 per cent of cases, the respiratory illness is severe enough to require intubation and mechanical ventilation. The white blood cell count is often decreased early in the disease, and many people have low platelet counts at the peak of the disease.

There is currently no cure or vaccine for SARS. According to the WHO, controlling outbreaks relies on containment measures including: prompt detection of cases through effective surveillance networks and including an early warning system; isolation of suspected cases; tracing to identify both the source of the infection and contacts of those who are sick and may be at risk of contracting the virus; quarantine of suspected contacts for ten days; exit screening for outgoing passengers from areas with recent local transmission by asking questions and temperature measurement; and disinfection of aircraft and cruise vessels having SARS cases on board using WHO guidelines. Personal preventive measures to prevent spread of the virus include frequent hand washing using soap or alcohol-based disinfectants. For those with a high risk of contracting the disease, such as health care workers, use of personal protective equipment, including a mask, goggles and an apron should be mandatory. Whenever possible, household contacts should also wear a mask. As we lamented at the beginning of this chapter, Peter Hotez's potentially world changing vaccine still languishes in that fridge, deprived of the funding which would test whether it would be effective in humans.

Abraham, Thomas, 2004. *Twenty-first Century Plague: The Story of SARS*

Fauci, Anthony, 'Pandemic Preparedness in the Next Administration: Keynote Address by Anthony S. Fauci'. YouTube video 14 February 2017.

Hixenbaugh, Mark, March 2020, https://www.nbcnews.com/health/health-care/scientists-were-close-coronavirus-vaccine-years-ago-then-money-dried-n1150091

Kahn, Joseph, 12 July 2007. 'China bars U.S. trip for doctor who exposed SARS cover-up'. *The New York Times*.

Low, Donald, 2004. Learning from SARS: Preparing for the Next Disease Outbreak: Workshop Summary.

The 'Swine Flu' of 2009

'In January 2010, Wolfgang Wodarg, then chair of the health committee at the Council of Europe, claimed major firms had organized a "campaign of panic" to put pressure on the WHO to declare a "false pandemic" to inflate sales of vaccines. Wodarg said the WHO's "false pandemic" flu campaign is "one of the greatest medicine scandals of the century".'

First described in April 2009, the virus, H1N1/09, appeared to be a new strain of H1N1 which resulted from a previous triple reassortment of bird, swine, and human flu viruses that further combined with a Eurasian pig flu virus, giving the name 'swine flu'. Criticism centred on how inappropriate names can, and do, confuse or mislead the public. In itself swine flu incorrectly implied that the disease is caused by contact with pigs or pig products.

Inappropriate naming and labelling of viruses generally gave rise to stigmatization and blame against certain communities, not least in this instance, Mexicans. Research published in 2013 concluded that Mexican Americans and Latino Americans had indeed been stigmatized due to the frequent use of term 'Mexican flu' in the news media.

Science ran an article with the title 'Swine Flu Names Evolving Faster Than Swine Flu Itself'. In April 2009 Azerbaijan imposed a ban on the importation of animal husbandry products from the entire Americas. The Indonesian government also halted the importation of pigs and initiated the examination of 9 million pigs. The Egyptian government left nothing to doubt and slaughtered all pigs on 29 April. Such are the consequences of sloppy, prejudicial naming.

The virus originated in Veracruz, Mexico, or in the south-western USA, and probably came directly from intensively-farmed pigs. It caught everybody by surprise because although warnings of a new plague had been issued regularly for years, it had been expected that the next pandemic would involve the highly pathogenic avian influenza virus H5N1, which had been recurring since 1997. Thankfully, the new virus turned out to be relatively mild.

Symptoms of infection were similar to seasonal influenza, albeit with a greater incidence of diarrhoea and vomiting. The virus was also found to preferentially bind to cells deeper in the lungs than seasonal viruses: this explained both why it was generally mild – it did not often penetrate that far – but also why it could be fatal, as it had the potentiality to cause severe and sudden pneumonia if it did penetrate deep enough, similar to the 1918 influenza. Binding to cells in the intestines also explained the uncharacteristic nausea and vomiting. It was also found that there were distinct high-risk groups, including pregnant women and the obese. Unusually and uncharacteristically, unlike most strains of influenza, the H1N1/09 virus does not disproportionately infect adults over age 60 .

Vaccine manufacture was initiated in June 2009; however, as happened with other pandemics, there was insufficient vaccine manufactured soon enough to deal effectively with the pandemic – even though similarities between this virus and the 1977 outbreak virus meant that most middle-aged people had pre-existing immunity to it, which either prevented infection, or reduced the severity of infections. This also meant that a single dose was sufficient in adults when it was initially thought that two injections would be required; vaccine stocks, therefore, went twice as far. In 2011, a study from the US Flu Vaccine Effectiveness Network estimated the overall effectiveness at 56 per cent. A CDC study released in 2013, estimated that the pandemic H1N1 vaccine saved roughly 300 lives and prevented about a million illnesses in the US. The study concluded that, had the vaccination programme started two weeks earlier, close to 60 per cent more cases could have been prevented.

While the disease may have been mild in most cases, and initially the death toll was considered low, by 2012 it was calculated that 300,000 or more people probably died, mainly in Africa and Southeast Asia. The virus has now become a normal seasonal strain, replacing the previously-circulating H1N1, but interestingly, has not replaced the H3N2 that has circulated since 1968.

As we have seen, there has been much criticism of the WHO and of big pharma companies relating to conflict of interest and attempts to cynically increase profits. In June 2010, Fiona Godlee, editor-in-chief of the *BMJ*, published an editorial which criticised the WHO, saying that an investigation had disclosed that some of the experts advising WHO on the pandemic had financial ties with drug companies which were producing antivirals and vaccines.

Caitjan Gainty, a historian of 20th-century medicine and technology at King's College London, has an interesting slant on the response to swine flue. She tells us that there were more than 18,500 lab-recorded deaths from swine flu during the pandemic, but statistical modelling suggests the true extent of deaths could have been as high as 570,000. She observes that the narrative around swine flu was closer to that of national security than healthcare:

'The language of preparedness and national security brought into common use during the cold war applied nicely to infectious disease. In the post 9/11 context, this language moved from useful metaphor to actual policy, quite explicitly in the US, where natural disasters and epidemic disease were placed in the remit of the Department of Homeland Security. Swine flu, like coronavirus today, was not just like a threat to national security. It was an official adversary.'

Chan, M., 8 June 2010. 'WHO Director-General's letter to BMJ editors'. World Health Organization.

Fineberg, H.V., April 2014. 'Pandemic preparedness and response – lessons from the H1N1 influenza of 2009'. *The New England Journal of Medicine*. 370 (14): 1335–42.

Flynn, P., 23 March 2010. 'The handling of the H1N1 pandemic: more transparency needed' memorandum, Social, Health and Family Affairs Committee, The Council of Europe.

MacKenzie, Debora, 29 April 2009. 'Swine flu: The predictable pandemic?'. *New Scientist*

Chapter 62

MERS: 2012 – Middle East respiratory syndrome coronavirus outbreak

'In 2014, a study published in the New England Journal of Medicine indicated that camel-to-human transmission of the virus was possible. In November 2013, a man became ill with MERS after tending to a sick camel. On 24 April 2014, a 25-year-old male from Jordan tested positive for the coronavirus. He had history of exposure to camels and had drunk camel milk.'

Ten years after the SARS pandemic, coronavirus hit again, this time in the guise of Middle East Respiratory Syndrome (MERS). MERS is a viral respiratory disease caused by a novel coronavirus (Middle East respiratory syndrome coronavirus, or MERS-CoV); it was first reported on 24 September 2012 by an Egyptian virologist, Dr. Ali Mohamed Zaki in Jeddah, Saudi Arabia.

In February 2013, the first UK case was confirmed in Manchester in an elderly man who had recently visited the Middle East and Pakistan; it was the tenth case globally. The man's son, whom he visited in hospital in Birmingham, was immuno-suppressed due to a brain tumour and contracted the virus, providing the first clear evidence for person-to-person transmission. He died on 19 February 2013. The second fatality was a 49-year-old Qatari man who had visited Saudi Arabia before falling ill. After forty-eight hours in a Qatari hospital he required intubation and ventilation and was transferred by air ambulance to London on 11 September. During transfer, he was clinically unstable, requiring manual ventilation. He was admitted to St Mary's Hospital and was later transferred to Guys & St Thomas's Hospital. As a result of a post by Ali Mohammed Zaki on Pro-MED, the novel coronavirus was quickly identified. He was treated for respiratory disease but, like the first patient in Saudi Arabia, died of kidney failure in October 2012.

Another patient who had been in Guys & St Thomas Hospital in the UK since September 2012 after visiting the Middle East died on 28 June 2013. A spokesperson for the hospital stated that 'Guys and St Thomas can confirm that the patient with severe respiratory illness due to novel coronavirus (MERS-COV) died on Friday 28 June, after his condition deteriorated despite every effort and full supportive treatment.'

As of April 2014, the European Centre for Disease Prevention and Control reported a total of four cases in the United Kingdom, three of which were fatalities.

Table 7: MERS Cases and Deaths, April 2012 to 15 November, 2013

COUNTRY	CASES (Deaths)
FRANCE	2 (1)
ITALY	1 (0)
JORDAN	2 (2)
OMAN	1 (0)
QATAR	8 (3)
SAUDI ARABIA	127 (53)
TUNISIA	3 (1)
UNITED KINGDOM (UK)	4 (3)
UNITED ARAB EMIRATES (UAE)	6 (2)
Total	154 (65) 42.2 per cent

Source: http://www.cdc.gov/coronavirus/mers/

Coronaviruses are a large family of viruses that can cause diseases ranging from the common cold to Severe Acute Respiratory Syndrome (SARS). Typical MERS symptoms include fever, cough and shortness of breath. Pneumonia is common, but not always present. Gastrointestinal symptoms, including diarrhoea, have also been reported. Some laboratory-confirmed cases of MERS-CoV infection are reported as asymptomatic yet they are positive for MERS-CoV infection following a laboratory test. Most of these asymptomatic cases have been detected following aggressive contact tracing of a laboratory-confirmed case. Approximately 40 per cent of reported patients with MERS-CoV infection have died.

Although most human cases of MERS-CoV infections are attributed to human-to-human infections in health care settings, current scientific research suggests that bats and dromedary camels may be major zoonotic reservoir hosts for MERS-CoV and an animal source of MERS infection in humans. On 4 June 2014, a study published in the *New England Journal of Medicine* indicated that camel-to-human transmission of the virus was possible. In November 2013, a man became ill with MERS after tending to a sick camel. DNA samples taken from the man, who eventually died of the virus, and the sick animal were virtually identical. This provided very strong evidence that the man had picked up the virus from the camel. On 24 April 2014, a 25-year-old male from Jordan tested positive for the coronavirus. He had history of exposure to camels and had drunk camel milk.

However, the World Organization for Animal Health (OIE) announced that 'currently there is no strong evidence that camels are source of infection for human cases of MERS'.

By May 2013, 10 of the 22 people who had died and 22 of 44 cases reported were in Saudi Arabia and over 80 per cent were male. This gender disparity may be because most women in Saudi Arabia wear niqabs that cover the mouth and nose, decreasing their chances of being exposed to the virus? Saudi health and religious officials were naturally very anxious about the six million or so Muslims from around the world who would potentially be exposed to the virus during the autumn Hajj. Not only might it infect pilgrims in Saudi Arabia but many of the pilgrims would be returning to numerous other countries with a potentiality to spread it back home.

Arabi, Y.M., 2017, Middle East respiratory syndrome. N Engl J Med.; 376:584–594

The Economist, 20 April 2013, An ounce of prevention: As new viruses emerge in China and the Middle East, the world is poorly prepared for a global pandemic'.

Khazan, O., 21 June 2013. 'Face Veils and the Saudi Arabian Plague'. *The Atlantic*.

Oh, M.D., 2018 Middle East respiratory syndrome: what we learned from the 2015 outbreak in the Republic of Korea, *Korean J Intern Med.*; 33, 233–246.

Chapter 63

Ebola virus disease 2013–16

'*The Ebola virus disease outbreak in west Africa is pivotal for the worldwide health system. Just as the depth of the crisis ultimately spurred an unprecedented response, the failures of leadership suggest the need for innovative reforms.*'
– Professor Lawrence O. Gostin, O'Neill Institute for National and Global Health Law, Georgetown University Law Center, Washington, DC

In 2013 the infectious disease medical community turned its focus to west Africa when outbreaks of Ebola occurred in Guinea, Sierra Leone and Liberia. The 2013–16 outbreak was the first to reach epidemic proportions. Earlier outbreaks had been brought under control much more efficiently but in 2013 extreme poverty, fragile healthcare systems, distrust of government after years of armed conflict, and a delay in responding for several months, all conspired to bring about a failure to control the epidemic. Other unhelpful factors included local burial customs which demanded washing the bodies of the deceased and the unprecedented spread of Ebola ravaging densely populated cities in the region. The sinister virus, however, had been around for some time already.

Ebola virus disease (EVD; also known as Ebola hemorrhagic fever, or EHF), or just Ebola, is a disease of humans and other primates caused by ebolaviruses. Ebolaviruses were first described in 1976 in two virtually simultaneous outbreaks, one in Nzara, South Sudan and the other in Yambuku, northern Democratic Republic of Congo. The one in Yambuku occurred in a village near the Ebola River from where the disease takes its name.

In 1990, Hazelton Research Products' Reston Quarantine Unit in Reston, Virginia, suffered a mysterious outbreak of fatal illness among a shipment of crab-eating macaque monkeys imported from the Philippines. A laboratory test known as an ELISA assay showed antibodies to Ebola virus. Soon afterwards, a US Army team at the United States Army Medical Research Institute of Infectious Diseases (USAMRIID) euthanized those monkeys which had not yet died, bringing the monkeys and those which had already died of the disease for study by the Army's veterinary pathologists and virologists, and eventual disposal under safe conditions. The Philippines and the United States had no history of Ebola infection, and upon further isolation, researchers concluded it was another strain of Ebola, or a new filovirus of Asian origin, which they named Reston ebolavirus (REBOV) after the location of the incident.

By 30 August 2007, 103 people (100 adults and three children) were infected by a suspected haemorrhagic fever outbreak in the village of Kampungu, Democratic

Republic of the Congo. The outbreak started after the funerals of two village chiefs when 217 people in four villages fell ill. The WHO sent a team to take blood samples for analysis and confirmed that many of the cases were the result of Ebolavirus. On 30 November 2007, the Uganda Ministry of Health confirmed an outbreak of Ebola in the Bundibugyo District. After confirmation of samples tested by the United States National Reference Laboratories and the Centers for Disease Control, the WHO confirmed the presence of a new species of Ebolavirus, which was tentatively named Bundibugyo. The epidemic came to an official end on 20 February 2008 but not before 149 cases of this new strain were reported, 37 of which were fatal.

On Christmas Day 2008, it was reported that the Ebola virus had killed 9 and infected 21 people in the Western Kasai province of the Democratic Republic of Congo. On 29 December, Médecins Sans Frontières reported 11 deaths in the same area, adding that a further 24 cases were being treated. In January 2009, Angola closed down part of its border with the Democratic Republic of Congo to prevent the spread of the outbreak.

Signs and symptoms typically begin between two days and three weeks after contracting the virus with a fever, sore throat, muscle pain and headaches. Then, vomiting, diarrhoea and rash usually follow, along with decreased function of the liver and kidneys. Some patients begin to bleed both internally and externally. The disease has a high mortality rate killing between 25 per cent and 90 per cent of those infected with an average of about 50 per cent. This is often due to low blood pressure from fluid loss, and typically follows six to sixteen days after symptoms first appear.

How is it spread? By direct contact with body fluids, such as blood, from an infected human or animals. It can also spread through contact with a recently contaminated item or surface. Airborne transmission has not been documented in either laboratory or natural conditions. If an infected person survives, recovery may be quick and complete. Prolonged cases, as we have seen with Post-Ebola Syndrome, are often complicated by long-term problems, such as inflammation of the testicles, joint pains, muscle pains, skin peeling or hair loss. Ophthalmological symptoms such as uveitis, light sensitivity, excess tearing, iritis, iridocyclitis, choroiditis and blindness have also been described and are particularly worrying given the shortage of ophthalmologists in west Africa.

We suspect that fruit bats are natural carriers of disease, able to spread the virus without being affected by it; they are a significant food source for both humans and wildlife. Bats are known to be carriers of at least ninety different viruses that can make the transition to a human host. Transmission is believed to be by contact with the blood and body fluids of those infected with the virus, as well as by handling raw bushmeat such as bats and monkeys, important sources of protein in west Africa. Infectious body fluids include blood, sweat, semen, breast milk, saliva, tears, faeces, urine, vaginal secretions, vomit and diarrhoea.

On 14 September 2015, the National Ebola Response Center confirmed the death of a 16-year-old female in a village in the Bombali district. Swabs taken from the body tested positive for the disease. The village was placed under quarantine. She had no history of traveling outside the village, and it is suspected that she contracted the disease from the semen of an Ebola survivor who was discharged in March 2015. A study published in *Lancet Global Health*, (August 2016) indicates that the virus may lurk in the semen of survivors for a year after recovering from the disease and, in one man's case, at least 565 days after he recovered from illness.

Breast milk may contain the virus for two weeks after recovery, and transmission of the disease to a baby may be possible. By October 2014, it was suspected that handling a piece of contaminated paper may be enough to contract the disease; this obviously has implications for medical record documentation and record keeping.

In July 2012, the Ugandan Health Ministry confirmed 13 deaths due to an outbreak in the Kibaale District. On 28 July, it was reported that 14 out of 20 (70 per cent mortality rate) had died in Kibaale. On 8 August, the Ugandan Ministry of Health recorded 23 probable and confirmed cases, including 16 deaths. Ten cases were confirmed by the Uganda Virus Research Institute as Ebola. During the incubation period of twenty-one days 185 people who came into contact with probable and confirmed Ebola cases were followed up.

On 17 August, the Ministry of Health of the Democratic Republic of the Congo reported an outbreak in the eastern region. By 21 August, the WHO reported a total of 15 cases and 10 fatalities. By 13 September 2012, the WHO revealed that the virus had claimed 32 lives and that the probable cause of the outbreak was tainted bush meat hunted by local villagers.

During 2013 the WHO reported a total of 1,716 cases in 24 outbreaks. The final death rate among hospitalised patients was 57–59 per cent; as of 8 May 2016, the WHO and the governments involved reported a total of 28,646 suspected cases and 11,323 deaths (39.5 per cent), though the WHO believes this figure to be seriously understated. Minor outbreaks occurred in Nigeria and Mali, and secondary infections of medical workers occurred in the United States and Spain. There were also isolated cases in Senegal, the United Kingdom and Italy. The case numbers peaked in October 2014 whereupon they began to decline gradually, following the commitment of substantial international resources.

Guinea

We now believe that a one or two-year-old boy, Emile Ouamouno fell ill on 2 December 2013 and died four days later in the village of Méliandou, Guinea. Researchers believe that the boy contracted the virus while he was playing near a tree that was a roosting place for free-tail bats infected with the virus. The boy's sister was ill next, followed by his mother and grandmother. Emile was the index case of the western African epidemic. Emile's midwife probably spread the disease to other villages. Local doctors and villagers knew about other fatal diseases such as Tai Forest virus in Côte d'Ivoire, and early cases were mis-diagnosed as other diseases more common to the area such as Lassa fever. The disease, therefore, had several months to spread before it became recognised as Ebola.

By 10 April 2014, 157 suspected and confirmed cases and 101 deaths had been reported in Guinea, 22 suspected cases in Liberia including 14 deaths, 8 suspected cases in Sierra Leone including 6 deaths, and 1 suspected case in Mali. By late May, the outbreak had spread to Conakry, Guinea's capital with about two million inhabitants. By late June 2014, the death toll had reached 390 with over 600 cases reported. By 23 July 2014, the World Health Organization had reported 1,201 confirmed cases including 672 deaths since the epidemic began in March. On 31 July 2014, WHO reported the death toll had reached 826 from 1,440 cases.

In August, Guinea's President Alpha Conde declared a national health emergency and, to control the Ebola virus, measures would include forbidding Ebola patients from leaving their homes, border control, travel restrictions and hospitalization for individuals suspected to be infected until cleared by laboratory results. He also banned transporting the dead between towns. Effective disease tracing was essential to prevent the outbreak from spreading. Previous Ebola outbreaks had occurred in remote areas making containment less problematic; the current outbreak struck in a highly-mobile and densely populated region which made tracking more difficult: 'This time, the virus is travelling effortlessly across borders by plane, car and foot, shifting from forests to cities and springing up in clusters far from any previously known infections. Border closures, flight bans and mass quarantines have been ineffective.'

Peter Piot, who co-discovered Ebola, said Ebola 'isn't striking in a "linear fashion" this time. It's hopping around, especially in Liberia, Guinea and Sierra Leone.' Infected people and those that they were in contact with evaded surveillance, moving around at will and concealing their illness while they infected others in turn. Entire villages, stricken by fear, closed themselves off, giving the disease an opportunity to strike in another area.

Containment was also difficult due to an irrational fear of healthcare workers. In some areas it was believed that health workers were spreading the disease on purpose, while others thought that the disease was a fabrication. Riots broke out in the regional capital, Nzérékoré; rumour had it that people were being contaminated when health workers sprayed a market area to decontaminate it. The frightening sight of healthcare workers wearing the obligatory protection outfits and taking those suspected of having Ebola, or of being contacts, to the treatment centre perhaps never to be seen again led to talk of organ harvesting and government and tribal plots. According to a September news report, 'Many Guineans say local and foreign healthcare workers are part of a conspiracy which either deliberately introduced the outbreak, or invented it as a means of luring Africans to clinics to harvest their blood and organs.' Another alarmist news report said:

> 'The health workers don't look like any people you've ever seen. They perform stiffly and slowly, and then they disappear into the tent where your mother or brother may be, and everything that happens inside is left to your imagination. Villagers began to whisper to one another—They're harvesting our organs; they're taking our limbs.'

To make matters even worse, many frightened people were not going to hospital for treatment for other ailments and were self-medicating with over the counter drugs from pharmacies.

Table 8: 2013–14 Ebola virus epidemic in West Africa

COUNTRY	CASES	DEATHS	END OF OUTBREAK
Liberia	10,675	4,809	9 June 2016
Sierra Leone	14,124	3,956	17 March 2016
Guinea	3,811	2,543	1 June 2016
Nigeria	20	8	19 October 2014
Mali	8	6	18 January 2015
United States	4	1	21 December 2014
Italy	1	0	20 July 2015
United Kingdom	1	0	10 March 2015
Senegal	1	0	17 October 2014
Spain	1	0	2 December 2014
Total	28,646	11,323	as of 8 May 2016

Things came to a tragic, bloody head when on 18 September, eight members of a health care team were murdered by local villagers in the town of Womey near Nzérékoré. The team consisted of Guinean health and government officials accompanied by journalists, who had been distributing Ebola information and performing disinfection work. They were attacked with machetes and clubs: their bodies were found in a septic tank. On 20 November, the local Red Cross in Kankan Prefecture sent blood samples via a courier whose taxi was hijacked by robbers. The bandits made off with the cooler bag containing the blood samples.

Sierra Leone

On 29 July, prominent virologist Sheik Umar Khan, Sierra Leone's only expert on haemorrhagic fever, died after contracting Ebola at his clinic in Kenema. Khan had spent years working on Lassa fever, a disease that kills over 5,000 a year in Africa. He had expanded his clinic to admit Ebola patients and is credited with treating over 100 patients before succumbing himself. Although Khan was fastidious in donning PPE in the clinical setting 'and I make sure my nurses are all in theirs' he was in the habit of embracing cured Ebola patients as they left his ward, to lift their spirits and mitigate the stigma Ebola patients faced.

For a number of reasons he was not offered a dose of the experimental drug ZMapp although one was available. ZMapp is an experimental biopharmaceutical preparation composed of three monoclonal antibodies produced in tobacco by molecular farming. Leaf Biopharmaceutical, a San Diego-based arm of Mapp Biopharmaceutical, is developing the composite drug.

The drug highlights the problems drug development and clinical trials have with allegations of racism. That ZMapp was first given to Americans and a European and not to Africans, according to the *Los Angeles Times*, 'provoked outrage, feeding into African perceptions of Western insensitivity and arrogance, with a deep sense of mistrust and betrayal still lingering over the exploitation and abuses of the colonial era.' However, Salim S. Abdool Karim, the director of an AIDS research centre in South Africa, added some context, perhaps, when, responding to a question on how people might have reacted if ZMapp and other drugs had first been used on Africans, he said: 'It would have been the front-page screaming headline: "Africans used as guinea pigs for American drug company's medicine".'

On 30 July, Sierra Leone declared a state of emergency and deployed troops to quarantine hot spots and in August enacted a law that subjected anyone harbouring someone believed to be infected to two years in jail. Prevention also included limiting the spread of disease from infected animals to humans by handling potentially infected bush meat only while wearing protective clothing and by thoroughly cooking it before it is consumed.

WHO estimated on 21 September, that Sierra Leone's capacity to treat Ebola cases fell short by the equivalent of some 532 beds. There were reports that political interference and administrative incompetence had hindered the flow of medical supplies into the country.

Sierra Leone imposed a three-day lockdown on its population from 19 to 21 September during which time 28,500 trained community workers and volunteers went door-to-door providing education on how to prevent infection, as well as setting up community Ebola surveillance teams. The campaign was named the 'Ouse to Ouse Tock' in Krio language; 80 per cent of targeted households were reached in the operation and at least 150 new cases were uncovered. During the lock-down a burial team was attacked.

By 2 October 2014, an estimated five people per hour were being infected with the Ebola virus in Sierra Leone. On 4 October, the country recorded 121 fatalities, the largest number in a single day. On 8 October, Sierra Leone burial crews went on strike. Before that there were reports of drunken grave-diggers making graves for Ebola patients too shallow with the result that wildlife was digging up and eating the corpses. There were also cases of bodies not being buried for days. Meanwhile, other diseases like malaria, pneumonia, and diarrhoea were going untreated because the health system was preoccupied with Ebola patients. Officials reported that very few pregnant women were surviving Ebola. Authorities struggled to maintain order in one town after a medical team trying to take a blood sample from a corpse was intercepted by an angry machete-wielding mob. When security forces arrived to protect the medical team, a riot ensued leaving two dead.

On 1 November, the United Kingdom announced plans to build three more Ebola laboratories in Sierra Leone. At the time, it took as long as five days to test a sample due to the volume involved. In Freetown food shortages and aggressive quarantines exacerbated the situation, according to the Disaster Emergency Committee. On 12 November, more than 400 health workers went on strike over salary issues at one of the few Ebola treatment centres in the country. On 12 December, Sierra Leone banned all public festivities for Christmas or New Year. In December Médecins Sans Frontières, in partnership with the Ministry of Health, carried out the largest-ever distribution of antimalarials in Sierra Leone. Teams distributed 1.5 million antimalarial treatments in Freetown and surrounding districts with the aim of protecting people from malaria during the disease's peak season. A spokesman said:

> 'In the context of Ebola, malaria is a major concern, because people who are sick with malaria have the same symptoms as people sick with Ebola. As a result, most people turn up at Ebola treatment centres thinking that they have Ebola, when actually they have malaria. It's a huge load on the system…'

The *New York Times* of 5 October reported that a shipping container full of protective gowns, gloves, stretchers, mattresses and other medical supplies had sat unopened on the docks in Freetown since 9 August. The $140,000 worth of equipment included 100 bags and boxes of hospital linens, 100 cases of protective suits, 80 cases of face masks and other items, all donated by individuals and institutions in the United States. Politics had again triumphed over public health. Government officials stated that the shipping container could not be cleared through customs, as proper procedures had not been followed. The Sierra Leonean government refused to pay the shipping fee of $6,500 even though, as the *New York Times* noted, the government had already received well over $40 million in cash from international donors to fight Ebola. In the two months that the container languished on the dockside in Freetown, health workers in Sierra Leone endured severe shortages of PPE, with some nurses forced to wear street clothes to work.

On October 21, the eastern town of Koidu saw Ebola related violence: local youths opened fire at police with shotguns after a former youth leader was refused health authority's permission to take her relative for an Ebola test. Several buildings were attacked and youth gangs roamed the streets shouting 'No more Ebola!' A local leader reported seeing two bodies with gunshot wounds in the aftermath. Police denied that anyone had been killed. Doctors reported two dead. The local district medical officer said he had been forced to abandon the local hospital because of the rioting.

Panic and superstition reigned: here are just three of the conspiracy theories:

- The Ebola outbreak was triggered by a bewitched aircraft that crashed in a remote part of Sierra Leone, casting a spell over three West African countries – but a strong alcoholic drink called 'Bitter Kola' can cure the virus.
- Ebola virus was a bad spirit, a devil or poisoning.
- Ebola virus did not exist: 'I thought it was a lie concocted to collect money because at that time I hadn't seen any people affected in my community.'

Here are some of the more tangible impacts of the virus in Sierra Leone, good and bad:

- The outbreak was noted for increasing hand washing stations, and reducing the prevalence of physical greetings such as hand-shakes. Liberia renounced its traditional finger-snap greeting.
- In June 2014 all schools were closed because of the spread of Ebola.
- In August 2014 the Sierra Leone Health Minister was removed from office.

- On 13 October the UN's International Fund for Agricultural Development reported that up to 40 per cent of farms had been abandoned in the worst Ebola-hit areas.
- In October 2014 Sierra Leone launched a 'school by radio program' transmitted on 41 of the local radio stations and on the only TV station.

Ebola in Liberia

In a *Los Angeles Daily News* (13 October 2014) article titled 'Some people would rather die of Ebola than stop hugging sick loved ones', the paper shows how in Liberia, Cokie Van der Velde, a sanitation specialist with Médecins Sans Frontières who organizes body collections in Monrovia said that in late September the main crematorium was running at full capacity, burning 80 bodies at a time on its mass pyre. In early October, the number of bodies had dropped to 30 or 40 a day. 'That means they're being kept hidden and buried in secret,' she said. Why would anyone hide contagious corpses or bury them secretly? For good reason: to honour the deceased and see them safely through to the next world, a *sine qua non* of the sequence of life. Because of Ebola, dignified rituals were replaced by an anonymous infection control team showing up in emergency hazmat suits, visors and masks to cart away your loved one for a soulless, utterly impersonal mass cremation and mass crisis burial.

Before the outbreak of Ebola Liberia was still reeling from a civil war that ended in 2003 leaving the country with few doctors for its population of 4.3 million. On 30 March 2014, Liberia confirmed its first two cases of Ebola; by 23 April, 34 cases and 6 deaths were recorded; by 17 June, 16 people had succumbed. Initial cases were misdiagnosed as malaria leading to doctors being infected with the Ebola virus. By 17 June 7 patients died from the disease at Redemption Hospital, including a nurse, along with other members of her household. On 2 July, the head surgeon of Redemption Hospital died from the disease; Redemption Hospital was shut down, and patients transferred or referred to other facilities in the area. On 21 July 4 nurses at Phebe Hospital in Bong County contracted the disease and on 27 July, Samuel Brisbane, one of Liberia's leading doctors, succumbed; a doctor from Uganda also died from the disease. Two US health care workers, Dr. Kent Brantly and a nurse, Nancy Writebol, were also infected with the disease. Both of them were missionaries and were medically evacuated from Liberia to the US for treatment where they made a full recovery.

By 28 July, most border crossings had been closed, with medical checkpoints set up at the remaining ports; there were quarantines in some areas. Some flights were suspended and schools were closed. On 27 August, wild dogs were seen eating unburied corpses, potentially making the dogs carriers of the disease. On 18 August, a mob of residents from the impoverished Monrovia suburb of West Point, raided a local Ebola clinic. The protesters turned violent, threatening the caretakers, releasing the infected patients, and looting the clinic of its supplies, as well as blood-stained bed sheets and mattresses. This raised fears of mass infections in West Point. Sanitation has always been an issue in most parts of Monrovia: there are four public toilets in the West Point area for its 70,000 inhabitants. The beach and the Mesurado River at

West Point are used as a toilet. The river is a source of drinking water, and the fish from the water are a primary source of food for many.

Bribery was rife either to falsify death certificates to hide Ebola as cause of death and thereby procure a traditional funeral for the deceased or else to dodge quarantine orders. A black market for the blood of Ebola survivors sprang up with buyers hoping to gain immunity or recovery via an ad hoc blood transfusion. For those who survived the procedure all they got was enhanced exposure to HIV/AIDS, malaria and other blood-borne diseases.

Despite increasing capacity with a new clinic in Monrovia, the WHO estimated that by 23 September, there were 3,458 cases, 1,830 deaths (52.9 per cent). All three Monrovia clinics were overrun with patients, some dying as they waited outside to be treated. There were cases in Monrovia where the bodies were dumped into the river. One woman used bin liners to protect herself as she cared for four other sick family members. On 3 October, at least eight Liberian soldiers died after contracting the disease from a female visitor to their barracks. On 10 October all journalists were banned from entering Ebola clinics. Liberia was declared free from the virus on 14 January 2016.

In addition to the three main areas of Sierra leone, Guinea and Liberia there were limited outbreaks in Senegal, Nigeria and Mali.

Cases outside Africa

Emory University Hospital in Atlanta was the first US hospital to admit patients exposed to Ebola. As we have seen, two American health care workers, Kent Brantly and Nancy Writebol, were exposed while treating infected patients in Liberia. Arrangements were made for them to be transported to Emory in a special aircraft. Emory Hospital boasts a purpose built isolation unit set up in collaboration with the CDC to treat people exposed to certain serious infectious diseases. The pair received the experimental drug ZMapp.

On 30 September 2014, the CDC declared its first case of Ebola. Eric Duncan became infected in Liberia and travelled back to Dallas, Texas. On 26 September, he fell ill but was sent home from hospital with antibiotics. He returned on 28 September and was placed in isolation and tested for Ebola; he died on 8 October having infected two nurses who had treated him; later they were declared Ebola-free. On 23 October Craig Spencer, an American physician who had returned to the United States after treating Ebola patients in western Africa, tested positive for the virus. Spencer recovered.

These imported cases in the United States, and in those in Spain, led to secondary infections of medical workers but did not spread further. On 5 August 2014, the Brothers Hospitallers of Saint John of God confirmed that Brother Miguel Pajares, who had been volunteering in Liberia, had become infected. He was evacuated to Spain and died on 12 August after being given ZMapp. On 21 September Brother Manuel García Viejo, another Spanish citizen who was medical director at the San Juan de Dios Hospital in Lunsar, was evacuated to Spain from Sierra Leone after being infected with the virus. He died on 25 September. In October, a nursing assistant, Teresa Romero, who had cared for these patients tested positive for Ebola, making this the first confirmed case of Ebola transmission outside Africa. By 19 October, Romero had recovered.

On 24 August 2014. William Pooley, a British nurse who contracted the disease while working in Sierra Leone as part of the relief effort for the Ebola virus epidemic was medically evacuated by the Royal Air Force on a specially-equipped C-17 aircraft. He was admitted to the high-level isolation unit at the Royal Free Hospital and discharged on 3 September 2014.

On 29 December 2014, Pauline Cafferkey, a British aid worker for Save the Children who had just returned to Glasgow from working at the treatment centre in Kerry Town, was diagnosed with Ebola at Glasgow's Gartnavel General Hospital. She was treated and declared free of infection and released from hospital on 24 January 2015. However, on 8 October, she was readmitted for serious complications caused by the virus. On 14 October, her condition was listed as 'critical' and 58 individuals were being monitored while 25 close contacts received an experimental vaccination. On 21 October, it was reported that she had been diagnosed with meningitis caused by the virus residing in her brain and replicating at a very low level until it had replicated to a degree capable of causing clinical meningitis: Post Ebola Syndrome? On 12 November, she was discharged from hospital after making a full recovery. On 23 February 2016, she was admitted for a third time, 'under routine monitoring by the Infectious Diseases Unit ... for further investigations'.

Dr Martin Deahl, a consultant psychiatrist who travelled back from Sierra Leone with Ms Cafferkey, criticised the screening process at Heathrow as 'a bit chaotic'. He said there were too few staff to deal with the returning health workers, the rooms in which they were processed were too small, and the processing team ran out of home-testing temperature kits to hand out. Dr Deahl described the quarantine advice as 'topsy turvy', adding he found it 'bizarre' that passengers were free to make their own way home from Heathrow but thereafter advised to minimise use of public transport.

On 17 March, it was reported that a UK military worker while working as a nurse had been repatriated from Sierra Leone for fear that she had contracted the virus through a needlestick injury while treating a patient in Kerry Town treatment centre. Corporal Anna Cross was taken in a specially adapted ambulance to the high level isolation unit at London's Royal Free Hospital. She tested positive for Ebola, and was the first person in the world to be treated with the experimental Ebola drug MIL 77; she made a full recovery.

These were not the first British cases: in 1976 Geoffrey Platt, a laboratory technician at the former Microbiological Research Establishment in Porton Down, Wiltshire, contracted Ebola in an accidental needlestick injury from a contaminated needle while handling samples from Africa. He was treated with human interferon and convalescent serum; he recovered fully.

As of 18 December 2014, the WHO and respective governments have reported a total of 19,078 suspected cases and 7,413 deaths, although WHO believes that this figure is substantially understated.

As noted above, the situation was not helped in any way by the fragility and inadequacies of some of the health care systems involved. Many of the seriously affected areas are extremely poor and have limited access to soap and running water for handwashing – given that there was barely enough clean water to drink. Traditional folk medicine and cultural practices came into play which involve physical contact with the deceased, especially funerary customs such as washing the body of the deceased. Some hospitals lacked basic supplies, particularly of PPE and were understaffed, which only increased the chance of staff catching the virus: in August, the WHO reported that 10 per cent of the fatalities were health care workers leading to the additional problem of recruiting foreign medical staff.

On 26 September WHO announced that '[the] Ebola epidemic ravaging parts of Western Africa is the most severe acute public health emergency seen in modern times' and its Director-General called the outbreak 'the largest, most complex and most severe we've ever seen'. In March 2015, the United Nations Development Group reported that a decrease in trade, closing of borders, flight cancellations, and drop in foreign investment and tourism activity fuelled by stigma, had caused vast economic consequences in both the areas directly affected in western Africa as well as other African nations with no cases of Ebola.

After a trial of an experimental Ebola vaccine involving 11,000 people in Guinea, Merck & Co, the vaccine's Darmstadt manufacturer, announced in 2019 that Ervebo, the first FDA-approved vaccine for the prevention of Ebola virus disease was found to be 'highly protective' against the virus. This confirmed the results of a study published in 2015 that awarded the vaccine 100 per cent effectiveness after tests on 3,537 people in Guinea who had been in close contact with Ebola patients. However, a study sponsored by the National Institutes of Health, the Food and Drug Administration and the US Department of Health and Human Services amongst others called the vaccine's effectiveness into question. Nevertheless, WHO approved the vaccine for use on 29 May 2017.

Ebolavirus was soon found to have a long tail and the destruction it had wreaked so far was by no means over. Far from it: in August 2015 the WHO held a meeting to work out a 'Comprehensive care plan for Ebola survivors' and identify the research that was now needed in the aftermath which was now regarded as 'an emergency within an emergency'. What was particularly worrying was research that revealed that some Ebola survivors experienced a so-called 'post-Ebola Syndrome', with symptoms so severe that survivors required further medical care for months and even years. Other serious long term social consequences were identified in December 2015 when the UN announced that 22,000 children had lost one or both parents to Ebola.

Given its lethal nature, Ebola is classified as a biosafety level 4 agent, as well as a Category A bioterrorism agent by the Centers for Disease Control and Prevention. It has the very real potential to be weaponized for use in biological warfare.

Infection control in the region specifically demands proper disposal of the dead through cremation or burial. Traditional burial rituals, especially those requiring embalming of bodies, should be discouraged or modified. For example, to the Kissi people who inhabit part of Sierra Leone, it is important to bury the bodies of the dead close by. Funeral ritual includes rubbing the corpses down with oil, dressing them in fine clothes, then having those at the funeral hug and kiss the corpse. Those that die from Ebola retain high concentrations of the virus in their body post mortem. As we saw the genesis of the outbreak in Sierra Leone was linked to a single funeral in late May of a traditional healer, who had been trying to cure others with Ebola in Guinea; WHO estimates as many as 365 died from Ebola disease after 14 people contracted the disease there.

The Government of the Democratic Republic of the Congo announced on 1 June 2020 that a new outbreak of Ebola virus disease is occurring in Wangata health zone, Mbandaka, in Équateur province. The announcement comes while the country also battles COVID-19 and the world's largest measles outbreak. The Ministry of Health confirmed that six Ebola cases have so far been detected in Wangata, of which four have died and two are under care. This is the Democratic Republic of the Congo's 11th outbreak of Ebola since the virus was first discovered in the country in 1976. Since 2019, 369,520 measles cases and 6,779 deaths have been reported. If confirmation were needed that Ebola has not left the region then this is it. New outbreaks of Ebola were expected. After nearly six months, and with 130 infections, the Democratic Republic of Congo (DRC) declared its eleventh Ebola outbreak over on 18 November 2020. The outbreak claimed the lives of 55 people.

In April 2017, Cafferkey announced she would return to Sierra Leone in May to raise funds for Ebola survivors and children orphaned by the disease.

In June 2019, Cafferkey gave birth to twin sons in a hospital in Glasgow, at the age of 43. In a statement, she said 'this shows that there is life after Ebola and there is a future for those who have encountered this disease.'

Bausch, D.G., 2007. 'Assessment of the Risk of Ebola Virus Transmission from Bodily Fluids and Fomites'. *The Journal of Infectious Diseases* 196

Bullard, Stephan Gregory, 2018. A Day-by-Day Chronicle of the 2013–2016 Ebola Outbreak. Berlin

Kibadi, Mupapa, 1999. 'Ebola Hemorrhagic Fever and Pregnancy'. *The Journal of Infectious Diseases*. 179 Suppl 1: S11–2

Parshley, Lois, 8 August 2014. 'ZMapp: The Experimental Ebola Treatment Explained'. *Popular Science*.

Chapter 64

The Zika Virus epidemic: 2015–2016

'The Zika virus was unexpected and caught us off guard, but it has taught us an important lesson. How many other neglected pathogens are out there, lurking in the shadows and waiting for the next 'perfect storm'? This is a scary question to ask. In a world with increasing globalization, international travel, urban crowding and global climate change, perhaps it is time for us to rethink our disease-control strategies, strengthen our research and public health infrastructures, and devise preventive measures against possible future disease outbreaks.'

– Jing-Wen Ai, (2016), Department of Infectious Diseases,
Huashan Hospital, Fudan University, Shanghai, China

Zika is a flavivirus transmitted mainly by *Aedes aegypti* and *Aedes albopictus* mosquitoes; *Aedes aegypti* mosquitoes are found through large swathes of the Americas, including parts of the United States, and also transmit Dengue and Chikungunya viruses. Chikungunya is an infection caused by the Chikungunya virus (CHIKV).

Zika was discovered in 1947 in Uganda by scientists conducting routine surveillance for yellow fever in the Zika forest; they isolated the Zika virus in samples taken from a Macaca monkey and in 1952 the first human cases were detected in Uganda and Tanzania. Two years later the virus was isolated from a young girl in Eastern Nigeria. In 1964 a researcher in Uganda fell ill while working with Zika strains isolated from mosquitoes providing the first proof that Zika virus causes human disease. Though a pink non-itchy rash lasting five days eventually covered most of his body, including the palms of his hands and soles of his feet, he reported his illness as 'mild'.

From the 1960s to 1980s, human infections emerged across Africa and equatorial Asia, including India, Indonesia, Malaysia and Pakistan, usually accompanied by mild illness. Researchers would later suggest that the clinical similarity of Zika infection with Dengue and Chikungunya may be one reason why the disease was so rarely reported in Asia. Another reason was because for more than fifty years since its initial discovery, Zika virus appeared to pose little threat to human beings. Zika virus infection is asymptomatic in about ~80 per cent of infected individuals, and in those who develop the disease, the symptoms are usually mild and rarely result in human fatality .

The first large outbreak of disease caused by Zika was reported from the Island of Yap in the Federated States of Micronesia in 2007; before this no outbreaks and only 14 cases of human Zika virus disease had been documented worldwide. House-to-house surveys among the island's population of 11,250 people identified 185 cases of suspected Zika virus disease, of which 49 are confirmed. An estimated 73 per cent of Yap residents over 3 years of age were infected with Zika virus although no deaths, hospitalizations, or neurological complications were reported. Travel or trade involving an infected person or mosquito in south east Asia are considered the most likely sources of this outbreak. In 2008 a US scientist working in Senegal fell ill with Zika infection on his return home to Colorado and infected his wife in what is probably the first documented case of sexual transmission of an infection usually transmitted by insects.

In 2013–14 the virus broke out in French Polynesia, Easter Island, the Cook Islands, and New Caledonia, the first generating thousands of suspected infections. Later investigations indicate a possible association between Zika virus infection and congenital malformations and severe neurological and autoimmune complications. An increase in the incidence of Zika infection towards the end of 2013 was followed by a rise in the incidence of Guillain-Barré syndrome, a rare condition in which a person's immune system attacks the peripheral nerves and which can progress to paralysis. In December 2013 on Tahiti Island a patient recovering from Zika presented with bloody sperm; Zika virus was isolated from his semen, lending support to the belief that Zika can be sexually transmitted. One person was found to have 100,000 times more virus in semen than blood or urine, two weeks after being infected. Oral, anal or vaginal sex can spread the disease.

On 20 March 2014 in French Polynesia two mothers and their newborns were found to have Zika virus infection acquired by transplacental transmission or during delivery. Eleven days later 1,505 asymptomatic blood donors were reported to be positive for Zika, alerting authorities to the risk of post-transfusion Zika fever. On 7 May 2015 Brazil's National Reference Laboratory confirmed that Zika virus was circulating in twelve states – the first report of locally acquired Zika disease in the Americas. On 17 July Brazil reported 49 cases confirmed as Guillain-Barré syndrome; all but two had a prior history of infection with Zika, Chikungunya or Dengue. In October 2015 Brazil reported a link between Zika and microcephaly, a rare condition associated with incomplete brain development at the more severe end of a spectrum of birth defects, sometimes referred to as Congenital Zika Syndrome (CZS).

On 5 October 2015 health centres in the Republic of Cape Verde began reporting cases of illness with skin rash, with and without fever, in the capital city of Praia, on the island of Santiago. By 14 October, 165 suspected cases were reported. Three days later Brazil reported the results of a review of 138 clinical records of patients with a neurological syndrome. Of these, 58 (42 per cent) had a previous history of viral infection. Of the 58, 32 (55 per cent) had symptoms that are said to be consistent with Zika or Dengue. On 8 October 2015 Colombia reported the results of a retrospective review of clinical records from which 90 cases were identified with clinical symptoms consistent with, but not proven to be, Zika infection. Colombia also confirmed 156 cases of Zika in thirteen municipalities, with most confirmed cases concentrated in the densely populated Bolivar department. On 5 November 2015 Colombia confirmed 239 cases of locally acquired Zika infection.

On 30 October 2015 Brazil reported an unusual and worrying increase in the number of cases of microcephaly among newborns since the August, numbering 54 by 30 October. On 11 November 2015 Brazil posted 141 suspected cases of microcephaly in Pernambuco state while further suspected cases were investigated in two other states. Brazil declared a national public health emergency when cases of suspected microcephaly continued to increase. It was helped in its dealing of Zika and associated conditions by:

> 'the high reach of the unified public health system, including hospitals in which more than 80% of babies are delivered. The public health obstetricians and neonatologists within this community, dealing with hundreds of childbirths per month, were the first to suspect something was amiss… the close network of practitioners and researchers working within the public health system, including doctors, midwives, epidemiologists, and other academics exchanging information and reporting new findings in a timely fashion. From November 2015, reports of suspected microcephaly cases increased 10-fold within just a few weeks.'[1]

On 12 November 2015 Panama announced cases with symptoms consistent with Zika. By 17 November 2015 Brazil reported Zika virus detected in amniotic fluid samples from two pregnant women whose foetuses were confirmed by ultrasound to have microcephaly. Altogether, 399 cases of suspected microcephaly were now being investigated in seven northeastern states. This soon rose to 739 cases of microcephaly under investigation. On 24 November 2015 El Salvador reported its first three confirmed cases.

French Polynesia posted the results of a retrospective investigation documenting an unusual increase in the number of central nervous system malformations in foetuses and infants from March 2014 to May 2015. At least 17 cases were identified with different severe cerebral malformations, including microcephaly and neonatal brainstem dysfunction.

On 25 November 2015: Mexico reported three confirmed cases of Zika infection, two of which were locally acquired; the third imported via Colombia; soon after Guatemala announced its first case; Paraguay reported six cases and Venezuela seven suspected cases, four of which tested positive by PCR. On 28 November 2015 Brazil detected Zika virus genome in the blood and tissue samples of a baby with microcephaly and other congenital anomalies who died within five minutes of birth.

It was on 25 November that the deaths started – Brazil declared three deaths among two adults and a newborn associated with Zika infection. On 2 December Panama reported three more confirmed cases with a further 95 showing compatible symptoms; but 6 December was especially significant when Cape Verde announced 4,744 suspected cases of Zika. On 16 and 21 December Honduras, French Guiana and Martinique posted their first confirmed cases.

---

1. Lowe, 2018

On 22 December 2015 Brazilian researchers published evidence, drawn from case reports in several countries, that the commonly held belief that Zika was 'a mild cousin of Dengue' may not actually be true, particularly for immunocompromised patients. At the end of the month Brazil reported 2,975 suspected cases of microcephaly while the United States revealed the first confirmed case in Puerto Rico. The new year began with the first diagnoses of intrauterine transmission of the Zika virus in two pregnant women in Brazil whose foetuses were, by diagnostic ultrasound, shown to have microcephaly, including severe brain abnormalities. Although tests of blood samples from both women were negative, Zika virus was detected in amniotic fluid. Later that month Brazilian ophthalmologists reported severe ocular malformations in three infants born with microcephaly. Guyana declared its first PCR confirmed case.

Brazil is the epicentre of the 2015–16 outbreak, and an estimated 440,000 –1,300,000 Brazilians were infected in 2015. Why Brazil? One contributing factor was that Brazil was host to the 2014 FIFA World Cup tournament and the 2015 international canoe-racing event, which may have been the main entry routes for Zika virus into the Americas. Most significant, though, is the fact that most of Brazil enjoys a tropical climate, and a large part of the Amazon rainforest is also located here, all of which promises a difficult battle against mosquitoes. In fact, the reported cases of Dengue fever, another arbovirus with transmitted *Aedes aegypti* the main vector, increased by 227.12 per cent in 2015 compared with 2014, highlighting the inadequate control of *Aedes* mosquitoes in Brazil. The absence of immunity for the Zika virus in Brazilians is perhaps the most compelling factor underlying the outbreak. In a country without a history of Zika virus disease, Brazilians offered total vulnerability to the virus thus further accelerating wide disease transmission.

The strongest evidence yet of a link between Zika infection and microcephaly came on 12 January 2016 when health officials in Brazil and the United States Centers for Disease Control and Prevention published laboratory findings of four microcephaly cases in Brazil – two newborns who died in their first 24 hours of life and two miscarriages – which indicated the presence of Zika virus RNA by PCR and by immunohistochemistry of brain tissue samples of the two newborns. Placenta of the two foetuses which miscarried during the first twelve weeks of pregnancy tested positive. All four women presented with fever and rash during their pregnancy. The United States then issued travel guidance for pregnant women which, 'out of an abundance of caution', advised pregnant women in any trimester to consider postponing travel to areas with ongoing local transmission of the virus, or to take precautions against mosquito bites if they must travel.

Ecuador reported its first eight cases of which three were imported from Columbia, and one from Venezuela. Barbados announced its first three cases while a case of microcephaly was reported in Hawaii, born to a woman who had lived in Brazil early in her pregnancy. Reports of first cases came in from Bolivia and Haiti (five cases). On 18 January 2016 France posted the first case in Saint Martin. Mid January saw El Salvador report an increase of Guillain-Barré syndrome: 46 cases were detailed, including two deaths. Of the 22 patients with a medical history, 12 (54 per cent) presented with fever and skin rash in the seven to fifteen days before the onset of symptoms, consistent with

Guillain-Barré syndrome. Brazil announced 3,893 suspected cases of microcephaly, including 49 deaths. In six cases, Zika virus was harvested from samples from newborns or stillbirths. The end of the month saw two confirmed cases of Guillain-Barré syndrome in Martinique, the first case in the United States Virgin Islands and Nicaragua's first two cases.

The Zika emergency was lifted in November 2016, but 84 countries still reported cases as of March 2017.

Zika left more than 3,700 children born with birth defects — the most severe of which, as we have noted, is microcephaly. Over 6,000 research papers have been published between 2015 and 2019 in a bid to beat this virus. A summary of the findings was published in Didier Musso's October 2019 paper in the *New England Journal of Medicine*.

Although there are no known cures for Zika, there have been promising developments in Zika vaccination. Three vaccines are showing high levels of protection against the virus. Scientists have conducted tests on the rhesus monkey, and human trials began in late 2016. However, it will take years before it is available for widespread usage.

Kineta, a Seattle-based biotech company, is actively working on treatments and has received funding from the National Institute of Allergy and Infectious Disease.

Enserink, M., 2015, Infectious Diseases. An obscure mosquito-borne disease goes global. United States: *Science*; 1012–3.

Jing-Wen, Ai, 2018, Zika virus outbreak: 'a perfect storm' *Int J Environ Res Public Health* 15(1): 96.

Kindhauser, Mary Kay, 2016, Zika: the origin and spread of a mosquito-borne virus. *Bulletin of the World Health Organization*

Liu, Z.Y., The evolution of Zika virus from Asia to the Americas. Nat Rev Microbiol 2019;17:131–139.

Musso, Didier, 2019, Zika Virus Infection — After the Pandemic, N Engl J Med 2019; 381:1444–1457

Chapter 65

COVID–19, 2019–

'*In our national fight against Covid-19, we are at a tipping point similar to where we were in March* [2020] *but we can prevent history repeating itself if we all act now... Earlier in the year we were fighting a semi-invisible disease, about which we had little knowledge, and it seeded in the community at great speed. Now we know where it is and how to tackle it – let's grasp this opportunity and prevent history from repeating itself.*'

– Deputy Chief Medical Officer Professor Jonathan
Van-Tam outlines the Covid-19 situation on 11 October 2020.

Is this the long-awaited brave new world approach to disease management? Let's hope so because, as this book clearly shows, the world has spent the last 2,600 years doing next to nothing to 'prevent history repeating itself...' Unfortunately, six or so months after Van-Tam's pronouncement we know that we failed to 'grasp this opportunity' and history is indeed 'repeating itself'.

We began the book with the eighth cohort of Mongolian health care workers boarding a plane to fight the COVID-19 outbreak in Wuhan. We approach the end with the report by WHO officials in March 2021 who travelled to Wuhan to investigate the causes and origin of the outbreak while Chinese authorities continue to insist that their hands are clean of any delay or opacity and that the virus originated elsewhere. In March 2021 the WHO concluded that it is 'highly unlikely that the coronavirus escaped from a lab at the Wuhan Institute of Virology' but that Huanan market may well be implicated when an intermediate animal – possibly one sold at the market – passed SARS-CoV-2 to humans after becoming infected with a predecessor coronavirus in bats.

The possible origin

Coronavirus disease 2019 (COVID-19) is a highly infectious disease caused by severe acute respiratory syndrome coronavirus 2 (SARS-CoV-2). It was identified in December 2019 in Wuhan, Hubei, China where it was first isolated from three people with pneumonia connected to the cluster of acute respiratory illness cases in Wuhan. We are all living through the ongoing pandemic it triggered.

A study of the first 41 cases of confirmed COVID-19, published in January 2020 in *The Lancet*, reported the earliest date of onset of symptoms as 1 December 2019 while the WHO reported the earliest onset of symptoms as 8 December 2019. *The Lancet* paper was authored by a large group of Chinese researchers from several institutions. Human-to-human transmission was confirmed by the WHO and Chinese authorities by 20 January 2020.

According to Chinese sources, of the initial 41 people hospitalized with pneumonia who were officially identified as having laboratory-confirmed SARS-CoV-2 infection, two-thirds were exposed to the Huanan Seafood Wholesale Market (one of 40,000 wet markets in China), which also sold live animals. Thirty-three out of 585 (5.64 per cent) environmental samples obtained from the market indicated evidence of COVID-19, according to the Chinese Center for Disease Control and Prevention.

The market occupied over 540,000 sq ft and had over 1,000 tenants. It is the largest seafood wholesale market in Central China, with wild animals including exotic game also sold there. *The South China Morning Post* reported on 29 January 2020 that the market had a section selling around '120 wildlife animals across 75 species' including badgers, giant salamanders and two kinds of crocodile. As coronaviruses (such as SARS-CoV and MERS-CoV) mainly circulate among animals and with a link between the pneumonia outbreak and the market having been established, it was soon suspected that the virus may have been passed from an animal to humans (zoonosis).

There is some disagreement over the conditions prevailing at the market. In late 2019, the market passed city official inspections according to *The Wall Street Journal*. However, this is contradicted by *Time* which reported 'unsanitary' conditions. It has narrow lanes and stalls close together where livestock was kept alongside dead animals. According to *Business Insider*, it was common to see animals openly slaughtered and carcasses skinned in the market. *The New York Times* reported that 'sanitation was dismal with poor ventilation and garbage piled on wet floors'.

Bats were initially thought to be the source of the virus, although we are not sure if bats were sold at the market. Later studies hypothesized that pangolins may be the intermediate host of the virus originating from bats, analogous to the relationship between SARS-CoV and civets. But pangolins are somewhat rare; researchers traced farmed animals at the Wuhan market back to three provinces in China where pangolins and bats carrying coronaviruses similar to SARS-CoV-2 had been found. The pangolin and bat viruses proved too distant to be the direct progenitors of SARS-CoV-2.

Despite the connection between the market and the pandemic, we do not know for sure whether the novel coronavirus outbreak started in the market. As we have said the earliest report of first symptoms was 1 December 2019 in a person who did not have any exposure to the market or to the remaining affected 40 people. Moreover, the data in *The Lancet* paper referred to above showed 13 of the initial 41 people (32 per cent) found with the novel coronavirus had no link with the market, a significant figure. In a later paper, *The Lancet* reported that of the first 99 people confirmed with COVID-19 in Wuhan Jinyintan Hospital between 1 and 20 January 2020, 49 (49.5 per cent) had recently been to the market.

On 1 January 2020, the Chinese health authorities closed the market to conduct investigations, clean and disinfect the location. The state-run Xinhua News Agency reported that it was being closed for 'renovations'. On 22 January 2020, a ban on the sale of all wild animal products in Wuhan was announced. In May 2020 the city banned eating wild animals and imposed limited hunting and breeding. On 24 February 2020, the

Chinese government declared that the trade and consumption of wild animals would be banned throughout China. The ban though did not extend to the ingestion of wild animal products in traditional Chinese medicine, according to the *New York Times*.

Something went wrong...

In 2020 if you were a German you had less than half the likelihood of dying from COVID than if you were British. A British person had 4,000 times the chance of dying than a Vietnamese. Pandemics are one of those scenarios where you make your own luck: China has a population 20 times the size of ours and a death toll a twentieth of ours. Clearly they were doing something we were not. In February 2020 SAGE reported that 'Currently Public Health England can cope with five new cases a week (requiring 800 contacts to isolate)'. SAGE explained that they had prepared for a pandemic – but for an influenza pandemic – where there are significant clinical differences and epidemiology. SAGE expected up to 50 new cases a week but 'when there is sustained transmission in the UK contact tracing will no longer be useful'. Compare this, which amounts to a capitulation to the disease, with South Korea's proactive and highly effective reaction. On 12 March Jenny Harries, deputy chief medical officer for England, after 1,200 deaths, declared that 'face masks are not a good idea'; she finally recanted on 1 April 2021. In September, when SAGE strongly advised a circuit-breaker, the Treasury, intent as it was to get 'office workers back to Pret a Manger' strongly opposed the move (*The Times*, 27 January 2021).

The world picture
as of 22 May 2021:

Global cases	165,069,258
Deaths	3,422,907 (2.05%)

as of 22 May 2021:

UK cases	4.5m
Deaths	128k (2.87%)

Source: JHU CSSE COVID-19 Data

Vaccinations
Percentage of population as of 22 May 2021 who have received at least one dose; doses administered in brackets:
Malta 66.4% (446k)
Israel 62.8% (10.5m)
Bhutan 62.5% (482k)
UK 55.2% (59.2m)
UAE 51.4% (11.6m)
People vaccinated in UK: first dose 37.5m; second dose 21.7m.

Source: Our World in Data and gov.uk

The hugely successful vaccination roll out, as of 26 April, shows 33,752,888 people have received their first jab with 12,897,123 having had both jabs. Vaccine hesitancy is falling with the percentage of black people disinclined to have the jab falling from 44% to 22% in late April.

How many people are in hospital? As of 22 May there were 913 people in hospital with COVID, of which 123 were on ventilators*.

There were 8,201 deaths from all causes in the week to 2 April, of which COVID-19 accounts for 4.9 per cent. The number of weekly deaths was 1,929 lower (24 per cent) for the five year average for the time of year *.

All figures where COVID mentioned on the death certificate.

Table 9: COVID–19, the national picture – cases and deaths

UK Cases 4.34m Deaths 127k as of 29 March		
LOCATION	**CASES**	**DEATHS**
England	3.8m	111k
Wales	221k	7,596
Scotland	209k	5,506
Northern Ireland	117k	2,115

Source: JHU CSSE COVID-19 Data

Pre-existing health conditions are a major factor in morbidity with 96-97% of deaths in the over 60s, 90% in the 40-60s and 86% in the 20-40s *.

Age is another significant factor in COVID-19 mortality; in total, there has been 150,841 deaths involving COVID-19 registered in the UK since the start of the pandemic up to 26 April 2021. People aged 75 years and over account for 77,245 of these: 74%. The average age of fatalities is 83 – 81 for males, 85 for females *.

Ethnicity too is crucial. Deaths after testing positive for COVID **:

White - population:	47,862, 900	deaths: 50,478	deaths per 100k: 105
Asian	4,336,440	4,337	99.3
Black	1,959,300	2,044	104.3
Mixed–	1,287,540	315	24

Place of death: as of 15 January, 65,443 deaths occurred in England and Wales hospitals (excluding psychiatric) (63%); 22,892 (22%) in care homes, 4662 at home, 1,277 in hospices *.

* Source ONS

** Source NHS England

Large extended families are at risk too because only 21 per cent of people who live with others are able to effectively separate. Many of these are unable to work from home so spread the virus into the workplace.

'the truth is we could have done better...any sensible risk register would have had the risk of a pandemic right at the top – above nuclear war or climate change.'

Sir John Bell, member of the advisory group to the government's
Vaccine Task Force and Regius Professor of Medicine, Oxford University

The pandemic continues to rage on around the world, so data relating to its insidious advance remain in a fast moving state of flux. Only now, the virus is fortified and invigorated in its new mutations, some of which may be more infectious and transmissible than its original form – some say up to 70 per cent more infectious. As yet its effect on illness severity, mortality and on the vaccines being rolled out or in trials is unclear. What is clear is that the world has a fresh challenge on its hands.

COVID 19 enjoys the status of a work in progress, a status not shared by this book which has an end date and a delivery date. Here, nevertheless, are some figures which give a picture of its relentless progress, at the time of writing on 27 April 2021.

As of 24 April we have the most reported deaths in Europe although we obviously do not have the biggest population. We lie 5th in the world after USA, Brazil, Mexico and India. Expressed in deaths per million population we have the unenviable record of reporting the second most deaths in the world with 1,876, just after Italy (1,958) and ahead of Brazil, Peru and Poland.

COVID-19 Variants

We know that viruses mutate in order to make themselves fitter and more agile, contagious and destructive. This, of course, presents serious challenges for scientists, clinicians, epidemiologists and policy makers – in fact anyone struggling to keep on top of the virus and its spread. Luckily COVID-19 has proved to be relatively stable but in the last few months a number of variants have emerged: the so-called Kent, South African, Brazilian and, most recently, the Indian. How virulent, vaccine resistant and pervasive these are is impossible to tell at the moment but acute surveillance and caution are essential. The carnage which is currently sweeping India is avoidable in other countries but only if we all maintain a high level of respect for the potential the virus has to wreak havoc.

COVIDspeak:

We now have, as we have seen, a whole new lexicon of words and phrases which, hitherto, were largely unknown to the average layperson: here are just a few of them:

Social distancing, hand hygiene and quarantine

Pandemic or epidemic viruses love a crowd; they mutate to make themselves work better within crowded environments and they ravage teeming populations. More specifically they decimate communities and have the ability to rip through established social units: religious communities, armies on the march and sailors confined in ships, servicemen in barracks, students and staff in schools and universities and health care workers in health care facilities have all felt the lethal ability of a virus to infect, prostrate and kill indiscriminately. One of the ways to thwart these virus reservoirs is to implement robust social distancing and rigorous quarantine measures. Sometimes, viruses are a victim of their own success: if they infect and kill enough people in a given population they find themselves with nowhere left to go. Their lethal work is done.

Social distancing is by no means new: such measures date back to at least the 5th century BC. As we have seen, the Bible contains one of the earliest known, and decidedly un-Christian, references to the practice in Leviticus 13:46: 'And the leper in whom the plague is... he shall dwell alone; [outside] the camp shall his habitation be.' During the Plague of Justinian of AD 541 to 542, the people of Constantinople tried it, while Justinian enforced his ineffective quarantine on the Byzantine Empire, by dumping bodies into the sea; keeping his holier than thou options open he blamed the outbreak on 'Jews, Samaritans, pagans, heretics, Arians, Montanists and homosexuals'. On anyone really, just not Justinian. Neolithic China and plague-struck Ragusa in 1377 were early exponents of quarantining.

More recently social distancing measures have been successfully implemented: for example in St. Louis, soon after the first cases of influenza were detected during the 1918 flu pandemic, authorities implemented school closures, bans on public gatherings and other social-distancing interventions. The influenza fatality rates in St. Louis were much lower than in Philadelphia, which had fewer cases of influenza but allowed a mass parade to continue and did not introduce social distancing until more than two weeks after its first cases on 17 September. The authorities pressed on with the planned parade bringing together more than 200,000 people on 28 September; over the next three days, the city's 31 hospitals were overrun. During the week ending 16 October, over 4,500 people died.

In the UK during the early days of COVID the government was equally hesitant and ambivalent, delaying effective lockdown and even allowing a UEFA Champions League match between Liverpool and Atlético Madrid (11 March) to proceed with Madrid supporters in mass attendance even though Spain was in lockdown; just as bizarrely the jam-packed 2020 Cheltenham Gold Cup was allowed to go ahead on 13 March. About 250,000 people attended the four-day event which ended 10 days before national lockdown measures began. Sir David King, the government's chief scientific adviser from 2000 to 2007, said it was 'the best possible way to accelerate the spread of the virus'.

The government says it followed the advice available at the time. Professor Tim Spector, from King's College London, said the two events – held from 16 to 19 March and on 11 March respectively – had 'caused increased suffering and death that wouldn't otherwise have occurred'. Liverpool's game was watched by around 52,000 people inside Anfield, including 3,000 visiting supporters who had travelled from Madrid – where such events had already been suspended. Aeroplanes from the four corners of the world continued, and astonishingly still do, to disgorge passengers in UK airports by the tens of thousands for months after airports should have been closed.

This may sound familiar: Bootsma and Ferguson (2007) analyzed social distancing interventions in sixteen US cities during the 1918 epidemic and found that the impact was often very limited because the interventions were introduced too late and lifted too early.

School closures were shown to reduce morbidity from the Asian flu by 90 per cent during the 1957–58 pandemic, and up to 50 per cent in controlling influenza in the U.S., 2004–2008. According to UNESCO, the widespread closure of primary, secondary, and post-secondary schools in more than 120 countries as of 23 March 2020, meant that more than 1.2 billion students were out of school due to school closures in response to COVID-19.

The UK prime minister was still bragging how he was still shaking hands in March 2020 – 'I was at a hospital the other night where I think there were a few coronavirus patients and I shook hands with everybody, you will be pleased to know, and I continue to shake hands,' he said. 'People obviously can make up their own minds but I think the scientific evidence is … our judgment is that washing your hands is the crucial thing.' SAGE begged to differ.

As of July 2020 one of the most successful attempts at quarantine was amongst the Xingu Amazon tribe who live in the protected indigenous territory in Brazil's Mato Grosso state. The 142 people in 16 families had warded off the virus but are in desperate need of medicines, soap, and fishing lines so that they can continue their self-imposed quarantine. The more they have to travel to get supplies the more they are at risk. The nearest medical facility is 100 or so miles away.

PPE and ventilators and when Hazmat suits became normal

The sight of healthcare workers lumbering around in what look like astronauts' standard issue has become an all-too familiar sight in the media; they lend a slow motion dystopian air to the COVID-19 horror story, terrifying patients (and potential patients) but at the same time offering reassurance that things are under control, however impersonal they render dedicated health care staff.

The following report shows a serious, compassionate, if extreme, angle to the issue: *Surrey Live* reporter Emma Pengelly tells us how a mother-of-four concerned for the wellbeing of her nine-week-old baby and elderly grandparents has worn a hazmat suit to Tesco in a bid to protect her family from COVID-19. Melissa Farry, from Langshott in Horley, has bought eight hazmat suits and also wears goggles, gloves and a face mask for protection. Mrs Farry has gone to such lengths because she fears infecting herself, her young family and her grandparents who are aged 76 and 77, one of whom has terminal cancer.

'I was walking around Tesco playing 'Ghostbusters' because when I walked in, I thought it felt so morbid,' she said. 'Everyone was walking around like it was their funeral.'

[https://www.getsurrey.co.uk/news/surrey-news/mum-four-wears-hazmat-suit-18017670]

In an article in *The Guardian*[1] reporter Sirin Kale (26 March 2020) cautions: 'You never want to be on the wrong side of a hazmat suit, because if you are, you

---

1. [https://www.theguardian.com/world/2020/mar/26/hazmat-suit-disease-deadly-viruses-danger-symbol-heroic]

know something's gone horribly wrong.' Kale goes on to reveal the hidden costs in supplying Hazmat suits: 'Getting a licence to produce hazmat suits is a costly and laborious undertaking. It can cost £63,000 to get the certificate to make one suit,'claims Pam Parker of PPS, a British hazmat suit manufacturer.

We have frequently described early attempts to protect against contagion based on the prevalent miasma theory of contagion. Before the use of hazmat suits, there were valiant attempts at PPE: the terrifying Venetian plague 'doctor' costume was, of course, one of the earliest attempts by medical people, (or those who masqueraded, literally, as medical people) to safeguard themselves during the frequent bubonic plagues. French doctor Charles de Lorme was the pioneer: his equipment featured a forbidding ankle length overcoat and a terrifying bird-like beak mask which had glass openings for the eyes. The mask had two small nose holes to act as a type of respirator which contained aromatic items such as dried flowers, herbs such as lavender and peppermint, spices, camphor, or a vinegar sponge. The purpose of the mask was to deflect bad smells, miasma, which were thought to be the principal cause of the disease before it was disproved by germ theory. Doctors believed the herbs would counter the 'evil' smells of the plague and prevent themselves from becoming infected. The kit was completed with gloves and boots, a distinctive wide-brimmed leather hat and a cane.

Sadly this early PPE probably made things worse. Lynteris points out the all-important shortcomings of such frightening garb: 'A permanent hazmat suit without removal protocols and disinfectant would be a vector of disease, rather than something that would stop it.'

We have already mentioned how the visionary preventative measures taken after the Manchurian plague of 1910 broke new ground and were world, and life, changing in the development of PPE serving us today in the struggle against COVID. 'Doctor Wu Lien-teh', says Lynteris, 'Insisted that all doctors, nurses and burial staff wore a simple gauze mask he designed. It was the first time we had a mask devised for use during an epidemic.' Another nail in the miasma coffin allowing scientists to fight pestilence without one hand tied behind their backs.

As is all too frequent in medical innovation down the years, Wu's measures were met with derision; however, sense and practicality prevailed and throughout the 20th century, the firefighting, chemical and nuclear sectors among others developed the modern hazmat suit, with medical versions coming into widespread use during the Ebola outbreaks of the 1990s.

Incredibly, it took months for some nations, including the UK, to make the wearing of face coverings mandatory in public places when its efficacy had been proven in other countries and in history.

Effective and well executed logistics of PPE supply and demand are vital too; to some extent all countries failed to stockpile adequately despite the warnings but, again, the UK was one of the most dilatory and ill-prepared with serial failures in procurement, supply and due diligence which has left warehouses full of millions of pounds worth of unusable masks. Much of our PPE was hurriedly bought at the top of the market when a modicum of foresight might have saved a lot of money and many a life, not least among health workers. The UK had 8,000 ventilators at the start of the pandemic; a further 14,000 were manufactured as part of the Ventilator Challenge Project.

There is nothing remotely romantic or tolerable about donning and doffing a hazmat suit – as any of the valiant healthcare workers fighting COVID-19 today will tell you. So next time you see a health care worker fitted out in a hazmat suit battling with COVID, remember that not only does the patient face the horrifying reality that, in Sirin Kale's word 'they are no longer just a person, but a vector of disease ... Because, although the person in a hazmat suit may seem far away, or even uncaring, they are doing the most humane thing imaginable: putting themselves in harm's way, to save a stranger's life'.

Source: Guardian News & Media Ltd

Psychological impact

Just as insidious as the virus itself are the psychological impacts the pandemic with all its ramifications – clinical and non-clinical – brings with it. In the UK in December 2020 some 19 per cent of adults reported symptoms of depression; up from 10 per cent in March. We need to put in place preventative measures which will support the lonely, the disabled and anyone self isolating for longer than two weeks.

Vaccines

As of December 2020 Britain had ordered stocks of seven different vaccines; they are listed in Table 10.

In all 395 million doses from seven companies producing four different types of vaccine. Other vaccines are available, including Russia's Sputnik V from Gamaleya and China's Coronavac from Sinovac and one from Sinopharm. The decision by GSK in mid December to halt human trials due to poor efficacy results is a stark reminder of how lucky the world is to have a choice of viable vaccines so quickly. Most vaccines fail so the apparent success of the BioNTech, Astra Zeneca-Oxford and and Moderna vaccines permit countries the luxury of an à la carte menu of jabs, each of which can be injected according to need.

mRNA vaccines

Conventional vaccines are produced using weakened forms of the virus, RNA vaccines, however, can be constructed quickly using only the pathogen's genetic code.

Many standard vaccines work by injecting a dead or weakened form of the pathogen into the body in preparations that are designed not to make you ill but rather to build immunity. The key to building this immunity is that the portion of the pathogen called the antigen trains the immune system to recognise and respond to the infectious agent.

Table 10: Some of the vaccines approved or in trials

Pfizer-BioNTech, USA/Germany (40m)	mRNA vaccine	£15 per dose
Moderna, USA (17m)	mRNA vaccine	£25 per dose
Oxford-Astra Zeneca, UK (100m)	adenovirus vaccine	£3 per dose
Janssen, Belgium (30m)	adenovirus vaccine	$10 per dose
Novavax, USA (60m)	protein subunit vaccine	$16 per dose
GSK- Sanofi Pasteur, UK/France (60m)	protein subunit vaccine	
Valneva, France (100m)	inactivated virus	
CureVac, Germany (60m)	mRNA vaccine	

RNA vaccines work by introducing a messenger RNA (mRNA) sequence into the body that contains the genetic instructions for the vaccinated person's own cells to make a harmless piece of what is called the "spike protein." and generate an immune response. The spike protein is found on the surface of the virus that causes COVID-19.

mRNA vaccines do not use the live virus that causes COVID-19.

Adenovirus vaccines

Made from a weakened version of a common cold virus (adenovirus) from chimpanzees. It has been modified to look more like coronavirus – although it can't cause illness. When the vaccine is injected into a patient, it prompts the immune system to start making antibodies and primes it to attack any coronavirus infection. It could be developed quickly because Oxford University researchers had already done a lot of work on developing a vaccine which could be adapted to tackle different diseases.

Protein subunit vaccines

These include harmless pieces (proteins) of the virus that cause COVID-19 instead of the entire germ. Once vaccinated, our immune system recognizes that the proteins don't belong in the body and begins making T-lymphocytes and antibodies. If we are ever infected in the future, memory cells will recognize and fight the virus.

Inactivated virus vaccine

These contain viruses whose genetic material has been destroyed by heat, chemicals or radiation so they cannot infect cells and replicate but can still trigger an immune response. This technology is well-established and has been used in seasonal flu, hepatitis A, polio and rabies vaccines.

The Covid-19 vaccines developed by Chinese companies Sinovac and Sinopharm, and India's Bharat Biotech, which have all been approved for emergency use in their countries, are also inactivated vaccines.

Testing, tracking and tracing – the *sine qua non* of disease control

The UK astonishingly suspended community testing on 12 March 2020 and boasted a 'world beating' track and trace app, which would be up and running in June to prevent a second wave and further lockdowns – effective track and trace sank without trace for many months and did not resurface for many months, during which time lives were being unnecessarily lost.

There was also a distinct and catastrophic lack of testing with unnecessary and avoidable deaths on a huge scale when the government released thousands of elderly hospital patients into care homes without testing them. The 'protective ring' the government promised to throw around care homes on 15 May failed to materialise. Indeed, on 28 January 2021 it was reported that elderly patients were being discharged from hospitals into care homes having tested negative, but tested positive at the care homes.

> *The UK 'faced an inevitable increase in community transmission and need a fully functioning' testing system in place.'*
> – Sir Jeremy Farrar, Director of the Wellcome Trust and
> SAGE Committee member, September 2020.

The Chinese mastered testing, tracking and tracing in the Neolithic Age; the Japanese in the 1st century AD – both civilisations quickly realising that the only way to overcome a spreading virus is to beat it at its own game, know where it is going and give it nowhere to go. The three t's are essential to achieve this and these are based on disease surveillance and vigilance and a policy of reporting disease outbreaks amongst the population at large: the fact that the UK, a year after COVID-19 was identified, had still to perfect a viable testing regime or a reliable track and trace programme, despite warnings by SAGE, is all the more jaw dropping when you realise that there is evidence for such procedures that is 5,000 years old. Did we learn nothing from SARS in 2002 either?

COVID-19 fake news

It is with some reluctance that I give space to the voluminous fake news that accompanies the COVID-19 pandemic, but here it is for the sake of completeness. Europol covers it in its 'Disinformation and Misinformation around COVID-19', describing it as a 'sneaky threat', pointing out how spreading misinformation can start: from individuals, such as criminals, after some sort of profit; from states and state-backed actors seeking to advance geopolitical interests; from opportunists looking to discredit official sources. It only gains traction if the public share it through social media.

Spreading disinformation and misinformation about COVID-19, though not always a criminal offence, has very serious repercussions, endangering public health and directly affecting people's lives. It puts people at risk by promoting fake products and services (e.g. fake COVID-19 tests and vaccines); promoting a false sense of security (e.g. misleading information about treatments); and promoting suspicion of the official guidelines and sources.

Anti-maskers – anti-vaxxers – anti-lockdowners

There were few anti-vaxxers in Glasgow, it seems, during a 1942 outbreak of smallpox when 'everybody is advised to get vaccinated. The clinics are thrown open and it is done free of charge, of course. By the weekend a quarter of a million people had been vaccinated'. Compliance it seems was caused not by fear of the smallpox but by fear that if it got worse then travel would be restricted and 'of course, holidays are near'. (Mass-observation Archive). In the Great Mask War during the flu epidemic of 1918 there was resistance and non-compliance even though it was largely accepted that those thick multi-layered gauze masks worked to limit or stall the spread of disease; mask-wearing was sometimes enforced with fines, arrests, jail and, in at least one case, gunfire. In Seattle mask-free people were banned from public transport, or fined by the police's (masked) 'Flu Squad'. These 'mask slackers' were reviled on a par with draft-dodgers. Violators of a new San Francisco law were fined between $5 and $100 and risked up to 10 days in jail: a *San Francisco Examiner* headline read, '1,000 Alleged Mask Slacker Cases in Jails.'

When the law was revoked 'citizens made bonfires of their muzzles in the streets' but it had to be reinstated after a later surge in flu cases, leading to the formation of the 2,000 member strong Anti-Mask League. A bomb filled with glass and buckshot was sent to San Francisco's public health chief.

The American experience is significant because it foreshadows the causes of the anti-mask debate today: fear, uncertainty, resentment of what is percieved as government meddling, restriction of civil liberties, scepticism surrounding the efficacy of masks. There are obviously good medical reasons why some people should be exempt from manadatory mask wearing but, despite all manner of creative excuses, those refusing to wear a mask to limit the spread of the disease are simply selfish.

The Lancet Digital Health (2.10) published 'The online anti-vaccine movement in the age of COVID-19' in which it reported that:

> 'A new report by the Centre for Countering Digital Hate (CCDH) has lambasted social media companies for allowing the anti-vaccine movement to remain on their platforms. The report's authors noted that social media accounts held by so-called anti-vaxxers have increased their following by at least 7-8 million people since 2019. "The decision to continue hosting known misinformation content and actors left online anti-vaxxers ready to pounce on the opportunity presented by coronavirus", stated the report. The CCDH warned that the growing anti-vaccine movement could undermine the roll-out of any future vaccine against COVID-19.'

The report noted that 31 million people follow anti-vaccine groups on Facebook, with 17 million people subscribing to similar accounts on YouTube. The CCDH calculated that the anti-vaccine movement could realise US$1 billion in annual revenues for social media firms. A paper published in *Nature* mapped online views on vaccination. They warned that in a decade the anti-vaccination movement could overwhelm pro-vaccination voices online. If that came to pass, the consequences would stretch far beyond COVID-19.

Post COVID Syndrome (Long COVID)

The NICE guidelines published on 30 October 2020 defines post-COVID syndrome as signs and symptoms that develop during or following an infection consistent with COVID-19 which continue for more than twelve weeks and are not explained by an alternative diagnosis. The definition says the condition usually presents with clusters of symptoms, often overlapping, which may change over time and can affect any system within the body. It also notes that many people with post-COVID syndrome can also experience generalised pain, fatigue, persisting high temperature and psychiatric problems.

On 2 April 2021 the ONS reported that 5% of people infected with COVID were suffering from long COVID, or 1.1m people by the week to 6 March 2021. Of these, 674,000 said the condition affected their day-to-day life – and 196,000 said it did so significantly. Rising rates of paediatric inflammatory multi-system syndrome (PIMS) are also giving cause for concern particularly as three quarters of patients are from an ethnic minority background. It currently affects one child in every 5,000.

[Source: https://www.england.nhs.uk/coronavirus/post-covid-syndrome-long-covid/]

Currently, one in twenty ex COVID patients experience long-term symtoms for at least a month.

> *'It is this generation's polio…large numbers of patients will have physical, cognitive and psychological disability post-critical illness that will require long-term management. We must plan ahead.'*
> – Professor Nicholas Hart, Clinical and Academic Director, Lane Fox
> Respiratory Service, Guy's & St Thomas's.

Bhagat, Abhishek, 2020, COVID-19 The Pandemic: its impact on health, economy and the world

Clarke, Rachel, 2021, *Breathtaking: Inside the NHS in a Time of Pandemic*, London

Horton, Richard, 2020, The COVID–19 Catastrophe: What's Gone Wrong and How to Stop It, London

Mackenzie, Debora, 2020, COVID-19: The Pandemic that Never Should Have Happened, and How to Stop the Next One, Bridge Street Press

Maxmen, Amy, 2021, WHO report into COVID pandemic origins zeroes in on animal markets, not labs; *Nature* 31 March 2021

Zhang, Wenhong, 2020, Covid-19: From Basics To Clinical Practice, World Scientific Publishing Co Pte Ltd

Epilogue or epitaph? It's up to us.

Are we going to learn? We had many opportunities to do so, but as we're all finding out, we did not take any major steps after the pandemics of 1958-1959, 1968, and 2009. Could it be different this time? Eliminating the risk is impossible but making adequate provisions for the next pandemic is not, and it is a far less costly alternative to scrambling after a crisis arrives. Is it too much to hope that companies would put the security of supply ahead of profits, that people will not insist on ceaseless flying and cruising, and that people accustomed to eating all kinds of wild animals will stop that practice and hence reduce the chances of a new animal virus jumping to people? We will see in a matter of months and years.

—Vaclav Smil, author of 'Global Catastrophes and Trends',
from which the above quotation is excerpted.

It doesn't have to be an epitaph, but it could be if decison makers and policy planners fail to remove their collective heads from the sands of procrastination, indecision and inertia. We simply must start listening to the lessons we can glean from history's struggles with pandemics and epidemics. Just as these pestilences have followed on from each other with frightening regularity and predictability, the smart money from the scientific world is on there being another destructive pandemic before the decade is through, with similar dislocating health and economic consequences. We owe it to the 127,000+ UK COVID-19 casualties and to future generations to minimise and mitigate that as much as possible. As the previous pages of this book clearly demonstrate and explicate, the history and the evidence is there; the lessons to be learned are all there: all we have to do is, for once, take note of them and act. That's what history and empirical evidence are for; that's why we do history.

Now is the time to start doing something about it, with decisive, transparent, honest and robust planning and ring-fenced investment and financing. Those people anxious and impatient for a return to 'normal' will surely be disappointed, and they will wait a long, long time. COVID-19 is not an annoying inconvenience which was sent from somewhere vaguely foreign to spoil *your* holiday, *your* shopping, *your* day on the beach, *your* nights out, or *your* Christmas; COVID-19 is not going to go away. It will probably diminish over time to tolerable and medico-socially acceptable levels, such as those we tolerate for flu, but we will still need to get used to living with it and with its effects and impact to some degree. In the UK an average of 10–15,000 people die per year from complications of flu.

Table 11:

Deaths due to coronavirus (COVID-19) compared with deaths from influenza and pneumonia, England and Wales: deaths occurring between 1 January and 31 August 2020

Of all death occurrences between January and August 2020, there were 48,168 deaths due to the coronavirus (COVID-19) compared with 13,619 deaths due to flu-related pneumonia and 394 deaths due to influenza.

Figure 1: There were more deaths due to COVID-19 between January and August 2020 than influenza or pneumonia.

Number of deaths due to influenza, pneumonia or COVID-19 by sex, England and Wales, occurring between 1 January and 31 August 2020 and registered by 5 September 2020

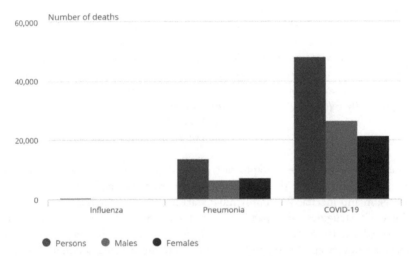

This graph compares deaths due to the coronavirus (COVID-19) with those due to influenza and pneumonia in the same period. Influenza and pneumonia are relatively well-understood causes of death involving respiratory infection and are likely to have somewhat similar risk factors to COVID-19. There is public interest in how deaths from these causes are similar and how they differ. We often count 'influenza and pneumonia' together because many cases of pneumonia are in fact caused by influenza.

Source: Office for National Statistics Statistical Bulletin 8 October 2020

Flu generates hundreds of thousands of GP visits and tens of thousands of hospital stays a year despite the universal availability of a vaccine, so the unequivocal message is 'get vaccinated'. The similarly unequivocal message relating to COVID-19 is 'get vaccinated'.

More than three times as many people died from COVID-19 than from flu and associated pneumonia in England and Wales in 2020, according to the Office for National Statistics. Between January and August 2020, there were 48,168 deaths due to COVID-19 compared to 14,000 from pneumonia-flu.

Quite simply, the better the planning, modelling and budgeting put in place today, the better we will all be able to cope with other viruses of similar or heightened virulence, viruses which are better equipped to destroy you, your family, your personal wealth if you have any, your society, your education, employment prospects and your community. And what about the long term effects on your children and your children's children?

Perhaps we should remind ourselves of the *Oxford English Dictionary* definition of disease. From 1623 it denoted 'an absence of ease (dis-ease), an uneasiness, an inconvenience, an annoyance'. Our experience of COVID-19 would certainly corroborate all of those (minor) things. So far so good, but in 1529 it was defined also as a derangement of the body or mind, an ailment, a morbid condition – all of which is closer to what we take from the word today. We need to embrace the entire spectrum of the word's meaning: yes, it is annoying and it worries us, but, at the same time, disease, and viruses, can be a morbid condition which kills us, with the added potential to destroy some of us psychologically along the way.

To many in the UK in February 2021 the policy decisions (or absence of decisions) made by the government since December 2019, vaccine development, production and roll out apart, amount to a pretty good blueprint for exactly how not to plan, prepare for or prosecute pandemic management. It would also do the UK no harm to adopt a more humble approach by looking at and adopting some of the measures applied by other nations who have been more successful in mitigating the effects of the disease. Taiwan is a case in point: they already had a Central Control Centre (after their SARS experience) which was highly proactive, alert and reflexive; they closed their borders; they have a planning programme which extends for the next twenty years and they constantly monitor epidemiological events in China (as you'd expect).

Here are just a few of the prerequisites for a modicum of preparedness, and something approaching efficient and decisive pandemic management for when the next virus hits:

1. Review systematically the lessons we (should have) learnt from previous epidemics and pandemics, especially recent pandemics of novel infections; namely AIDS, SARS, MERS, Zika and Ebola.
2. Insist on clear, accurate, understandable and up-to-date public information based on the latest science by the most authoritative sources and routinely delivered by the Prime Minister supported by credible and authoritative public health experts/scientists/practising physicians. Stop 'following the science' selectively, just when it suits. Just follow it. End the 'chumocracy'; insist on the best people for the job. Sir Paul Nurse, Head of the Francis Crick Institute, London, said 'I get a sense the UK has been rather too much on the back foot, increasingly playing catch up, firefighting through successive crises'. He urged 'a much clearer publicly presented strategy as to what we're trying to do, and the evidence upon which it is based'. This was in April; nothing much has changed: consequently, on 20 December 2020 Matt Hancock, Health Secretary, had no choice but to declare that the new strain of the virus was 'out of control'. The clear decision not to follow the science and not declare a circuit break in September 2020 clearly cost many lives.

3. Urge better, more reflexive reaction by the WHO. Their hesitation in declaring a pandemic until March when the writing was clearly on the wall in January caused costly confusion and complacency. If their protocols don't permit this then urge that the protocols are modified and modernised so that they do allow this. 'The WHO itself needs to gain teeth, they have no sticks. They are a carrot organisation,' according to Devi Sridhar, Chair of Global Public Health, University of Edinburgh.

4. Ensure prudent local manufacture and stockpiling of PPE bought forward at reasonable market prices. End the just in time/just too late mentality; reduce the need to import. It cost lives in 2020 when health care providers turned into patients. Ditto respirators and other essential ICU or COVID ward equipment, routine and otherwise. UK procurement in 2020 of essential items has been nothing short of embarrassingly inept; we need to end once and for all this shady allocation of contracts prefererential to government cronies.

5. Likewise, stockpile or manufacture locally the drugs conceivably required in COVID care; many of the most critically prescribed life-saving drugs are manufactured in China or India. End this dangerous virtual monopoly and spread out the manufacture of critical pharmaceuticals. Most if not all are generics, so are relatively inexpensive to manufacture. When China and India are in lockdown or quarantine, exports of vital pharmaceuticals will slow down or even stop, which is potentially catastrophic when there are pronounced surges in global demand. Likewise, we now need no reminding just how vulnerable the Suez Canal is as a major commercial artery.

6. Drugs, vaccines and equipment should be regarded as global public goods with corresponding unfettered global access for all nations. The world will not be sufficiently COVID-free until all countries are COVD-free. Progress has been made by CEPI, Gavi and the WHO having launched COVAX to ensure equitable access to COVID-19 vaccines and to end the acute phase of the pandemic by the end of 2021. Their work, and the work of other like-minded organisations must not end in 2021. Gavi is an international organisation created in 2000 to improve access to new and underused vaccines for children living in the world's poorer countries. 'Gavi is co-leading COVAX, the vaccines pillar of the Access to COVID-19 Tools (ACT) Accelerator. This involves coordinating the COVAX Facility, a global risk-sharing mechanism for pooled procurement and equitable distribution of COVID-19 vaccines.'

7. Invest heavily in long term research to learn more about why COVID positive BAME communities are more likely to suffer serious illness and die.

8. Invest more, a lot more, in the Coalition for Epidemic Preparedness Innovations (CEPI) – a global partnership launched in 2017 to develop vaccines to mitigate future epidemics. 'COVID-19 has brought the world to its knees. Now is the moment to unite and break the cycle of panic and neglect that has characterised our response to epidemic and pandemic disease. CEPI has a $3.5 billion plan of action to substantially reduce global epidemic and pandemic risk.' Parallel this with ramped up local vaccine research. The global scientific community has demonstrated that it can safely condense hitherto cumbersome regulatory procedures as well as co-operate in borderless research and work on a truly global, apolitical basis. Médecins sans frontières et recherche médicale sans frontières. Currently there are no fewer than 184 potential vaccines undergoing

trials with 79 at phase 1–3. Thirteen have been approved of which 5 are already in phase 4 and are being monitored in the wider population.

9. End the puerile 'vaccine nationalism' which is particularly evident and triumphalist in the UK, EU and Russia; vaccine development is not a race, nor is vaccine roll-out. They are both the result of stunning global efforts with global co-operation for the global good.

10. The UK government has appointed a minister with special responsibility for vaccine roll out, working astride the departments of health and business in which he already acts as business secretary. While this is a major step forward it does smack of yet more of the UK's characteristic short-termism and just in time policy making: we have known about imminent vaccines for months – he could have been appointed and set to work months ago. Oddly the minister is responsible only for England; the post is an interim appointment. What is required is a permanent position in Cabinet firmly rooted in health and social care without the conflicting tensions involved in trying to balance the business and public health requirements of the country. The brief should include all aspects of epidemic and pandemic management including disease surveillance. For economic and logistic reasons the mandate should of course extend to all nations of the UK. Being better preparared for the next pandemic is a long term, progressive and continuous task which, if pursued properly, will save money, safeguard the economy and avoid many deaths.

11. Research, research, research: on a national and international level. We need to invest much more heavily, most notably in staff and research grants, if only to allow those scientists seconded to COVID vaccine research and development to return to their usual work. We must attract the best scientists from all around the world and make it easy for them to enter and work in the UK.

According to *The Times*,

> The UK research and innovation budget faces an effective cut of nearly a quarter over the next year…they amount to 'a devastating reduction which would reverse two years of intended increases and mean that the ambition for Britain to be a science superpower would be deferred for much of this parliament'.
>
> The cuts to UK Research and Innovation (UKRI), the agency for funding scientific research, come despite the government pledging to more than double public funding for research and development to £22 billion by 2024–25.
>
> - Rhys Blakely, 26 March, 2021

How confusing and ambivalent is that? Tom Whipple adds:

> The mooted £2 billion cuts, which account for almost a quarter of the public research budget, come on top of £120 million of research funding already lost from the overseas aid budget.
>
> 'The shortfall will hit many of the teams who worked on the coronavirus response and also jeopardise government plans to make Britain a "science

superpower", the researchers, who included the head of the Royal Society, the Academy of Medical Sciences and Universities UK, said'.

12. International aid to poorer nations should be ramped up, not, as in the UK for example, cut; this astonishingly myopic decision is another manifestation of the UK's perception of pandemic management as a short term task which can be peremptorily dealt with and then filed away for good. Cuts in international aid will impact on education which is pivotal to mitigating epidemic disease in poorer countries influencing as it does behaviour, hygiene and compliance. Cuts in international aid will be detrimental to vaccine availability and roll out as well as to PPE distribution – all of which are pivotal in the fight against the spread of disease within developing countries and to the outside world.

13. Insist on more 'out of the box' preventative measures. The recent announcement that prophylactic high dose vitamin D which may have a protective effect in COVID 19 infection will be made available to high risk COVID groups is the sort of enlightened thinking we need much more of.

14. Lobby for stricter enforcement of the Convention on International Trade in Endangered Species (Cities) laws which would prevent a bat ever meeting a pangolin, or in the case of SARS, a civet. Lobby for a law allowing temporary international travel bans as soon as a potentially pandemic pathogen is discovered.

15. Acknowledge the role climate change and ecology play in triggering pandemics: when we clear a forest we destroy natural habits of countless animals, insects and birds which migrate into established human populations and bring with them the potential to act as vectors to virgin human communities. Moreover, the way we keep animals, in factory-like conditions, facilitates the creation of bio-weapons and bioterrorism. Some experts predict that the next pandemic will be a bird flu, H7N9, which so far has killed 40 per cent of people infected, making it 100 times deadlier than COVID-19. It will start in battery chicken farms; one way to head it off to some extent would be to consume less cheap, factory-farmed meat and eggs and eat more plant-based alternatives.

16. Most importantly assess what all of this will cost and establish whether it adds up to more or less than the totality, direct and indirect, of the potential financial burden on the economy if we turn out to be as ill prepared in the next destructive pandemic as we are for COVID-19. Everyone knows that prudent pre-emptive action can often be far less costly in the long-term than scrabbling around at the last minute fighting an established and raging pandemic.

17. COVID-19 has laid bare many of the defects and inequalities in societies around the world, none more so than in the UK. The present government claims to be committed to levelling up our society, drastically reducing the yawning gap between the well-off and the poor, the haves and the have-nots; closing the gulf between investment and infrastructure in the south and in the north and in the devolved nations; and establishing real universal equal opportunities between women and men, BAME and white, able and disabled, between people with physical and mental special needs and the sound of mind and body, between immigrants and British. COVID, like death, its comrade in arms, is an

efficient leveller but it also adumbrates where, as a nation, we are not level and where we are deficient, as in all those areas listed above. More than anything else, COVID demonstrates how the poor and disadvantaged and those discriminated against have suffered disproportionately in terms of morbidity and mortality. Now is the time, yes mid-pandemic, to lay the foundations for this levelling up: it will be money well and wisely spent, because in flattening out the disparities in our society there will be fewer casualties next time round as there will be fewer poor and vulnerable people.

18. Ventilation is crucial in the fight against the virus: good ventilation reduces the concentration of the virus in the air and therefore reduces the risks from airborne transmission by up to 4 times – that's why we are less vulnerable outside, that's why we are urged to open windows and ventilate a room. But it goes much further than that. Professor Cath Noakes of the University of Leeds School of Civil Engineering is a leading expert on the way pathogens spread inside buildings – particularly where large numbers of people gather – such as in hospitals, care homes or other public buildings and is a member of the SAGE group. One of her current research projects – HECOIRA – is a partnership between industry and two NHS trusts to develop new ways of designing and monitoring healthcare environments to improve infection control – and also to make them more effective spaces for patient and staff wellbeing. It is vital we take this important work into account when designing or adapting such facilities in the future.

19. What are we doing about copper? The coronavirus causing the COVID-19 pandemic survives for days on glass and stainless steel but dies within hours after landing on copper. Jim Morrison on Smithsonianmag.com (14 April 2020) tells how Bill Keevil, at the University of Southampton, has studied the antimicrobial effects of copper for over 20 years: he began with the bacteria that causes Legionnaire's Disease and then turned to drug-resistant killer infections like MRSA; he tested viruses that caused pandemics such as MERS and the Swine Flu (H1N1) pandemic of 2009. In each case, copper contact killed the pathogen within minutes.

Michael G. Schmidt, at the Medical University of South Carolina who researches copper in healthcare settings, has focused his research on whether using copper alloys in frequently touched surfaces reduces hospital infections. On any given day, about one in thirty-one hospital patients has at least one healthcare-associated infection, according to the Centers for Disease Control, costing as much as £35,000 per patient. Schmidt's landmark study, funded by the Department of Defense, looked at copper alloys on surfaces including bedside rails, tray tables, intravenous poles, and chair armrests at three hospitals around the country. That 43-month investigation revealed a 58 per cent infection reduction compared to routine infection protocols.

A two-year study published in 2020 compared beds in an intensive care unit with plastic surfaces and those with copper. Bed rails on the plastic surfaces exceeded the accepted risk standards in nearly 90 per cent of the samples, while the rails on the copper bed exceeded those standards on only 9 per cent. 'We again demonstrated in spades that copper can keep the built environment clean from microorganisms,' Schmidt says.

Keevil and Schmidt have found that installing copper on just 10 per cent of surfaces would prevent infections and save £800 a day.

Keevil says France and Poland are beginning to put copper alloys in hospitals. In Peru and Chile, which produce copper, it's being used in hospitals and the public transit systems. 'So it's going around the world, but it still hasn't taken off,' he says.

'Viruses are global; our response has not been. And it needs to be.'
– Devi Sridhar, Chair of Global Public Health, University of Edinburgh

China crisis: China's response to the outbreak

This is an ongoing controversial issue which, it was hoped, the January-February 2021 WHO delegation to Wuhan would be able to clarifiy to some degree. It remains a work in progress. The situation as currently understood is that on 23 January 2020, China imposed a lockdown for 57 million people in Wuhan and other cities in Hubei in an effort to quarantine the epicentre of an outbreak of COVID-19. The World Health Organization (WHO) welcomed the move, calling it "unprecedented in public health history". That was the good news; the bad news was that as long before as 8 January 2020, that new coronavirus, by now known as SARS-CoV-2, was identified as the cause of an outbreak of pneumonia by Chinese scientists. The first death and 41 clinically confirmed infections triggered by the coronavirus were reported as early as 10 January; in the intervening weeks the Chinese authorities insisted that there was no human-to-human transmission.

The outbreak had gone unnoticed until 26 December 2019, when Zhang Jixian, director of the Department of Respiratory Medicine at Hubei Xinhua Hospital, noticed a cluster of patients with pneumonia of unknown origin, several of whom had connections to the Huanan Seafood Market. She subsequently alerted the hospital, as well as municipal and provincial health authorities, which issued an alert on 30 December.

A retrospective analysis published in *The Lancet* in late January, found that the first confirmed patient started experiencing symptoms on 1 December 2019; the *South China Morning Post* later reported that a different retrospective analysis showed the first case may have been a 55-year-old patient from Hubei province as early as 17 November.

The WHO issued its first report on the outbreak on 5 January 2020. Professor Zhang Yongzhen of Fudan University completed sequencing of the novel virus on the same day and published the results to the online database GenBank on 11 January. It showed striking similarities to SARS. On 14 January, the blind-sided WHO tweeted:

'Preliminary investigations conducted by the Chinese authorities have found no clear evidence of human-to-human transmission of the novel coronavirus (2019-nCoV) identified in Wuhan, China'.

The already dire scenario was made much, much worse by the week-long mass movement of hundreds of millions of Chinese people for the lunar new year celebrations – annually the biggest migration in the world. Another super-spreader was a 19 January mega banquet for thousands of families thrown in the Baibuting district of Wuhan. On

20 January, 224 cases had been reported of pneumonia caused by the novel coronavirus. China finally relented and admitted human to human transmission: 'It [coronavirus] is most likely transmitted to humans from wild animals. However, now it appears that we have human-to-human transmission'.

This in turn produced the following terrifying, if tentative, pronouncement to the world from the WHO:

It is clear that at least some human-to-human transmission exists from the evidence we have, but we don't have clear evidence that shows the virus has the capacity to transmit among humans easily.

And the rest, as they say, is history. By 22 January, the novel coronavirus had spread to major cities and provinces in China, with 571 confirmed cases and 17 deaths reported. Confirmed cases were also reported in Hong Kong, Macau, Taiwan, Thailand, Japan, South Korea, and the United States. The first UK cases were in York on 20 January when two Chinese nationals were quarantined and transferred to an isolation unit at Newcastle's Royal Victoria Infirmary. They recovered.

The cover up

But there had clearly been a cover up which belied the 'openness, transparency and responsibility' vaunted by President Xi Jinping. The subterfuge was revealed by a group of senior medical professionals who risked surveillance and arrest and were advised 'not to tell the truth' which every doctor now knew, namely that the virus enjoyed human to human transmission. Passports were confiscated and internet access was curtailed amongst the medical community.

What we can do immediately

All countries need to learn the lessons of the past but the UK in particular has been particularly averse, projecting an attitude through cabinet ministers that we know best because we are the best. COVID-19 has eloquently demonstrated the foolishness and arrogance of such a belief: Britain was clearly not ready and was unprepared; more dangerously, the government thought they *were* prepared – and this from a team seen at some meetings totting up COVID cases on their phones from scribbles on whiteboards dragged into Downing Street.

It may be instructive to remind ourselves of some of the failings and to project future positive and joined-up action from that platform, while at the same time learning the lessons history has bequeathed to us at one time or another.

1. Britain has the worst overall COVID-19 death toll in Europe
2. Britain has the second worst excess death rate per capita in Europe, twice that of France and eight times that of Germany.
3. It failed to protect its old and vulnerable, sentencing care home residents to death in shocking numbers. Professor Sir Brian Jarman told *The Times* (4 July, 2020) ['Health chiefs] watched unfolding events like Roman spectators watching gladiators thrown to the lions'. Brian Jarman was formerly Professor of Primary Health Care from

1983–98 at Imperial College School of Medicine and President of the British Medical Association.

4. It failed to contain the disease in local outbreaks, allowing it to spread nationally.

5. It locked down too late and eased the lockdown too early. Professor Sir Ian Boyd who sits on the SAGE Committee says that locking down a week or two earlier would have made a big difference to the coronavirus death rate.

6. It closed its borders far too late. They remain alarmingly porous.

7. It has an equivocal, non-transparent attitude to being 'guided by the science'.

8. It nurtures a 'chumocracy' in the appointment of senior staff and in PPE procurement. A case in point is the monumental debacle that is Randox Science, responsible for much of our testing. Their organisation is said to be 'shabby' with a frighteningly cavalier approach to cross-infection amongst its workforce and to delivering the results on time, or, sometimes, at all. On 7 August 2020, the United Kingdom Medicines and Healthcare Products Regulatory Agency requested Randox to recall the Randox COVID-19 Home Testing Kit due to safety concerns in a measure it described as precautionary. Randox has been awarded nearly £500 million by the UK government to provide private-sector testing without having to compete for a tender.

9. It set silly targets which could not be met (eg. tracking and tracing); it vaunted policies which were unrealistic (eg. education).

10. It developed 'world beating' programmes which were flawed (eg. the IOW App in August). Mass tracing was advised on 12 February but dismissed. Public Health England requested a ten-fold increase in its testing capacity. And then there was the GCSE and A level algorithm...

11. It fosters an unhealthy, triumphalist nationalism, presenting the development and roll out of vaccines as a kind of school race which Britain won because 'we are the best' and better than everybody else. Oh dear, just look at points 1–10 again...

12. We had our eye on the wrong ball: influenza, when the most successful anti COVID nations – Hong Kong, South Korea, Singapore, Taiwan – threw all their resources at combating the type of respiratory virus COVID turned out to be. We took little, if any, heed of their experience, particularly how they navigated through SARS in 2003.

13. It has created 'a picture of a country whose systemic weaknesses were exposed with appalling brutality, a country that believed it was stronger than it was and that paid the price for failures that have built up for years'. (Tom McTague in The Times, 15 August 2020, itself an edited version of a piece first published in The Atlantic – after conversations with diplomats and officials from Britain and other European governments.)

14. It needs to deploy more and better economics and social psychology experts; for example, the much vaunted 'eat out to help out' was nothing like the success it was said to have been: it actually caused more infections and, overall, most restaurants and cafés saw very little economic benefit. The money would have been much better spent on shoring up the tracking and tracing. One virologist suggested it should be renamed 'Eat out to help the virus out'.

15. We need to reboot our vaccine production capacity and supply chain after 10 years of government running it down to inadequate levels. We need to have a system that can produce at pace and scale according to demand.'*It's not Astra Zeneca's fault - it's a national legacy issue, and it's one of the things we've got to fix*', says Sir John Bell.

16. The Royal College of GPs tells us that 40,000 retired doctors and nurses applied to help with vaccinations but many were daunted by the absurd bureaucracy involved. The 21 point checklist included:

passport and proof of right to work
highest education certificate
conflict resolution level 1
fire safety level 1
preventing radicalisation level 1

'*The reality is, there has been a major systemic failure*'
   - Ian Boyd, Professor of Biology, St Andrew's University and member of SAGE

I list these serious shortcomings not to apportion blame but to set clear and simple objectives which we should strive to achieve next time. We need more success stories, for example:

1. The NHS rising to the enormous challenge it suddenly faced
2. The economic safety nets
3. The new Nightingale hospitals which sprang up as if from nowhere even though they were not needed in the end
4. The sterling work of the scientists from home and abroad who identified new therapies and did so much to progress and roll out a vaccine in record time.

As Peter Frankopan, Professor of Global History at the University of Oxford, points out: 'how governments understand and deal with the medical and economic legacy of COVID will shape the future. So, as we already knew, high levels of infection are associated with social deprivation but they go back over 100 years and still come back to haunt us. As recently as 3 March 2021 it was disappointing and worrying to hear Rishi Sunak, Chancellor of the Exchequer, defending his budget with the fallacious statement that this [COVID] 'is a once in a century event' when we all now know that there has already been six other such events since 2000. Such a mindset does not augur well for the planning for and management of future calamities.

The core theme of this book is that pandemics and epidemics have often changed the course of history; what the world needs to do now is, through effective and timely pandemic planning and management, change the predictable course of history before it happens, so to speak. In other words, do not allow the predictable, the 'COVID experience' if you like, to recur in the first place.

History is watching us. Let's return the compliment.

Choi, Bernard C.K., 2005, What could be future scenarios ? Lessons from the history of public health surveillance for the future, *AIMS Public Health*, 2, 27–43

Frankopan, Peter, 2020, Covid can be the catalyst for a safer and better world, *The Times* 12 December 2020

Osterholm, Michael T., 2020, *Deadliest enemy, our war against killer germs*, London

Whipple, Tom, 2020, The world must prepare now to fight the next pandemic, *The Times* 14 November 2020.

Endword

'*He knew that this happy crowd was unaware of something that one can read in books, which is that the plague bacillus never dies or vanishes entirely, that it can remain dormant for dozens of years in furniture or clothing, that it waits patiently in bedrooms, cellars, trunks, handkerchiefs and old papers, and that perhaps the day will come when, for the instruction or misfortune of mankind, the plague will rouse its rats and send them to die in some well-contented city.*'

– Albert Camus, *The Plague*, 1947.

We have, after all, had fair warning about international outbreaks of disease, with 13 since the millennium...I certainly hope that the world has seen that we need to put funding into planning for pandemics...a disease in one country is of interest to, and the responsibility of, the world.

– Carina Tyrell, Clinical Fellow at the Medical Research Council Epidemiology Unit, University of Cambridge

India April-May 2021 – Watch out world...

As this book goes to press the tragic and truly catastrophic situation assailing India delivers a sobering and timely shock, illustrating graphically what can happen when we get things wrong.

The 400 or so pages in this book tell us where we have gone wrong in the past and how crowd diseases have wreaked unrelenting and merciless havoc across the globe. The prodigious death toll down the years is beyond belief. By the same token, though, the book provides us all with a programme of lessons on how *not* to repeat the mistakes of the past.

Nevertheless, in our haste to get back to 'normal' and to open up lockdowns as soon as possible, ever shortening that vital safe social distance, we run the danger of unravelling all the good, life-saving work our prudent pandemic strategies and effective vaccine programmes have afforded us.

Ask the government of India whether it now believes that its brief re-acquaintance with crowds and crowding – in the sacrosanct name of religion, political rallies and sport – was really worth it when the people they are supposed to be looking after see their loved ones dying in the streets, in makeshift ambulances outside overflowing hospitals, gasping for oxygen when, irony of ironies, it's there all around but, cruelly, not in a form that the Indian government is able to deliver.

As we cautioned at the very beginning of this book, quoting Pasteur, '*Gentlemen, it's the microbes which will have the last word.*'

But only if we let them.

Appendix 1

The Antonine Plague reaches Hadrian's Wall

...send away the noisy clatter of raging plague...

In 1807 evidence emerged which confirmed the existence of the plague at Housesteads on Hadrian's Wall (*RIB* 1579). It comes in the form of a funerary slab with the inscription: 'To the gods and goddesses according to the interpretation of the oracle of Clarian Apollo the First Cohort of Tungrians (set this up).' While this is formulaic (we know of at least ten others) and would have been trotted out by all units, it seems likely that it was a reaction to a general order from Marcus Aurelius to invoke Apollo in a bid to safeguard their forts and cities from rampant smallpox. An identical inscription has been found at Ravenglass.

The Romans were no stranger to plagues but, just to be on the safe side, they turned to that age old precautionary measure, the oracle. Indeed, in total eleven dedications 'To the gods and goddesses according to the interpretation of the oracle of Clarian Apollo' have been found built into walls to ward off the plague. Our Tungrians had more to fear than the one in W.H. Auden's delightful *Roman Wall Blues*:

Over the heather the wet wind blows,
I've lice in my tunic and a cold in my nose.

The rain comes pattering out of the sky,
I'm a Wall soldier, I don't know why.

The mist creeps over the hard grey stone,
My girl's in Tungria; I sleep alone.

Aulus goes hanging around her place,
I don't like his manners, I don't like his face.

Piso's a Christian, he worships a fish;
There'd be no kissing if he had his wish.

She gave me a ring but I diced it away;
I want my girl and I want my pay.

When I'm a veteran with only one eye
I shall do nothing but look at the sky.

Another oracle from Claros, once preserved on a stone in Pergamum, told people to 'beg from immortals a good remedy against the plague, so that it may travel far to the land of hostile men'.

In 2011 Roger Tomlin provided more evidence for the plague's spread to Britannia when he published research on an amulet found in 1989 at Vintry in the City of London: it gives us 30 lines of Greek and was written for a man with the Greek name Demetri(o)s. It translates as '...send away the noisy clatter of raging plague, air-borne... penetrating pain, heavy-spiriting, flesh-wasting, melting, from the hollows of the veins. Great Iao, great Sabaoth, protect the bearer. Phoebus [Apollo] of the unshorn hair, archer, drive away the cloud of plague....! Lord God, watch over Demetrios.'

Life in the Limes (pp.197–205)

Appendix 2

Contracts for the boys and girls

The UK government, perhaps in panic, perhaps due to a lack of procurement skills, perhaps to inculcate a climate of 'chumocratic' government, has a reputation for inept and dubious practice in the appointment of senior staff and in PPE procurement. A case in point is the monumental debacle that is Randox Science, responsible for much of our testing. Their organisation is said to be 'shabby' with a frighteningly cavalier approach to cross-infection amongst its workforce and an alarming lack of concern for delivering results on time, or, sometimes, at all. On 7 August 2020, the United Kingdom Medicines and Healthcare Products Regulatory Agency requested Randox to recall the Randox COVID-19 Home Testing Kit due to safety concerns in a measure it described as precautionary.

Randox has been awarded nearly £500 million by the UK government to provide private-sector testing without having to compete for a tender. In March 2019 former cabinet minister and Conservative MP Owen Paterson, a consultant to Randox, had lobbied the government to seek contracts for them thus violating rules stating that an MP may not lobby on behalf of a paying client. When asked if Paterson had lobbied on behalf of the company, a spokesman for DHSC said they were 'unable to comment on the personnel matters of other organisations'.

The hapless Baroness Harding, Chair of NHS Improvement, has sat on the board of Cheltenham Racecourse. Her husband is Tory MP politician John Penrose who has served as the United Kingdom Anti-Corruption Champion since 2017; she is a jockey and racehorse owner, owning the 1998 Cheltenham Gold Cup winner, 'Cool Dawn'. And then there was the astonishing, lethal, decision to allow the 2020 Cheltenham Gold Cup to go ahead, in a time of COVID...

She was appointed the first CEO of TalkTalk in 2010, when Carphone Warehouse split its telecoms business from its retail operation. In October 2015, TalkTalk was hit by a cyber-attack, during which personal and banking details of up to four million customers, not all of which were encrypted, were thought to have been accessed. *City A.M.* described her responses as 'naïve', noting that early on, when asked if the affected customer data was encrypted or not, she replied: 'The awful truth is that I don't know.' Her inflexible line on termination fees was also criticised. *Marketing* ran a headline, 'TalkTalk boss Dido Harding's utter ignorance is a lesson to us all.' *The Evening Standard* noted that 'It has been a tough week for TalkTalk boss Dido Harding, facing complaints from customers and calls for her head.' The company admitted the incident had cost it £60 million and lost it 95,000 customers. Fining the company £400,000, the Information Commissioner Elizabeth Denham blamed a 'failure to implement the most basic cyber security measures'.

Other multi-million-pound beneficiaries include Serco (£410m) who redacted part of the document explaining how the government would monitor their performance before publication. In July 2019, a fine of £19.2m was imposed on Serco for fraud and false accounting over its electronic tagging service for the Ministry of Justice. The company has also been accused of an extensive cover-up over sexual abuse of immigrants at Yarl's Wood Immigration Removal Centre in Bedfordshire, and of failing to develop a strategy for managing Higher Active Radioactive Waste at the Atomic Weapons Establishment.

Serco's failures include the deplorable handling of pathology labs and fatal errors in patient records. At St Thomas' Hospital, the increase in the number of clinical incidents arising from Serco non-clinical management has resulted in patients receiving incorrect and infected blood, as well as patients suffering kidney damage due to Serco providing incorrect data used for medical calculations.

And there is Concentrix, who in 2016 was criticised by a cross-party parliamentary committee on welfare for incorrectly closing the claims of tens of thousands of claimants, leaving them without money for essentials. A government report disclosed that of 36,000 appeals against Concentrix, 87 per cent were upheld. In September 2016, HMRC announced that it would not renew the contract, due to expire in 2017, although the Treasury has resisted calls for a full inquiry so far. As a result of Concentrix's failings, thousands of claimants are also due to receive back-payments for incorrectly stopped claims. Processing the resultant case reviews cost HMRC £43 million.

The government connives at reckless behaviour by its own, weakening national compliance; Dominic Cummings's cavalier trip to Barnard Castle dented compliance badly and, ultimately, probably resulted in unnecessary deaths.

Space does not permit more in this astonishing litany; however, if we are to navigate our way through subsequent pandemics then this self-serving, squalidly unprofessional behaviour has got to be eradicated. The best companies, the best people, the demonstrably transparent and efficient need to be in place in times when we need the highest integrity and reliability.

Appendix 3

Eyam, plague village

T he depredations of the 1965-1666 'Great Plague of London' (see page 163) were not, of course, confined to the capital. The insidious plague infiltrated many other cities, towns and villages throughout the kingdom; one of them was Eyam, a hitherto unassuming Derbyshire Peak District village betwixt Chesterfield and Buxton.

It was on 1 November 1666 that farm labourer Abraham Morten passed away as the last of 260 Eyam villagers to die from bubonic plague. They had signed their death warrant in July of that year when the entire village astonishingly agreed to impose quarantine on itself in a valiant bid to stop the spread of the Great Plague in its tracks.

Abraham was one of 18 Mortens who succumbed and were listed as plague victims on the parish register. His death, and the deaths of all the others began 14 months earlier, with the arrival of a bale of cloth sent from London, where the rampant disease had already slain thousands of inhabitants. No one could know that the bale of damp cloth was home to deadly fleas, vectors of the plague.

A tailor's assistant by the name of George Viccars opened the bale and draped the cloth in front of the hearth to dry, unwittingly activating the disease-ridden fleas incubating in the parcel's contents. George Viccars became the first plague victim in Eyam: he was just visiting the village to help make clothes for Wakes Week and sadly never got to leave. From Viccars the contagion tore through the community. Between September and December 1665, 42 villagers succumbed and by the spring of 1666, many, quite naturally, were on the verge of fleeing their homes and abandoning their livelihoods in order to save themselves.

That was when the new rector, William Mompesson, stepped in. He was of the fervent belief that it was, as a man of the church, his duty to prevent the plague spreading to the nearby villages and the populous towns of Sheffield and Bakewell; he decided that the village should be quarantined.

Persuading his parishioners to sacrifice their lives in an act of unalloyed altruism was going to be hard enough, but Mompesson had another problem in that he was already deeply unpopular with the villagers. He had been posted to Eyam in April 1664 after the previous rector, Thomas Stanley, a Cromwell supporter, was removed. Stanley had refused to acknowledge the 1662 Act of Uniformity, which made the use of the Book of Common Prayer, introduced by Charles II, compulsory in religious services. Stanley reflected the pro-Puritan leanings of the people of Eyam and so remained influential with the villagers; his support, therefore, was crucial if Mompesson's scheme was to succeed.

Stanley, now ostracised to the edge of the village, agreed to meet and the two men formulated their remarkable and groundbreaking plan which was revealed to the parishioners on 24 June 1666. Mompesson pronounced that the village must be enclosed, with no-one allowed in or out, adding that the Earl of Devonshire, who lived nearby at Chatsworth, had offered to send food and supplies if the villagers agreed to be quarantined.

In a bid to offer reassurance to his flock and touching on their Christian faith, Mompesson said that if they agreed to stay – effectively choosing to die – he would do everything he could to alleviate their suffering and remain with them, explaining that he was willing to sacrifice his own life rather than see neighbouring communities afflicted.

His wife, Catherine, noted in her diary that there were many misgivings over the wisdom of his plan, but she concluded that with help from Stanley – who had asserted that a cordon sanitaire was the most effective way of dealing with the plague – the doubters reluctantly agreed to the plan.

August 1666 saw the peak in the number of victims with five or six deaths a day. The weather was uncommonly hot that summer making the fleas particularly industrious, so the pestilence spread unchecked throughout the village; hardly anyone broke the cordon though.

The same month, Elizabeth Hancock buried six of her children and her husband close to the family farm. They had all perished in just eight terrible days and she was forced to drag the bodies of her children one by one to a field where they could be buried. Another survivor who also had to bury his family was Marshall Howe who assumed the role of village undertaker. He was infected during the early stages of the outbreak, but survived, believing that the immunity this conferred meant that he could not be infected twice. We can perhaps understand why he loved such a morbid job when we learn that he often helped himself to the victims' possessions as his reward.

Cases fell in September and October and by 1 November the disease had gone. The cordon had worked. Eyam's mortality rate was higher than that suffered by the plagued citizens of London. In little over a year, 260 Eyam inhabitants died from 76 different families; the total population of Eyam is estimated at somewhere between 350 and 800 before the plague struck.

Mompesson left Eyam in 1669 to work in Eakring, Nottinghamshire, but such was the stigma and reputation of the 'plague village' he was reduced to living in a hut in Rufford Park until the residents got over their fears.

Carew, Jan, 2004, *Eyam: Plague Village*, Nelson Thomas, Cheltenham

Race, Philip 1995, 'Some Further Consideration of the Plague in Eyam, 1665/6', *Local Population Studies* 54, 56-65.

Wallis, Patrick, 2006, 'A Dreadful Heritage: Interpreting Epidemic Disease at Eyam, 1666–2000', *History Workshop Journal*, Vol.61, No.1, 31–56.

Whittles L.K. & Didelot, X. 2016, 'Epidemiological Analysis of the Eyam Plague Outbreak of 1665–1666', *Proceedings of the Royal Society B: Biological Sciences*, Vol.283, No.1830

Further reading

Allen, Arthur, 2014, *The Fantastic Laboratory of Dr Weigl: how two brave scientists battled typhus and sabotaged the Nazis*, New York

Attwood, Margaret, 2009, *Year of the Flood*, London

Boeckl, Christine M., 2000, *Images of Plague and Pestilence: iconography and iconology*, Truman State University Press, Kirksville, Missouri

Bray, R.S., 1996, *Armies of Pestilence: The impact of disease on history*, New York

Camus, Albert, 1947, *The Plague* (*La Peste*); trans. Robin Buss, 2001, Harmondsworth

Cartwright, Frederick F, 1972, *Disease and History*, New York

Choi, Bernard C.K., 2005, *What could be future scenarios? Lessons from the history of public health surveillance for the future*, AIMS Public Health, 2, 27-43

Chrystal, Paul (in press 2021), *Bioterrorism*, Barnsley

Crawford, Dorothy H., 2018, *Viruses: A Very Short Introduction* [2nd edition], Oxford

Crawshaw, Jane L. Stevens, 2016, *Plague Hospitals: Public Health for the City in Early Modern Venice*, London

Defoe, Daniel, 2003, *A Journal of the Plague Year*, Harmondsworth

Frankopan, Peter, 2020 Covid can be the catalyst for a safer and better world, *The Times* 12 December 2020

Giordano, P. 2020, *How Contagion Works*, London

Hays, J.N. 2006, *Epidemics and Pandemics: Their Impact on Human History*. ABC CLIO

Hempel, Sandra, 2020, *The Atlas of Disease*, London

Hirst, Leonard Fabian, 1953, *The conquest of plague: a study of the evolution of epidemiology*, Oxford

Honigsbaum, Mark, 2020, *The Pandemic Century: A History of Global Contagion from the Spanish Flu to Covid-19*, London

Iqbal, Akhtar Khan, 2004. '*Plague: the dreadful visitation occupying the human mind for centuries*'. Transactions of the Royal Society of Tropical Medicine and Hygiene. 98 (5): 270–277

Kaufmann, Miranda, 2017, *Black Tudors: The Untold Story*, London

Lyons, Albert S. 1987, *Medicine: An Illustrated History*, New York

Ma, Ling, 2019, Severance, London

Mack, Arien, 1992, *In Time of Plague: the history and social consequences of lethal epidemic disease*, New York

Mandel, Emily St John, 2015, *Station Eleven*, London

Marquez, Gabriel Garcia, 1989, *Love in the Time of Cholera*, London

Martin, Sean, 2015, *A Short History of Disease*, Harpenden

Mayhew, Henry, 1985 repr., *London Labour and the London Poor*, London
McMillen, Christian, W. 2016, *Pandemics: A Very Short Introduction*, Oxford
McNeil, William H. 1998, *Plagues and People*, New York
Michie, Jonathan, 2020 'The Covid-19 crisis – and the future of the economy and economics.' International Review of Applied Economics. 34 (3): 301–303.
Morens, D.M., G.K. Folkers, and A.S. Fauci. 2004. The Challenge of Emerging and Re-emerging infectious diseases. Nature 430: 242–249.
Oldstone, Michael B. 2009, *Viruses, Plagues, and History: Past, Present and Future: Past, Present and Future*, Oxford
Osterholm, Michael T., 2020, *Deadliest Enemy, our war against killer germs*, London
Paul, David, 2012, *Eyam: plague village*, Stroud
Peckham, Robert, 2016, *Epidemics in Modern Asia*, Cambridge
Pepys, Samuel, 2020, *The Diary of Samuel Pepys: The Great Plague of London & The Great Fire of London*, 1665-1666
Porter, Katherine Ann, 1939, *Pale Horse, Pale Rider*, Harmondsworth
Rajgor, Dimple D. (27 March 2020). 'The many estimates of the COVID-19 case fatality rate'. *The Lancet* Infectious Diseases
Saracci, Rodolfo, 2010, *Epidemiology: A Very Short Introduction*, Oxford
Smil, Vaclav, 2012, *Global Catastrophes and Trends: The Next Fifty Years*, Cambridge MA
Watts, Charlotte H.; Vallance, Patrick; Whitty, Chris (18 February 2020). 'Coronavirus: global solutions to prevent a pandemic'. Nature. 578 (7795): 363
Whipple, Tom, 2020, The world must prepare now to fight the next pandemic, *The Times* 14 November 2020.
Williamson, Stanley, 2007, *The Vaccination Controversy: The Rise, Reign and Fall of Compulsory Vaccination for Smallpox*, Liverpool
Wohl, Anthony S, 1983, *Endangered lives: public health in Victorian Britain*, London
York Archaeological Trust, 2009, *Plague, Poverty, Prayer*, York
Ziegler, Philip, 2003, *The Black Death*, Stroud
Zinsser, Hans, 1935, *Rats, Lice and History*, London

Index